Comprehensive Approach to NCLEX-RN, HAAD and DHA Examinations

Comprehensive Approach to NCLEX-RN, HAAD and DHA Examinations

Renjith Augustine RN RP MSc (Psychiatric Nsg)
MSc (Psychology) PGDBS PG Diploma in Diabetic Educator

RN Educator
EEZEE English Group of Institutions
Irinjalakuda, Kerala, India

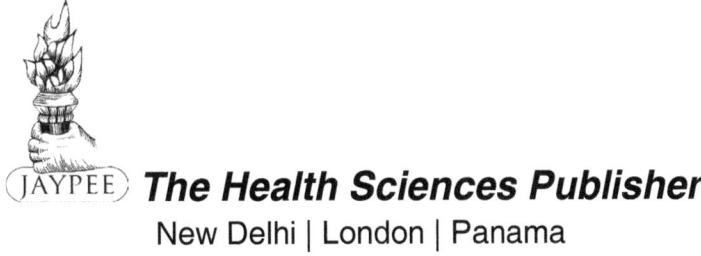

JAYPEE *The Health Sciences Publisher*
New Delhi | London | Panama

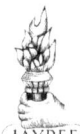 **Jaypee Brothers Medical Publishers (P) Ltd**

Headquarters
Jaypee Brothers Medical Publishers (P) Ltd.
4838/24, Ansari Road, Daryaganj
New Delhi 110 002, India
Phone: +91-11-43574357
Fax: +91-11-43574314
E-mail: jaypee@jaypeebrothers.com

Overseas Offices

J.P. Medical Ltd.
83, Victoria Street, London
SW1H 0HW (UK)
Phone: +44-20 3170 8910
Fax: +44(0)20 3008 6180
E-mail: info@jpmedpub.com

Jaypee-Highlights Medical Publishers Inc.
City of Knowledge, Bld. 235, 2nd Floor, Clayton
Panama City, Panama
Phone: +1 507-301-0496
Fax: +1 507-301-0499
E-mail: cservice@jphmedical.com

Jaypee Brothers Medical Publishers (P) Ltd.
17/1-B, Babar Road, Block-B, Shaymali
Mohammadpur, Dhaka-1207
Bangladesh
Mobile: +08801912003485
E-mail: jaypeedhaka@gmail.com

Jaypee Brothers Medical Publishers (P) Ltd.
Bhotahity, Kathmandu, Nepal
Phone: +977-9741283608
E-mail: kathmandu@jaypeebrothers.com

Website: www.jaypeebrothers.com
Website: www.jaypeedigital.com

© 2017, Jaypee Brothers Medical Publishers

The views and opinions expressed in this book are solely those of the original contributor(s)/author(s) and do not necessarily represent those of editor(s) of the book.

All rights reserved. No part of this publication may be reproduced, stored or transmitted in any form or by any means, electronic, mechanical, photo-copying, recording or otherwise, without the prior permission in writing of the publishers.

All brand names and product names used in this book are trade names, service marks, trademarks or registered trademarks of their respective owners. The publisher is not associated with any product or vendor mentioned in this book.

Medical knowledge and practice change constantly. This book is designed to provide accurate, authoritative information about the subject matter in question. However, readers are advised to check the most current information available on procedures included and check information from the manufacturer of each product to be administered, to verify the recommended dose, formula, method and duration of administration, adverse effects and contraindications. It is the responsibility of the practitioner to take all appropriate safety precautions. Neither the publisher nor the author(s)/editor(s) assume any liability for any injury and/or damage to persons or property arising from or related to use of material in this book.

This book is sold on the understanding that the publisher is not engaged in providing professional medical services. If such advice or services are required, the services of a competent medical professional should be sought.

Every effort has been made where necessary to contact holders of copyright to obtain permission to reproduce copyright material. If any have been inadvertently overlooked, the publisher will be pleased to make the necessary arrangements at the first opportunity.

Inquiries for bulk sales may be solicited at: jaypee@jaypeebrothers.com

Comprehensive Approach to NCLEX-RN, HAAD and DHA Examinations

First Edition: **2017**

ISBN: 978-93-86150-66-0

Dedicated to

All Nurses and Nursing Students who are going to attend competitive exams

Preface

Nursing is not a static, unchanging profession but is continuously growing and evolving as society changes. A nurse should understand the various concepts in a broad and comprehensive way in order to qualify national and international competitive exams.

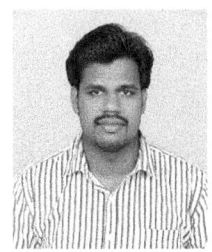

The various competitive exams are getting tougher every year. To succeed, you will need a wide knowledge of the subject. This is a huge curriculum and it is difficult to know whether you have gathered all the necessary facts and have reached the right standard. This is precisely where this book comes from. There is no predetermined syllabus or criteria for testing the nursing knowledge.

During my teaching experience, I have found out that there is a lack of study material which caters to the student requirements in order to pass these exams. The students have often sought recommendations for a publication which caters to their complete syllabus. For lack of such a book on nursing, there has always been a high demand for prepared notes which could be used for their preparation. This edition is a genuine effort to mitigate their hardship and also to stimulate academic interest and build an appreciation of the relevance of nursing practice and engaging the students to write in internationally based exams, like HAAD, DHA, RN, MOH and PROMETRIC.

I am confident that this book would provide good teaching material for all the instructors and students, who are going to write a competitive exam. Suggestions for improvement will be gratefully acknowledged.

Renjith Augustine

Acknowledgments

I would like to express a deep sense of gratitude to the "Almighty", who is continuously giving the moral support and guidance required in all my deeds.

I would like to express my sincere thanks to Dr Manoj P Jose, MD, Senior Consultant Physician, Little Flower Hospital and Research Centre, Angamaly, Kerala, India for giving his valuable assistance in accomplishing this task.

I would like to acknowledge and thank all my family members—especially my wife Mrs Tindu Thomas, my father Mr TD Augustine and my brother Mr Ajith Augustine, who lent their support in accomplishing the task.

I would like to express my gratitude to Mr Asish Paul; Mr Tony Antony—Director of EEZEE English Group of Institutions, Irinjalakuda, Kerala, India; and to all my students who gave continuous cooperation and valued assistance in bringing out this book.

I would also like to thank Shri Jitendar P Vij (Group Chairman), Mr Ankit Vij (Group President), Ms Chetna Malhotra Vohra (Associate Director—Content Strategy), and Ms Ruby Sharma (Project Manager) of Jaypee Brothers Medical Publishers, New Delhi, India for helping me in bringing out this book.

About the Exam

To NCLEX-RN Examination

NCLEX-RN examination is a licensure examination to assess the quality of a nursing personal to rule his or her competency in their professional area. The full form of NCLEX-RN is National Council Licensure Examination for Registered Nurses. This is an entry examination for the nurses to United States and Canada from the years 1994 and 2015. NCLEX examination can be of two types: NCLEX-RN examination and NCLEX-PN examination; RN is for registered nurse and PN for practical nurse. The questions will be in same format, multiple choices with options. The entire syllabus for this exam is categorized into: Nursing fundamentals, medical nursing, surgical nursing, pediatric nursing, psychiatric nursing and maternity nursing. The number of questions varies from 75 to 265 and the time of examination from 2 hours to 6 hours. There is no scoring for the exam, only pass or fail. The questions will not be direct questions as you studied in nursing institutions; however, they all are in applied aspect based on the patient picture. Once you qualify the exam, the computer will automatically stop displaying the subsequent questions.

To HAAD Examination

HAAD examination is a licensure examination to nurses who want to work in Abu Dhabi. The aim of the test is to check your competence in nursing profession in order to render high quality patient care. The full form of HAAD is Health Authority of Abu Dhabi. There are about 150 questions and the candidates are given 180 minutes (3 hours) to respond for all the questions. The questions will be in applied aspect from the entire nursing syllabus, nursing fundamentals, medical nursing, surgical nursing, pediatrics, psychiatric nursing and gynecology. The passing percentage is nearly 85–90%. Examinees are given three attempts (in three separate applications) to pass the HAAD examination. If the candidate failed all the three attempts, he or she will have to wait 12 months from the last exam to be able to retake the exam.

To DHA Examination

DHA examination is a licensure examination for all nurses to work in Dubai. DHA is Dubai Health Authority, previously known as DOH. The questions are almost same as that of NCLEX-RN and HAAD exam, only the passing criteria are different. The syllabus and format are also same as that of HAAD exam. The validity of DHA is one year from the exam. The duration of exam is 2 hours and the total number of questions is 70. Out of 70 questions, the candidate has to get 70% (65–70%). Examinees are given three attempts (in three separate applications) to pass the DHA examination. If the candidate failed all the three attempts, he or she will have to wait 12 months from the last exam to be able to retake the exam.

How to face Test Strategies?

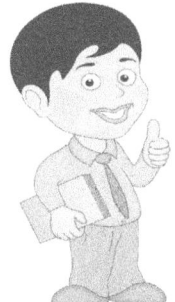

Time for Exam

- Make a study list of the entire syllabus
- Take the keynotes
- Study well for exam, cover the entire topic
- Create a positive attitude toward exam as I will pass surely ....
- Relax properly on the day before exam, do not study ....
- Prepare your mind and body for exam ....
- Take proper foods, and snacks ....
- Focus on the questions ....
- Go slow ....
- Do your best ....

Contents

1. **Nursing fundamentals** 1
   - Explain nursing process
   - Ethical issues in nursing
   - Acid-base imbalance
   - Nutrition and vitamins
   - Laboratory values
   - Positions
   - Drug calculation
2. **Integral aspects** 10
   - Explain modes of nursing care delivery
   - Nursing innovations and telemedicine
   - Discuss nursing research and evidence-based practice
   - Disaster nursing
   - Performance appraisal, delegation, recruitment
   - Crisis intervention
   - Geriatrics
3. **Neurological system** 23
   - Keynotes in the neurological system
   - Anatomy of the nervous system
   - Various diagnostic measures
   - Disorders in the nervous system
4. **Respiratory system** 33
   - Keynotes in the respiratory system
   - Anatomy of the respiratory system
   - Oxygen administration
   - Various diagnostic measures
   - Mechanical ventilation
   - Disorders in the respiratory system
5. **Cardiovascular system** 43
   - Keynotes in the cardiovascular system
   - Anatomy of heart
   - Various diagnostic measures
   - ECG
   - Disorders in cardiovascular system
   - Vascular disorders
6. **Endocrine system** 69
   - Keynotes in the endocrine system
   - Endocrine and exocrine glands
   - Diagnostic measures
   - Endocrine disorders
   - Diabetes mellitus
   - Pancreatitis

7. **Gastrointestinal system** 81
   - Keynotes in the gastrointestinal system
   - Anatomy of gastrointestinal system
   - Various diagnostic measures
   - Disorders in the gastrointestinal system

8. **Renal system** 98
   - Keynotes in the renal system
   - Anatomy of renal system
   - Various diagnostic measures
   - Disorders in the renal system
   - Dialysis

9. **Musculoskeletal system** 107
   - Keynotes in the musculoskeletal system
   - Anatomy of musculoskeletal system
   - Various diagnostic measures
   - Tractions
   - Disorders in the musculoskeletal system

10. **Hematological system** 119
    - Keynotes in the hematological system
    - Composition of blood
    - Various diagnostic measures
    - Disorders in the hematological system

11. **Integumentary system** 126
    - Keynotes in the integumentary system
    - Anatomy and structure
    - Disorders in the integumentary system
    - Burns
    - Shock

12. **Oncology** 132
    - Keynotes in the oncology
    - Staging and grading of cancer
    - Chemotherapy and radiation therapy
    - Type of cancers

13. **Eye and ear** 136
    - Keynotes in eye and ear
    - Anatomy and structure
    - Disorders in eye
    - Disorders in ear

14. **Immune system** 141
    - Keynotes in the immune system
    - Immunity
    - Immune disorders
    - AIDS

15. **Pediatric nursing** 144
    - Keynotes in pediatric nursing
    - Theories and principles of growth and development
    - Common disorders in newborn

- Common disorders in pediatric neurological system
- Common disorders in pediatric respiratory system
- Common disorders in pediatric gastrointestinal system
- Common disorders in pediatric cardiovascular system
- Common disorders in pediatric genitourinary system
- Common disorders in pediatric musculoskeletal system

16. Psychiatric nursing 168
- Keynotes in the psychiatric nursing
- Theories of personality
- Psychotherapy and ECT
- Classification of disorders

17. Maternity nursing 196
- Keynotes in maternity nursing
- Anatomy of female reproductive system
- Antepartum disorders
- Intrapartum period
- Postpartum changes

18. Previous questions and answers 212

Index.. 279

CHAPTER 1

Nursing Fundamentals

Chapter Objectives

- Explain nursing process
- Ethical issues in nursing
- Acid-base imbalance
- Nutrition and vitamins
- Laboratory values
- Positions
- Drug calculation

INTRODUCTION

The era of modern nursing commences with the work of Florence Nightingale in the Crimean war (1854-1856). She was born in Italy in 1820. She was the second daughter of wealthy English parents. In 1851, Nightingale entered the Deaconess school in Kaiserswerth. She was 31 years old and her family and friends were strongly opposed to her becoming a nurse. After her graduation in 1853, she became superintendent of charity hospital for the government.

In 1854, the Crimean war began. Her dedicated service both during the day and at night, when she and some other nurses made their rounds carrying oil lamps, created a public image of the lady with the lamp. In time, the 'Nightingale lamp' or the "Lamp of learning" became a symbol of nursing and nursing education. Todays, many schools of nursing display a model of the lamp or a picture of Florence Nightingale carrying a lamp.

In 1860, Nightingale opened the first nursing school outside a hospital. The nursing course was 1 year in length and included both classroom and clinical experience, a major innovation at that time.

Modern nursing is a dynamic, therapeutic and education process in meeting the health needs of the individuals, the family and the community. Nursing is one of the health professions which functions in conjunction with other health care agencies in assisting individuals, families and communities to achieve and maintain desirable standards of health.

NURSING

"The unique function of the nurse is to assist the individual, sick or well, in the performance of those activities contributing to health or its recovery (or to peaceful death) that he would perform unaided if he had the necessary strength, will or knowledge and to do this in such a way as to help him gain independence as rapidly as possible."
—Henderson, 1966

"Nursing is the protection, promotion and optimizing of health and abilities, prevention of illness and injury, alleviation of suffering through the diagnosis and treatment of human response and advocacy in the care of individuals, families, communities and population."
—The American Nurses Association, 2003

NURSING PROFESSION

Profession has been defined as an occupation that requires extensive education or a calling that requires special knowledge, skill and preparation. A profession is generally distinguished from other kinds of occupations by:

a. Its requirement of prolonged, specialized training to acquire a body of knowledge pertinent to the role to be performed.
b. An orientation of the individual toward service, either to a community or to an organization.
c. Ongoing research
d. A code of ethics

e. Autonomy
f. Professional organization

NURSING PROCESS

A process is a series of steps that is used to perform any activity to meet the desired outcome. Nursing process is a five step process for providing professional and quality nursing care to the patients.

Steps in Nursing Process

- Assessment
- Diagnosis
- Planning
- Implementation
- Evaluation

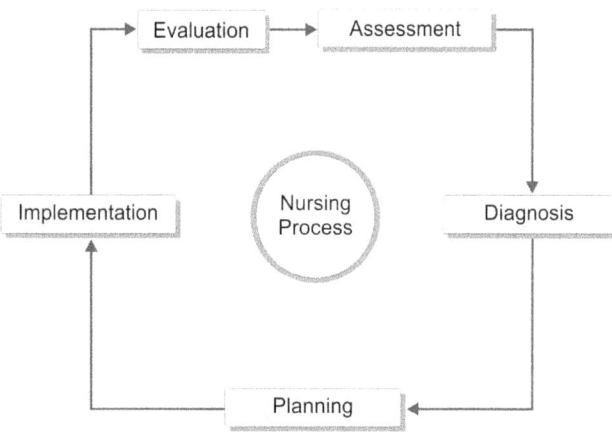

Assessment

Assessment is the first step in nursing process. In this phase the nurse assess the condition of the patient by collecting data from the patients or relatives. The data is collected by variety of means such as personal interview, physical examination, health history, family history, and so on. There are two types of data, subjective data and objective data. Subjective data are data from patient's point of view or verbal report, e.g. I have fever. Objective data are observable and measurable data, what the nurse observes, e.g. monitoring temperature to assess the severity of fever.

Diagnosis

Diagnosis is the second step in nursing process. In this phase the nurse makes a judgment about the potential or actual problems based on the assessment findings. Multiple diagnosis are sometimes made for a single patient, among that we have to pick the most priority one first. After analyzing the collected data (high temperature), we will come to the conclusion that patient is having fever. The diagnosis is a critical step as it is used to determine the course of treatment.

Planning

Planning is the third step in nursing process. Once a patient and nurse agree on the diagnosis, a plan of action can be developed. If multiple diagnosis need to be addressed, the head nurse will prioritize each assessment and devote attention to severe symptoms and high risk factors. Each problem is assigned a clear, measurable goal for the expected beneficial outcome. After selecting the diagnosis (fever) nurse plan the actions to reduce the fever such as cold sponge, medications, fluids, diets, etc.

Implementation

Implementation is also called as working phase. The nurse works through the desired plan. This plan is specific for each person and focus on the achievable outcome. Implementation can take place over the course of hours, days, weeks or even months. After planning the activities for the desired diagnosis (fever) nurse implement the plan such as administering medications, health education, fluids, etc.

Evaluation

Evaluation is the last step of nursing process. Once all nursing intervention actions have taken place, the nurse completes an evaluation to determine the goals for patient wellness has been met. The possible patient outcomes are generally described under three terms: patient's condition improved (fever decreased), patient's condition stabilized and patient's condition deteriorated, died or discharged.

ISSUES IN NURSING

Ethical Issues

Ethics

Ethics are the rules or principles that govern right conduct and are designed to protect the rights of human beings.

A code of ethics is a set of ethical principles that are accepted by all members of a profession.

ICN Code of Ethics for Nurses

In 1953 ICN adopted its first code of ethics for nurses and was revised in 2000. The four principle elements contained within the ICN code involve standards related to nurses and people, practice, profession and co-workers.

ICN recommended that nurses have four fundamental responsibilities, i.e. to promote health, to prevent illness, to restore health and to alleviating suffering. And also inherent in nursing is respect for human rights, like right to life, to dignity and to be treated with respect. And the care should not be restricted by age, sex, color, creed, culture or nationality.

Nurses and People

The nurse's primary responsibility is to those people who require nursing care. The nurse in providing care promotes an environment in the values, customs and spiritual beliefs of the individual are respected. The nurse holds in confidence personal information and uses judgment in sharing this information.

Nurses and Practice

The nurse carries personal responsibility for nursing practice and for maintaining competence by continual learning. The nurse maintains the highest standard of nursing care possible within the reality of a specific situation.

Nurses and Co-workers

The nurse maintains a cooperative relationship with co-workers in nursing and other fields. The nurse takes appropriate action to safeguard the individual when his care is endangered by a co-worker or any person.

Nurses and the Profession

The nurses play a major role in determining and implementing desirable standards of nursing practice. The nursing is active in developing a core of professional knowledge. The nurse acting through the professional organizations participates in establishing and maintaining equitable social and economic working conditions in nursing.

Key Principles of Ethics in Healthcare System

- *Autonomy*: The right of self-determination, independence and freedom. Right to health care decision.
- *Justice*: Obligation to be fair with all people.
- *Fidelity*: Obligation of an individual to be faithful to the commitment made to himself and to others. It is the main support of accountability.
- *Veracity*: The duty to tell the truth.
- *Beneficence*: Doing good for the client. What exactly is good for one person may not be the same for others.
- *Maleficence:* Maleficence is the requirement that health care providers do no harm to their client either intentionally or unintentionally.

Common Ethical Issues

- Physician assisted suicide (PAS)
- Do not resuscitate order (DNR)
- Refuse to treat by nurses
- Refusal of treatment by patient
- Genetic research

Legal Issues

- Legal: Established by or founded upon law or official or accepted rules.
- Law: It means a body of rules to guide human action.

Legal Liability in Nursing

Statutory Law is created by elected legislative bodies such as state or provincial legislatures, the U.S. Congress, administrative bodies such as state boards of nursing or the Canadian Parliament.

Common Law is created by judicial decisions made in courts when cases are decided.

Criminal Law is concerned with relationships between individuals and governments and with acts that threaten society and its order. Misuse of controlled substances is an example of criminal conduct for nurses. A crime is an offense against society that violates a law. Criminal acts are prosecutes in the criminal justice system. A **felony** is a crime of a serious nature that usually carries a penalty of imprisonment or death.

Civil Law is concerned with the relationships among people and the protection of a person's rights. Although violations of civil law might cause harm to an individual or property, society as a whole is usually not affected. For example, defamatory statements made about an individual might lead to interpersonal problems, but they do not threaten society as a whole.

Legal Issues

- Torts
- Assault
- Battery
- Invasion of privacy
- Defamation of character
- Negligence
- Malpractice

Torts: A tort is a civil wrong committed against a person or property. Torts may be subtle and difficult to define; they may be classified as intentional or unintentional. Unintentional torts include negligence. Malpractice is one example of an unintentional tort or negligence. Intentional torts are willful acts that violate another's rights. Examples are assault, battery and defamation, invasion of privacy, false imprisonment and fraud.

Assaults: Assault is any willful attempt or threat to harm another, coupled with the ability to actually harm the other person. The victim believes harm will come as a result of the threat. Assault may be subtle; for example, a nurse might attempt to coerce a client into taking a drug he or she does not wish to take. A more blatant example might involve a nurse handing an uncooperative client in the emergency room, e.g. "If you don't take off those filthy clothes, I am going to rip them off you!" and moves toward the client, a claim of assault could be made.

Battery: Battery is any intentional touching of another's body or anything the person is touching or holding without consent. Injury is not a requirement. There have been instances of battery of confined clients by personnel in mental institutions.

Invasion of privacy: Clients have claims for invasion of privacy when their private affairs, with which the public has no concern, have been publicized. A client is entitled to confidential health care. All aspects of care should be free from unwanted publicity or exposure to public scrutiny.

Defamation of character: Defamation of character is the holding up of a person to ridicule, scorn or contempt within the community. There are two types of defamation: **slander** and **libel**. For example, if a nurse tells a client that his physician is incompetent; the nurse could be held liable for slander. If the nurse writes such a comment, the charge would be libel. The important issues in a claim of defamation of character are whether the information was shared with third persons (other than the client) and if harm has been done to the reputation of the plaintiff (legal short hand).

Negligence: Negligence is conduct that falls below the standard of care. It is established by law for the protection of others against unreasonable risk of harm and it is characterized chiefly by inadvertence, thoughtlessness or inattention.

If nurses give care that does not meet appropriate standards, they may be held liable for negligence. Negligence may involve carelessness, such as failing to check a client's arm band and then administering the wrong drug. Another example of negligence may be administering a medication even when it has been documented that the client has an allergy to that medication. For example:
- Intravenous therapy errors resulting in infiltrations or phlebitis.
- Burns to clients
- Falls resulting in injury to clients.
- Failure to use aseptic technique where required.

Malpractice: Malpractice is one type of negligence. It is defined as professional misconduct, unreasonable lack of skill or fidelity in professional duties, evil practice or illegal or immoral conduct. In a malpractice lawsuit against a nurse, the following criteria must be established.
1. The nurse (defendant) owned a duty to the client (plaintiff).
2. The nurse did not carry out that duty.
3. The client was injured.
4. The client's injury was a result of the nurse's failure to carry out his or her duty.

ACID-BASE IMBALANCES

There are mainly four acid-base imbalances.
1. Respiratory acidosis
2. Respiratory alkalosis
3. Metabolic acidosis
4. Metabolic alkalosis

RO/ME
Respiratory – Opposite direction
Metabolic – Equal direction

Respiratory acidosis	pH ↓	PCO_2 ↑	HCO_3 ↑
Respiratory alkalosis	pH ↑	PCO_2 ↓	HCO_3 ↓
Metabolic acidosis	pH ↓	PCO_2 ↓	HCO_3 ↓
Metabolic alkalosis	pH ↑	PCO_2 ↑	HCO_3 ↑

Respiratory Acidosis

- Hypoventilation
- Asthma
- Pneumonia
- Pulmonary edema
- Pulmonary embolism
- CNS depressants
- Brain trauma

Nursing care: Administer oxygen

Respiratory Alkalosis

- Hyperventilation
- Fever
- Hysteria
- Pain
- Hypoxia
- Mechanical ventilation

Nursing care: Limit oxygen

Metabolic Acidosis

- Diabetic ketoacidosis and DM
- Severe diarrhea
- Renal failure
- Renal insufficiency
- High fat diet
- Excessive ingestion of acetyl salicylate acid (aspirin)
- Malnutrition
- Insufficient metabolism of carbohydrate

Nursing care: Administer sodium bicarbonate

Metabolic Alkalosis

- Diuretics
- Excessive vomiting
- GI suction
- Hyperaldosteronism
- Infusion of sodium bicarbonate
- Massive transfusion of whole blood

Nursing care: Administer chloride

NUTRITION

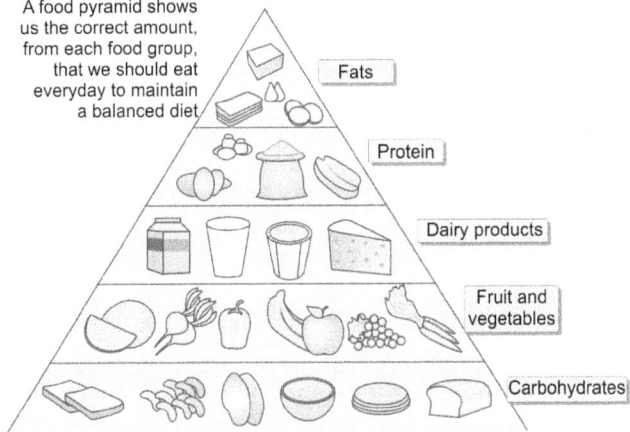

A food pyramid shows us the correct amount, from each food group, that we should eat everyday to maintain a balanced diet

The energy sources are carbohydrates, fats and protein. Carbohydrates are the base of food pyramid and fats are the top of food pyramid.

Carbohydrate-Rich Foods

Potatoes, whole grains, citrus fruits, berries, water melon, nuts and legumes, cereals, dried fruits, bread, banana and green leafy vegetables.

Protein-Rich Diets

Eggs, milk, yogurt, fish and sea foods, soya, nuts, meats, chicken, etc.

Indications of High-Protein Diet

- Burns
- Mild to moderate liver diseases
- Cystic fibrosis
- Under nutrition
- Pregnancy
- Nephrotic syndrome

Indications of Low-Protein Diet

- Liver failure
- Kidney failure

Fat-Rich Diets

Beef, poultry, butter, cream, milk, cheese, etc.

Total Parenteral Nutrition

Total Parenteral Nutrition (TPN) is feeding the patient intravenously; nutrients are infused directly into the veins through a central line catheter.

The contents are hypertonic solutions, amino acids, vitamins, lipids, etc.

Nursing Care

- Monitor RBS every 4 hours.
- Monitor for any complications (Hyperglycemia, Hypertension, Infection).
- Fat emulsions (lipids) contain egg yolk; phospholipids should not be given to client with egg allergies.
- Insulin and heparin may be added in the TPN solution.
- When TPN disconnects, never discontinue abruptly, it will cause hypoglycemia. So, the flow rate should be decreased gradually.
- Do not write on a plastic IV bag with a marking pen as the ink may be absorbed into the solution. So use a label and place the label on to the bag.

VITAMINS

There are two categories:
- Fat-soluble vitamins (A, D, E, K)
- Water-soluble vitamins (B, C)

Vitamin A	Retinol	Vitamin C	Ascorbic acid
Vitamin B_1	Thiamine	Vitamin D_3	Cholecalciferol
Vitamin B_2	Riboflavin	Vitamin E	Tocopherol
Vitamin B_3	Niacin/Nicotinic acid	Vitamin K	Phylloquinone
Vitamin B_5	Pantothenic acid	Vitamin P	Citrin
Vitamin B_6	Pyridoxine		
Vitamin B_7	Biotin		
Vitamin B_9	Folic acid		
Vitamin B_{12}	Cyanocobalamin		

Vitamin A
- It is also called as retinol.
- Rich sources are fish liver oil, animal fat, egg yolk, liver, dark green leafy vegetables and milk.
- Deficiency will leads to blindness.

Vitamin B_1
- It is also called as thiamine.
- Rich sources are cereals, pulses, nuts, green vegetables, yeast, egg and meat.
- Deficiency will leads to beri-beri.

Vitamin B_2
- It is also called as riboflavin.
- Rich sources are yeast, grains, green leafy vegetables, pulses, egg, liver and milk.
- Deficiency will lead to sore throat, glossitis and cheilosis.

Vitamin B_3
- It is also called as nicotinic acid.
- Rich sources are meat, grains, liver, fish, cheese and pulses.
- Deficiency will lead to pellagra.

Vitamin B_6
- It is also called as pyridoxine.
- Rich sources are yeast, liver, egg yolk, peas and soybean.
- Deficiency will leads to changes to skin, nervous system and erythropoiesis.

Vitamin C
- It is also known as ascorbic acid.
- Rich sources are citrus fruits, fresh vegetables, tomato, potato, green chillies and cabbage.
- Deficiency will leads to scurvy.

Vitamin D
- It is also called as calciferol (D_2) or cholecalciferol (D_3).
- Rich sources are fish liver oil, egg yolk, butter, milk, milk and milk products and sunlight.
- Deficiency will leads to rickets and Osteomalacia.

Vitamin E
- It is also called as Tocopherol.
- Rich sources are germ oil, cereals, nuts, egg yolk and green leafy vegetables such as spinach.
- Deficiency of vitamin E produces sterility in animals and Hemolysis.
- It is also called antioxidant and beauty vitamin.

Vitamin K
- It is also called as Phylloquinone or coagulation vitamin.
- Rich sources are dark green leafy vegetables.
- Also produced by the normal flora of intestine.
- Deficiency will leads to bleeding disorders.

MINERALS
Calcium
- Rich sources are sardines, milk and milk products.
- Deficiency will leads to osteoporosis and rickets.

Phosphorus
- Rich sources are milk, cheese and egg.
- Deficiency will leads to rickets.

Magnesium
- Rich sources are milk, cheese, legumes, etc.
- Deficiency will leads to renal problem and tremor in alcoholics.

Sulfur
- Rich sources are milk, fish, poultry, etc.
- It is a constituent of keratin in skin.

Iron
- Rich sources are liver organ meat, poultry and dark green leafy vegetables.
- Deficiency will leads to anemia.

Iodine
- Rich sources are iodized salt e.g. sea foods.
- Deficiency will leads to goitre and cretinism.

Potassium

- Rich sources are orange, banana, dry fruits and fresh fruits.
- Deficiency will lead to muscle cramps, arrhythmias.

Types of Diet on the Basis of Consumption

Clear Liquid Diet

- Not nutritionally adequate
- Foods included are water, apple juice, frozen ice, carbonated beverages.

Full Liquid Diet

- Can be nutritionally adequate
- Used as a transition between clear liquid and soft diet.
- Foods included are clear liquid plus, milk and milk products, fruit juices, cooked and stained foods.

Soft Diet

- Used as a transition between full liquid diet and regular diet.
- Foods allowed are full liquid diet plus foods low in fiber, cooked vegetables, boiled eggs and meats.

Bland Diet

- Diet promotes wound healing, healing of gastric ulcer.
- Foods allowed are soft diet without spices, low residual diet.

LABORATORY VALUES

Normal CSF volume	125–150 mL
Normal CSF pressure	50–175 mm H$_2$O (6–13 mm Hg)
Normal CSF glucose	50–80 mg/dL
Normal CSF protein	15–45 mg/dL
Normal ICP	5–15 mm Hg
Normal IOP	10–21 mm Hg
Normal CVP	4–10 cmH$_2$O (3–8 mm Hg)
Normal GFR	125 mL/minute
Serum sodium	135–145 mEq/L
Serum potassium	3.5–5.1 mEq/L
Serum bicarbonate	22–29 mEq/L
Serum chloride	98–107 mEq/L
Normal CT	8–15 minutes
Normal PT	9.6–11.8 seconds
Normal APTT	20–36 seconds
Normal ESR	0–30 mm/hr

Contd...

Contd...

Normal platelet	150000–450000 cells/mm^3
Normal Hemoglobin	12–14 gm/dL
Normal Hematocrit	42–52%
Serum iron	65–175 mcg/dL
Normal RBC count	4.5–6.2 million cells/microliter
Serum bilirubin Total	< 1.5 mg/dL
Serum bilirubin direct	0–0.3 mg/dL
Ammonia	10–80 mcg/dL
Serum cholesterol	140–199 mg/dL
LDL	< 130 mg/dL
HDL	30–70 mg/dL
Triglycerides	< 200 mg/dL
Serum protein	6–8 mg/dL
Serum albumin	3.5–5 gm/dL
Serum globulin	2.5–4.5 gm/dL
Serum uric acid	3–8 mg/dL
Fasting blood sugar	70–110 mg/dL
PPBS	< 140 mg/dL
Serum creatine	0.6–1.2 mg/dL
Blood urea Nitrogen	8–25 mg/dL
Serum calcium	8.6–10 mg/dL
Serum magnesium	1.6–2.6 mg/dL
Serum phosphorus	2.7–4.5 mg/dL
Serum TSH	0.2–5.4 micro IU/L
Serum Thyroxine (T4)	5–12 mcg/dL
Serum Triiodothyronine (T3)	80–230 ng/dL
Normal WBC	4000–11000 cells/mm^3
Normal serum lithium	0.5–1.2 mEq/L

POSITIONS

Condition/procedure	Position
Tonsillectomy	Prone or side line position
Liver biopsy	Right sided position
CA mouth	Side line position
Hiatal hernia	Sitting position before and after meals
Dumping syndrome	Supine position for half hour after meals
Cyanotic heart disease	Squatting/frog-like position
Colostomy irrigation	High Fowler's position
Pancreatitis	Knee chest position
Pulmonary embolism	Fowler's position

Contd...

Contd...

Condition/procedure	Position
Prevent hip contractures	Prone position
Kidney biopsy	Prone position
Seizures	Side line position
Enema	Left lateral position
Lumbar puncture	Lateral recumbent position
Abdominal Aneurysm surgery	Fowler's position
Air embolism	Left side
Appendicitis	Semi-Fowler's position in case of rupture
Asthma	Sitting position
Autonomic dysreflexia	High Fowler's position
Bronchoscopy	Semi-Fowler's
Cataract surgery	Semi-Fowler's
Cerebral aneurysm	Semi-Fowler's
Cleft lip	Supine
Cleft palate	Prone
Congestive cardiac failure	High Fowler's position
Craniotomy	Semi-Fowler's for supratentorial Flat for infratentorial
CVA	Elevate the head
Hypophysectomy	Elevate the head
Increased ICP	Elevate the head of bed
Laryngectomy	Semi-Fowler's position
Epistaxis	Leaning forward to prevent aspiration
Lobectomy	Semi-Fowler's
Mastectomy	Elevate with pillow, the extremity of affected side
Placenta previa	Sitting position
Pulmonary edema	Fowler's
Pyloric stenosis	Right side lying
Shock	Modified trendelenburg
Thoracentesis	Fowler's position
Thyroidectomy	Semi-Fowler's
Total parenteral nutrition	Trendelenburg position
Varicose vein	Elevate the legs
Lung biopsy	Prone/supine/decubitus position
Self-enema	Sims' position

Same-sided position is given for pneumonectomy, liver biopsy, myringotomy, retinal detachment

CALCULATIONS AND PROBLEMS

1 drain = 60 grains
1 ounce = 30 mL
1 liter = 1000 mL
1 grain = 60 mgm
1 pint = 500 mL
1 kg = 2.2 lbs
1 mgm = 1000 mcg
1 teaspoon = 4–5 mL
1 teaspoon = 60 drop
1 mL = 16 drop
1 inch = 2.5 cm
qd = everyday
qod = every other day
d = daily
bid = twice a day
tid = three times a day
qid = four times a day
q4h = every 4 hrs
q6h = every 6 hrs
q8h = every 8 hrs
q4–6h = every 4–6 hrs
prn = as needed

Formulas

$C = (F - 32) \times 5/9$ (For converting Fahrenheit to Celsius)
$F = (C \times 9/5) + 32$ (For converting Degree to Fahrenheit)

Young's Formula

Child's dose = [(Age of child/(Age of child + 12)] × Average adult dose

Example:
A 10 year old girl/60 Lbs with 300 mg Average adult dose is given for the girl. Calculate the child's pediatric dose.
Given,
Age of child = 10 years
    Average Adult dose = 300 mg
To find,
Child's pediatric dose

Solution:
Child's dose = [(Age of child/(Age of child + 12)] × Average adult dose
    = [10/(10 + 12)] × 300 mg
    = (10/22) × 300 mg
    = (0.45454545454) × 300 mg
    = 136.363636364 mg

Clark's Formula

Child dose = (weight in pounds/150) × adult dose.
    Clark's rule uses Weight in lbs, NEVER in kg.
    Adult dose × (Weight ÷ 150) = Child dose

Example:
11-year-old girl/70 lbs, adult dose is 500 mg
500 mg × (70 ÷ 150) = Child's dose
500 mg × (.47) = Child's dose
500 mg × .47 = 235 mg

Other Formulas

Pulse pressure = Systolic BP–Diastolic BP
MAP (mean arterial pressure) = [(Systolic BP + 2 (Diastolic BP)]/3
Cerebral perfusion Pressure (CPP) = MAP–ICP
Drops per minute = (order dose/overdose) × drop factor

Drop Factor

- The drop factor is the number of drops contained in 1 milliliter.
- Macrodrip tubing administers a larger drop and may be used for 10 gtts/mL, 15 gtts/mL or 20 gtts/mL.
- Microdrip tubing administers 60 gtts/mL

Problems and Solutions

1. Prepare 250 cc of 4% solution of boric acid.
   (4% solution means 4 gms of boric acid in 100 cc)
   4:100 = X: 250
   100X = 1000 (cross multiplication)
   X = 1000/100 = **10**

2. A child is to receive dexona (dexamethasone) intravenously at the ordered dosage of 7.6 mg. The drug concentration in the vial is 4 mg/mL. Which of the following amounts should the nurse administer?
   4 mg: 1 mL = 7.6 mg: XmL
   4 X = 7.6 × 1
   X = 7.6/4 = **1.9 mL**

3. Choral hydrate 1000 mg has been ordered. It is available in a syrup containing 0.5 g/5 mL. How many milliliters should the nurse give?
   0.5 g = 500 mg
   1000 mg/X mL = 500 mg/5 mL
   X = (1000 × 5)/500 = **10 mL**

4. The client is prescribed Dynapar 15 mg IM. The nurse has a 1 mL preloaded syringe of Dynapar labeled 30 mg/mL. How many milliliters of medication should the nurse administer?
   30 mg/1 mL = 15 mg/X mL
   X = (15/30) = **0.5 mL**

5. A client has been diagnosed with acute prostatitis. The physician order 1 gm of chloramphenicol every 4 hours. The pharmacy has 250 mg capsules available. How many capsules should the nurse administer every 4 hours?
   1 gm = 1000 mg
   250 mg: 1 capsule = 1000 mg: **X** mL
   250 × X = 1000 × 1
   X = 1000/250 = **4 capsules**

6. A client is admitted with dehydration and oliguria. The physician order 1000 mL of 5% dextrose IV to be infused within 8 hour period. The IV set delivers 15 gtt/mL. The nurse should regulate the flow rate so, it delivers how many drops of fluid per minute?
   Order dose = 1000 mL
   Over time = 8 hours
   Drop factor = 15
   Flow rate = (order/over) × drop factor
   = (1000/8 × 60) × 15
   = **30 gtt/minute**

7. A nurse is assessing a client with brain injury. What is a client's cerebral perfusion pressure (CPP) when the blood pressure (BP) is 90/50 mm Hg and the intracranial pressure (ICP) 21?
   CPP = MAP–ICP
   MAP = (systolic + (2 × diastolic))/3
   MAP = (90 + 100)/3 = 63.3
   CPP = MAP–ICP
   CPP = 63.3-21 = **42.3 mm Hg**

8. The doctor order cholecalciferol 600000 units IM has been ordered. The nurse have available 1 mL prefilled syringe labeled 600000 units/mL. How many milliliters should the nurse administer?
   600000 units/1mL = 600000/X mL
   X = 600000/600000 = **1 mL**

CHAPTER 2

Integral Aspects

Chapter Objectives

- Explain modes of nursing care delivery
- Nursing innovations and telemedicine
- Discuss nursing research and evidence-based practice
- Disaster nursing
- Performance appraisal, delegation, recruitment
- Crisis intervention
- Geriatrics

MODES OF NURSING CARE DELIVERY

Nursing service is the part of the total health organization which aims at satisfying the nursing needs of the patients and community. In nursing services, the nurse works with the members of allied disciples, such as dietician, medical social service, and pharmacy in supplying a comprehensive program of patient care in the hospital.

Methods of Patient Assignment

There are five methods of nursing assignment:
1. Primary nursing
2. Functional nursing
3. Team nursing
4. Modular nursing
5. Case management method

Primary Nursing (One Nurse to One Patient or 24 Hours' Nursing Care)

The "primary nurse" is responsible for coordinating all aspects of care for the same group of patients throughout their stay in a given area. It is also called 24 hours nursing care delivery.

Primary nursing method is a method of nursing assignment, in which each nurse is given total responsibility of planning, executing and evaluating nursing care for a small case load of 4 to 6 patients (One nurse provides complete care for a small group of inpatients within a nursing unit of a hospital).

Merits
- There is opportunity for the nurse to see the client and family as one system.
- The nurse is able to use a wide range of skills, knowledge, and expertise.
- The scene is set for increased trust and satisfaction by the client and nurse.

Demerits
- The nurse may be isolated from colleagues.
- An inadequately prepared or educated primary nurse may be incapable of co-ordinating a multidisciplinary team.

Functional Nursing (Based on Function)

Functional method of nursing assignment consists of separating the task involved in each patients care and assigning each staff member to perform one or two care tasks or functions for all patients in the unit. It is suitable only for short-term use. For example, bed-making nurse, bed bath nurse, IV nurse, etc.

Team Nursing (A Group of Nurses)

Team nursing is a method of nursing assignments that binds professional, technical and auxiliary nursing personnel into small teams to mutually suppressive workers, there by combining the superior knowledge and skill of professional workers with lower personnel costs of technical and auxiliary workers.

Modular Nursing (Based on Area or Small Group)

Modular nursing is a combination of team nursing and primary nursing because her professionals are cooperatively taking care of the patients and each pair of nursing personnel is responsible for the care of the patients in their case load from admission to discharge.

Case Method (Based on Case)

Case method is a method of nursing assignment otherwise known as nursing care management. It is the set of activities undertaken by a single nurse to mobilize, monitor, and evaluate all resources used by a patient during the total course of an illness.

NURSING INNOVATIONS

The word innovation means "introduction of something new" or a new way of doing something.

"Innovation is change that creates a new dimension of performance". Many successful innovations improve on an existing product to make it faster, cheaper or more efficient.

Purpose of Innovation

- Innovation is central to maintaining and improving quality of care.
- Nurses innovate to find new information and better ways of promoting health, preventing disease and better ways of care and cure.

Role of a Nurse

- Assess the need in hospital—patient care
- Understand the clients need
- Identify the areas of opportunity to introduce the innovative process
- Formulate the growth strategy—tools and validation
- Enact the growth strategy
- Use correct evidence-based practices

TELENURSING AND TELEMEDICINE

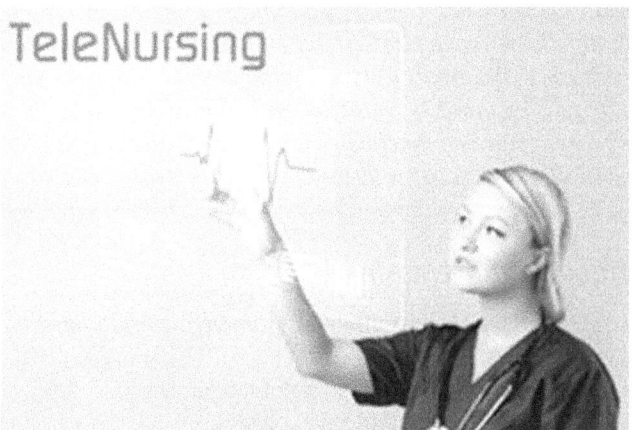

Tele-nursing is a latest innovation in nursing (*Tele* is a prefix meaning "at a distance". So *telenursing* means "care of patients at a distance").

Telemedicine

Telemedicine is defined as "the practice of health care delivery, diagnosis, consultation, treatment, transfer of medical data, and education using interactive audio, visual, and data communications."

Telehealth

Telehealth is "the use of electronic information and telecommunication technologies to support long-distance clinical health care, patient and professional health-related education, public health and health administration."

Telenursing

The American Nurses Association has defined telenursing as "a subset of telehealth in which the focus is on the specific profession's practice".

Telenursing is one of the fastest growing areas in healthcare, in which nurses deliver, manage, and coordinate patient care and services via telecommunication technology. Telenursing is achieving a large rate of growth in many countries.

Telenursing is the delivery, management, and coordination of care and services provided via telecommunications technology within the domain of nursing. Telenursing is the use of telemedicine technology to deliver nursing care and conduct nursing practice by the removal of time and distance barriers for the delivery of health care services.

Example: One of the most distinctive telenursing applications is home care and care of elderly patients. For example, patients who are immobilized, or live in remote or difficult to reach places or patients with chronic diseases, such as COPD, heart failure or other neural disorders may stay at home and be "visited" and assisted regularly by a nurse via video conferencing, internets or videophones. The specialist doctors in the distant place can see the patient and give treatment. It functions mostly with the help of satellites.

Purposes of Telenursing

- Telenursing is cost efficient, time saving and increases patient's ability to self-care.
- It helps to reduce the length of hospital stay.
- Reduce distances and save travel time.
- Improvement of resource and time allocation
- Greater degree of job satisfaction among telenurses
- Helps to keep patients out of hospital

Drawbacks

- Lack of ability to touch or direct delivery of care to a patient by nurse.
- Technical skill is needed by nurses.
- Network connection error/failure/delay.

ELECTRONIC MEDICAL RECORD

It is a computerized patient record system.

An electronic medical record (EMR) can be defined as the legal patient record created in hospitals and ambulatory environments that is the data source for the EMR (electronic health record).

An electronic medical record is a computerized medical record created in an organization that delivers care, such as a hospital and doctor's surgery. It includes demographics, medical history, medication and allergies, immunization status, laboratory test results, radiology images, and billing information.

Purposes

- Improves the quality of patient care by minimizing the errors
- Helps to reduce the medical errors
- Promote evidence-based medicine
- Used widely in all areas
- Greater storage and security of data
- Speed of transferring patient pictures
- Easy accessibility and affordability of data even in any areas.

NURSING RESEARCH

The word research comes from the Re-search, i.e. Re-Again and Again. Search—finding out something new.

Research in nursing is a careful, critical, exhaustive investigation of a problem or to discover new fact or verifying the old facts through hypotheses testing.

Research
"Research is a process of systematically search for new facts and relationship."

Nursing Research
"Nursing research is systematic inquiry designed to develop knowledge about issues of importance to the nursing profession, including nursing practice, education, administration and informatics" (Polit & hungler).

Purposes

1. **Identification**
   To examine the phenomena about what is known and what is unknown
2. **Description**
   To understand the nature of nursing phenomena and sometimes the relationship among these phenomena
3. **Explanation**
   To explain the nature of relationship
4. **Exploration**
   To explore the relationship about the phenomena and identifies the extend of the relationship
5. **Prediction and Control**
   Research helps to predict and control to produce desired outcome

Kinds of Research

Quantitative Research and Qualitative Research

Quantitative Research
In this type of research, data are collected in numerical form and analyzed by using descriptive and inferential statistics. It involves analysis of numerical data (Quantity).

Qualitative Research
In this type of research, data are collected in descriptive form and analyzed in words, pictures, diagrams or objects.

Applied Research and Basic Research

Applied Research
Research designed to solve particular circumstances, such as determining the cause of low moderate in a given department.

Basic Research

Basic research is designed to understand the underlying principles behind a human behavior.

Exploratory and Confirmatory

Exploratory research is research into the unknown.

Confirmatory research means you have a good idea what is going on next (i.e. you have a theory and objective of the research is to find out if the theory is supported by the fact.)

Scope of Nursing Research

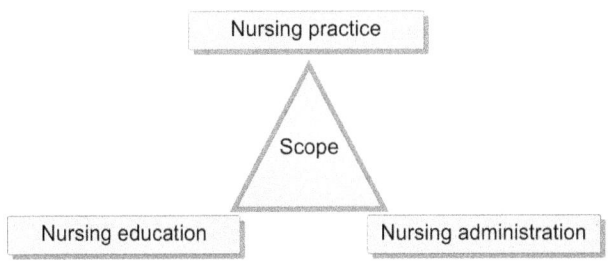

- Nursing research helps in improving the broad professional knowledge.
- Helps in providing evidence-based practice
- Helps in improving high quality nursing care based on theoretical knowledge
- Helps in improvement in payment system in health care system
- Helps in improvement in nursing procedure and nursing care
- Helps in development of specialized area in nursing service
- Helps in research utilization, i.e. theory into practice
- Helps in planning nursing care.

Problems in Conducting Research in Nursing

The common problems in conducting nursing research are:
1. **Research characteristics**
   - Lack of research design application
   - Problems in sample selection
   - Problems in data collection method
   - Problems in data analysis
2. **Nurses' characteristics**
   - Lack of skill of the nurses
3. **Organization characteristics**
   - Lack of support from the organization
   - Lack of qualified supervisors
   - Lack of proper guidance
4. **Characteristic of nursing profession**
   - Nonrelevance of the problem

Roles of a Nurse in Research

The roles of a nurse are as follows:
1. Principal investigator
2. Member of research team
3. Identifier of research problem
4. Evaluator of research finding
5. User of research findings
6. As a client advocate during the studies
7. As a subject in studies

Principal Investigator

Nurse can act as a principal investigator in scientific investigations. To be a principal investigator, a special research preparation is necessary.

Member of Research Team

Nurse can serve as a member of a research team. Nurse may act as a data collector or the person who administer the experimental intervention of the study.

Identifier of Research Problem

Nurse can identify the research problem or the problems which are relevant to the nursing profession.

Evaluator of Research Finding

A nurse researcher can evaluate what are the research findings and, based on the finding or evidence, she can practice.

User of Research Findings

The primary goal of the research finding is better patient care. After evaluating the research finding, nurse should use relevant finding in their practice.

As a Client Advocate during the Studies

One of the most important responsibilities of the nurse is to act as a client advocate in research study. This involves making sure that the ethical aspects of the research are upheld.

As a Subject in Studies

Nurses may act as a subject or participant in the research study. Sometimes the study is conducted in the nurses or some nurses are involved in the long-term survey program, i.e. nurses are the inevitable part of the research process.

EVIDENCE-BASED PRACTICE

Evidence-based practice (EBP) is a strategy that integrates research and practice. Evidence is information acquired through scientific evaluation of practice. Evidence-based nursing practice refers to the incorporation of evidence from research, clinical expertise, client preferences and other available resources to make decisions about the client. In nursing practice, evidence comes from both experimental and nonexperimental studies. Reflecting upon the development of nursing practice showed that, it has moved from theory based on 1950s followed by the extended growth of research in nursing in the 1980s and now in 21st century evidence-based practice has been adopted and utilized in the nursing practice.

Evidence-based practice (EBP) has been described as "the integration of best research evidence with clinical expertise and patient values."

Importance

- Evidence-based nursing practice helps to improve quality of nursing care and is best service to the patient.
- Evidence-based nursing practice promotes practices that have better outcome and are scientifically proven to be effective.
- It aims to eliminate unsound or risky nursing practices, thus promote patient safety.
- It helps to keep nurses knowledge up to date.
- It enhances professional practices.
- It achieves cost-effective nursing care.
- It optimizes patient outcomes.

Role of a Nurse

Step I: Asking the Questions

Searching the research evidence requires a structured approach. When a problem or questions has been identified, it must be phrased as questions that can be answered.

For example, nurse might wonder whether placing items, such as call bells and urinals in a stroke—patients unaffected visual field is more effective than placing them in the affected visual field.

Step II: Locating the Resources

When a clinical question is formulated the search for answers began with locating resources that will provide the evidence to address the clinical question.

The skills required for achieving these steps are:
- Computer skills
- Library resources
- Electronic data device
- Internet resources
- Sharing resources (from other specialties)

Step III: Critically Appraising the Evidence

Reviewing each of the relevant references and decision must made whether the intervention good or not. Eliminate irrelevant fact.

Step IV: Integrating Information to Implement a Decision

Integrate all the relevant facts. It should be based on clinical experiences and the patient references.

Step V: Evaluating the Outcome

When a decision is made regarding the recommendation for practice and the next step is to recommend implementing the interventions.

DISASTER NURSING

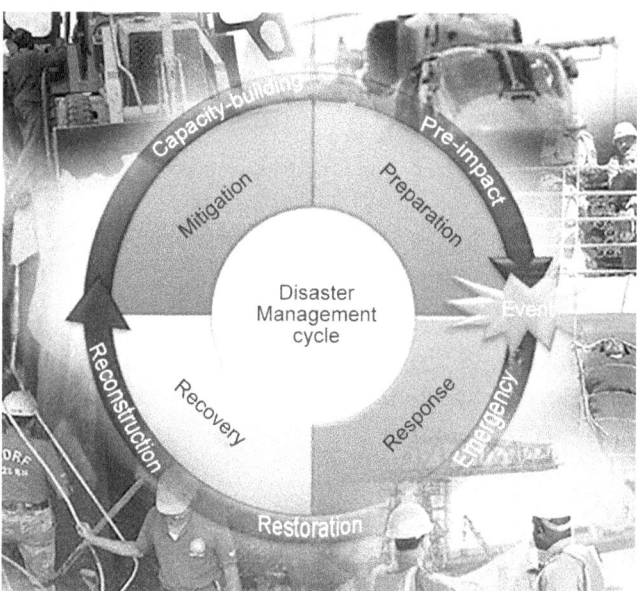

Disaster management cycle

Definition

It can be defined as the adaptation of professional nursing skills in recognizing and meeting the nursing, physical and emotional needs resulting from a disaster. The overall goal of disaster nursing is to achieve the best possible level of health for the people and the community involved in the disaster.

Disaster

A disaster can be defined as any occurrence that cause damage, ecological disruption, loss of human life, deterioration of health and health services on a scale, sufficient to warrant an extraordinary response from outside the affected community or area. A disaster is a sudden catastrophic event which disrupt the natural harmony.

Types of Disasters

1. Natural disasters
2. Man-made disasters

Natural disasters: These are unavoidable. The impact can be extremely powerful and can cause substantial, physical disruption, social disruption, and many secondary stressors, such as loss of both home and income (e.g. flood, hurricane, drought, earthquakes, tsunami, etc.).

Man-made disasters: Violence, war.

Phases of Disaster

The life cycle of disaster is generally referred to as disaster continuum, and is characterized by three major phases, namely:
1. Pre-impact phase (before)
2. Impact phase (during)
3. Post-impact phase (after)

Phases of Disaster Management

1. Disaster preparedness
2. Disaster impact
3. Disaster response
4. Rehabilitation
5. Disaster mitigation

Disaster preparedness: Disaster preparedness is an ongoing multisectoral activity. This consists of strengthening the capacity of a country to manage efficiently all types of emergencies, so that the resources should be able to provide assistance to the victims and bring back the life to normal. The preparedness should start from the community people because many times the external agency may not arrive for days to the affected area, especially if transportation and communication are affected.

Disaster impact: Medical treatment for large number of causalities is likely to be needed only after certain type of disaster. Most injuries are sustained during the impact, and thus, the greatest need for emergency care occurs in the first few hours. The management of mass causalities can be further divided into search and rescue, first aid, triage and stabilization of victims, hospital treatment and redistribution of patients to other hospital if necessary.

Search, rescue and first aid: After a major disaster, the need for search, rescue and first aid is likely to be so great that organized relief services will be able to meet only a small fraction of the demand. Most immediate help comes from the uninjured survivors.

Field care: Most injured person's coverage spontaneously to health facilities, using whatever transport is available, regardless of the facilities, operating status. Providing proper care to the casualties requires that the health service resources be redirected to this new priority. Bed availability and surgical services should be maximized. Provisions should be made for food and shelter. A center should be established to respond from inquiries from patient's relatives and friends. Priority should be given to victim's identification and adequate mortuary space should be provided.

Triage: When the quantity and severity of injuries overwhelm the operative capacity of health facilities, a different approach to medical treatment must be adopted. The principle of "first come, first treated", is not followed in mass emergencies. Triage consists of rapidly classifying the injured on the basis of the severity of their injuries and the likelihood of their survival with prompt medical intervention. It must be adapted to locally available skills. Higher priority is granted to victims whose immediate or long-term prognosis can be dramatically affected by simple intensive care. Triage is the only approach that can provide maximum benefits to the greatest number of injured in a major disaster situation.

Although different triage systems have been adopted and still in use in some countries, the most common classification uses the internationally accepted four color code system.

Red indicates high priority treatment or transfer, yellow signals medium priority; green indicates ambulatory patients and black for dead or moribund patients.

Triage should be carried out at the site of disaster, in order to determine transportation priority, and the admission to the hospital or treatment centers, where the patient's needs and priority of medical care will be reassessed. Ideally, local health workers should be taught the principles of triage as part of disaster training.

Person with minor or moderate injuries should be treated at their own homes to avoid social dislocation and the seriously injured should be transported to hospital with specialized treatment facilities.

Tagging: All patients should be identified with tags stating their name, age, place of origin, triage category, diagnosis, and initial treatment.

Identification of dead: Taking care of the dead is an essential part of the disaster management. A large number of deaths can also impede the efficiency of the rescue activities at the site of the disaster.

Disaster response: Immediately following a disaster, the most critical health supplies are those needed for treating casualties, and preventing the spread of communicable diseases. Following the initial emergency phase, needed supplies will include food, blankets, clothing, shelter, sanitary engineering equipments and construction material. A rapid damage assessment must be carried out in order to identify needs and resources. It includes the epidemiological surveillance and disease control, vaccination, nutrition, etc.

Rehabilitation phase: Rehabilitation starts from the very first moment of a disaster. In first weeks after disaster, the pattern of health needs will change rapidly, moving from causality treatment to more routine primary health care. Services should be recognized and restructured. Priorities also shift from health care toward environmental health measures.

Disaster mitigation: This involves lessening the likely effects of emergencies. These include depending upon the disaster, protection of vulnerable population and structure (e.g. improving structural qualities of schools, houses and other buildings so that medical causalities can be minimized). This mitigation compliments the disaster preparedness and disaster response activities.

Role of a Nurse in Disaster Management

Disaster Preparedness

- Facilitate preparation with community, initiate disaster plan
- To provide updated record of vulnerable populations within community
- Aware and report unsafe equipments
- Understand community resources

Disaster Response

- Community assessment
- Case finding and referring, prevention, health education and surveillance
- Work a member of assessment team
- Involved in ongoing surveillance

Disaster Recovery

- Provide health education
- Provide psychological support
- Referrals to hospital as needed
- Remain alert for environmental health

PERFORMANCE APPRAISAL

Performance appraisal is the assessment of how a staff member is doing his or her job. Performance review program consists of a series of periodic performance appraisals, feedback interviews and goal planning session between a supervisor and his subordinates.

Performance appraisal means the systematic evaluation of the performance by an expert or his immediate superior.

Importance of Performance Appraisal

- Performance appraisal helps the management to take decision about the salary increase of an employee.
- The continuous evaluation of an employee helps in improving the quality of an employee in job performance.
- The Performance appraisal brings out the facilities available to an employee.
- It minimises the communication gap between the employer and employee.
- Promotion is given to an employee on the basis of performance appraisal.
- The training needs of an employee can be identified through performance appraisal.
- The decision for discharging an employee from the job is also taken on the basis of performance appraisal.
- Performance appraisal is used to transfer a person who is misfit for a job to the right placement.
- The grievances of an employee are eliminated through performance appraisal.
- The job satisfaction of an employee increases morale. This job satisfaction is achieved through performance appraisal.
- It helps to improve the employer and employee relationship.

DECISION-MAKING

Decision-making is the process of selecting one course of action from alternatives.

Stages for Decision-making

Developed by B Aubrey Fisher, there are four stages that should be involved in all group decision-making. These stages, or sometimes called phases, are important for the decision-making process to begin.

- **Orientation stage:** This phase is where members meet for the first time and start to get to know each other.
- **Conflict stage:** Once group members become familiar with each other, disputes, little fights and arguments occur. Group members eventually work it out.
- **Emergence stage:** The group begins to clear up ambiguity in opinions is talked about.

- **Reinforcement stage:** Members finally make a decision, while justifying themselves that it was the right decision.

Steps in Decision-making

The decision-making task can be divided into 7 steps which are stated in order of sequence are as:
1. Establishing goal and objectives
2. Making the diagnosis
3. Analyzing the problem
4. Searching alternative solution
5. Selecting the best possible solution
6. Putting the decision into effect
7. Following up the decision

DELEGATION

Delegating is a major element of the directing function of nursing management. It is an effective nurse management competency by which nurse managers get the work done through their employees.

Delegation is the process of assigning responsibility and authority to coworker and ensuring his accountability.

Purposes of Delegation

- **Assignment of duties:** As one person cannot perform all the tasks, he must allocate a part of his to subordinates for the purposes of accomplishment by them.
- **Grant of authority:** Delegation of authority means division of authority and powers downward to the subordinates. If the delegated duty is to be discharged by subordinates, they must be entrusted with requisite authority for enabling them to make such work performance.
- **Creation of accountability:** Delegation of duties implies accountability from side of subordinates. Because of this accountability, the manager must keep for himself some reserved authority and duties for directing, regulating and controlling the course of work undertaken by his subordinates.

Role of a Nurse Manager

- Train and develop subordinates.
- Control and coordinate the work of subordinates.
- Develop ways of measuring the accomplishment of objectives with communication, standards, measurements, and feedback to prevent errors. Nursing employees want to know the nurse manager's expectations of them. They understand expectations from clearly defined jobs, work relationships, and expected results.
- Visit subordinates frequently. Spot potential problems of morale, disagreement and grievance. Coordination to prevent duplication of effort.
- Solve problems and think about new ideas. Emphasize employees solving their own problems.
- Know subordinate's capabilities and match task or duty to the employee. Be sure the employee considers it important.
- Agree on performance standards (Relate managerial references to employee performance).
- Give appropriate tasks.
- Do not take back delegated tasks.

RECRUITMENT

The success of any organization will depend ultimately on the caliber of its recruit and by the effectiveness of its recruitment and selection procedures. It is the part of selection procedures concerned with finding the applicants and providing an audience with them. Recruitment is a process in which the right person for the right post is procured.

Recruitment involves seeking and attracting a pool of people from which qualified candidates for job vacancies can be chosen.

Purposes of Recruitment

- To seek out, evaluate and obtain commitment from an individual
- To place and orient the person for successful conduct of work of an organization
- To find out the source of manpower to meet the requirement
- To bring linkage activity among those with jobs and those seeking jobs
- To stimulate people to apply for job
- To precede the selection process
- To attract the man power in adequate numbers
- To facilitate effective selection of an efficient working force

Sources of Recruitment

1. *Internal sources* (recruitment from within the organization)
   - Present permanent employees
   - Present temporary employees
   - Retired employees
   - Dependent of diseased, disabled and present employees
2. *External sources* (these sources lie outside the organization)
   - New entrants
   - Unemployed

Methods of Recruitment

According to Runn and Stephens, the recruitment method are of three categories, they are:

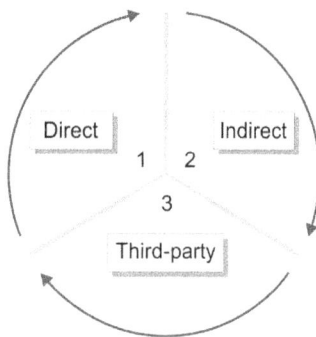

Direct Method

This includes sending recruiters to educational institutions and professional institution, employee contacts with public, manned exhibits and waiting list.

Indirect Method

This includes advertising in mass media like news paper, radio, TV, net in trade and professional journals and brochures.

Third-party Method

This includes:
- Private employment agencies
- State public employment agency
- Friends and relatives
- Trade unions
- Schools and colleges
- Voluntary organization

Commonly used methods of recruitment are:
- Professional or trade associations
- Advertisements
- Employment exchange
- Campus recruitment
- Walk-ins, write-ins and talk-ins
- Consultants
- Contractors
- Radio and television
- International recruiting

LEADERSHIP

Leadership is the ability to influence other people. Leader is a part of management and one of the most significant elements of direction. A leader may or may not be manager but a manager must a leader. A manager as a leader must lead his subordinates and also inspire them to achieve organizational goals.

Role of a Leader
- Motivation of the subordinates
- Creating confidence in subordinates
- Building morale
- Helps to achieve goals in organizations

Types of Leadership
- Autocratic leadership: Taking decision by himself
- Democratic leadership: Take suggestions from others
- Free rein or laissez-fair: Give complete freedom to others.

BARRIER NURSING

Barrier nursing or isolation technique is intended to confine the micro-organisms within a given and recognized area. There are number of isolation techniques and precautions used to prevent the spread of infection.

General Precautions
- Maintain high degree of cleanliness
- Health teaching
- Minimize the number of visitors
- Emphasize on hand washing
- Keep all articles separate for each person
- Immunization against communicable diseases
- Persons with lowered resistance
- Patients should be nursed in separate rooms

Methods
- Cleaning of articles
- Hand washing
- Gown technique
- Face masks
- Gloves

CRISIS INTERVENTION

Human beings has to maintain balance in life, whenever he is exposed to stressor or stressful situations he will try to overcome it by his own way of dealing with problems, by adopting adequate coping strategies, with the help of situational support, he will try to overcome it. Eustress is always essential for an individual to lead qualitative life. *Crisis intervention* is a short-term therapy focused on solving the immediate problem. It is usually limited to 6 weeks. The goal of crisis intervention is for an individual to return to a pre-crisis level of functioning.

Crisis

A state of disequilibrium resulting from the interaction of an event with the individuals or familys' coping mechanisms, which are inadequate to meet the demands of the situation, combined with the individuals or familys' perception of the meaning of the event.

Manifestations of Stress

- Heavy burden of free floating anxiety, e.g. heightened emotional tension
- Depression, anger, guilt, tension, fear
- Neglects in performing self care activities
- Helplessness, hopelessness, uselessness
- Low self esteem, uncontrollable crying
- Lack of confidence
- Withdrawal behavior, aloofness
- Lack of self-control.

Nursing Care

- Encourage the client to express openly the problems affecting
- Always work with feelings of the client
- Help the person to confront with crisis by talking about present denial feelings and recognize denial as a normal reaction to crisis
- Motivate the person to talk about the losses and changes involved in crisis
- Explain the relationship between crisis and this present behavior
- Give the person time to experience the feelings and to fully express them
- Avoid giving the false reassurance
- Do not encourage the client to blame as others are responsible for the occurrence of crisis, situation.

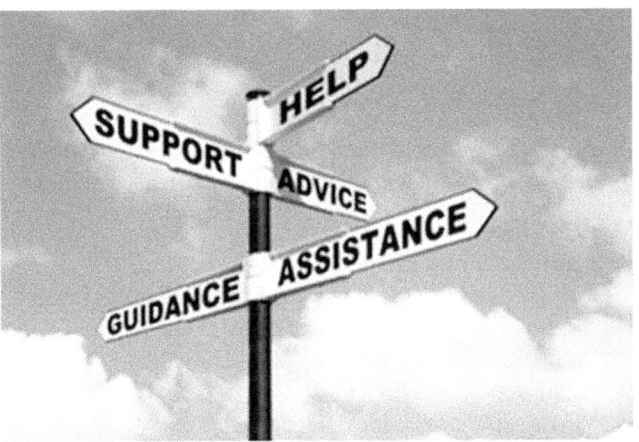

Assessment

The first step of crisis intervention is assessment. At this time, data about the nature of crisis and its effect on the patient must be collected. From these data, an intervention plan will be developed.

During this phase, the nurse begins to establish a positive working relationship with the patient. A number of balancing factors are important in the development and resolution of a crisis and should be assessed:
- Precipitating event or stressor
- Patient's perception of the event or stressor
- Nature and strength of the patient's support systems and coping resources
- Patient's previous strengths and coping mechanisms

Planning and Implementation

The next step of crisis intervention is planning, the previously collected data are analyzed and specific interventions are proposed. Dynamics underlying the present crisis are formulated from the information about the precipitating event. Alternative solution to the problem is explored, and steps for achieving the solutions are identified.

Evaluation

The last phase of crisis intervention is evaluation, when the nurse and patient evaluate whether the intervention resulted in a positive resolution of the crisis.

Techniques of Crisis Intervention

- *Catharsis:* The release of feelings that takes place as the patient talks about emotionally charged areas (e.g. tell me about how you have been feeling since you lost your job).
- *Clarification:* Encouraging the patient to express more clearly the relationship between certain events (e.g. I have noticed that after you have an argument with your husband you become sick and cannot leave your bed).
- *Suggestion:* Influencing a person to accept an idea or belief, particularly the belief that the nurse can help and that the person will in time feel better (e.g. many other people have found it helpful to talk about this and I think you will too).
- *Reinforcement of Behavior:* Giving the patient the positive responses to adaptive behavior (e.g. that is the first time you were able to defend yourself with your boss and it went very well. I am so pleased that you were able to do it).
- *Support of Defense:* Encouraging the use of healthy, adaptive defenses and discouraging those that are

unhealthy or maladaptive. (e.g. going for a bicycle ride when you were so angry was very helpful because when you returned, your wife were able to talk things through).

- *Raising Self-esteem:* Helping the patient regain feeling of self-worth (e.g. you are a very strong person to be able to manage the family all this time. I think you will be able to handle this situation, too).
- *Exploration of Solution:* Examining alternative ways of solving the immediate problem (e.g. you seem to know many people in the computer field. Could you contact some of them to see whether they might know of available jobs?).

GERIATRICS

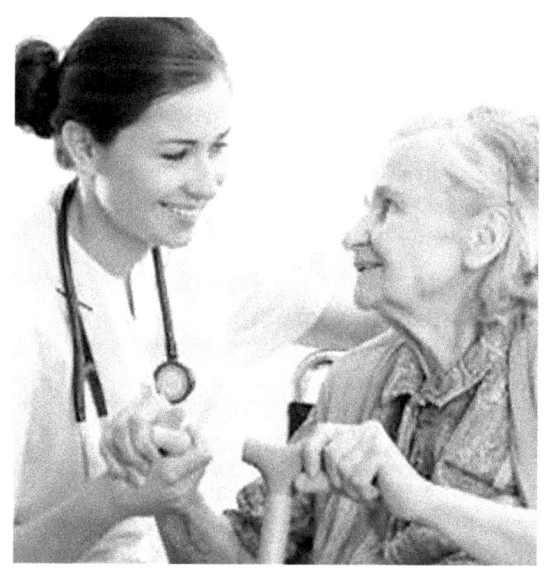

Geriatrics is the study of old age, includes the physiology, pathology, diagnosis, and management of the diseases of older adults. The broader field of **gerontology**, or the study of the aging process, draws from the biologic, psychological, and sociologic sciences. Because hospitalized patients are being discharged to home "quicker and sicker" than ever before, nurses in all settings, including hospital, home care, rehabilitation, and outpatient settings, need to be knowledgeable about geriatric nursing principles and skilled in meeting the needs of elderly patients.

Aging is a normal process of time-related change, begins with birth and continues throughout life. It is a time when people move away from previous more desirable situations. By the year 2030, the future elderly population will be especially diverse and increase by 25%. Aging is an inevitable phenomenon in all biological beings and this reality, along with the varied lifestyles, environmental conditions, and life histories characteristic of older adults, creates the need for highly individualized nursing care.

Healthy aging is considered as everyone's goal and an achievement to be celebrating by society as a whole. Therefore, WHO during 1999 had chosen the theme for world health day is "Active aging makes the difference" to coincide with the international year of the older persons.

Geriatric Nursing

Geriatric nursing is comprehensive source of clinical information and management advice relating to the care of older adults.

Gerontological nursing is defined as a health services that incorporates generic nursing methods and specialized knowledge about the aged to establish conditions within the patient and within the environment.

—Gunter and Estes in 1979

Purpose of Geriatric Nursing

- To optimize an older person's ability to enjoy good health.
- To improve their overall quality of life.
- To reduce the need for hospitalization and intuitional.
- Enable them to live independently for as long as possible.
- Detection of disease at early stage.

Changes in Elderly

General Changes
- Rule out the physical changes and disease process
- Most physiological functions decline with age
- Diminished ability to respond to stress
- Changes in posture, weakness of muscle
- Problem in role adjustment is a major psychological change in old age based or Erikson's development theory, integrity vs despair

Integumentary System
- Decreased in dermal vascularity and density, decreased immune response
- Decreased vitamin D production
- Prolonged wound healing
- Appearance of Pruritis and eczema
- Impaired mobility, lack of physical activity, impaired skin integrity, risk of development of pressure ulcer

Nursing Care
- Administer emollients to the skin
- Topical corticosteroid creams in case of any pruritis
- Provide adequate lighting to prevent risk for fall
- Paint the edge of the bed or stairs with bright color for notice
- Provide assistance in ADL

- Place a bell near the bed to call the duty staff for assistance
- Provide nonslippery and correct fitting shoes without heels

Musculoskeletal System
- Lean body mass, decreased muscle strength
- More risk for getting pelvic fracture
- Increased risk for osteoporosis
- Increased chance of osteoarthritis

Nursing Care
- Assess the muscle strength and BMD
- Encourage to perform exercises as tolerated
- Provide calcium supplements and milk
- Administer calcium and calcitonin intranasal sprays
- Administer NSAIDs and vitamin D
- Provide proper nutritious diet
- Provide proper rest periods

Cardiovascular System
- Decreased beta adrenergic response, heart rate, cardiac output
- Impaired myocardial diastolic function
- Stiffness of major arteries
- Increased afterload and systolic pressure
- Chance of getting cardiac disorders, such as angina, dysrhythmia
- Decreased peripheral circulation

Nursing Care
- Monitor blood pressure intermittently
- Assess the extremities for proper blood supply
- Monitor the capillary refill
- Administer oxygen in case of angina attack

Respiratory System
- Decreased lung compliance, collapse of airways, reduced vital capacity
- Difficulty breathing after exercises
- Decreased reaction to hypoxia and hypercapnia
- Increased ventilation-perfusion imbalance
- Increased chance of getting asthma, COPD, pneumonia and tuberculosis infections

Nursing Care
- Monitor the respiratory status
- Assess the vital status, vital capacity, sputum production
- Assess any chance of getting aspiration pneumonia
- Administer oxygen
- Check the cough reflex

Gastrointestinal System
- Changes in the gum, tooth loss
- Decreased peristalsis and develop constipation
- Decreased gastric acid secretion and decreased small intestinal villous
- Decreased liver and pancreatic function
- Decreased number of enzymes in the small intestine, simple sugars is absorbed more slowly
- Decreased fluid intake and mobility cause constipation
- Physiological anorexia

Nursing Care
- Monitor the frequency of bowel and bladder emptying
- Provide more fiber rich diet and adequate fluids
- Encourage the person to take proper food

Genitourinary System
- Decreased GFR, tubular secretion and bladder capacity
- Uninhibited bladder contractions, nocturnal sodium and fluid excretion
- Increased risk for renal failure, UTI
- Urinary incontinence, post voidal dribbling in adults
- Chance of BPH in males

Nursing Care
- Monitor intake and output
- Assess for any BPH in male, monitor PSA test
- Assess the renal function

Reproductive System
- Decreased production of estrogens, androgens and precursors
- Decreased vaginal secretion resulting in atrophic vulvovaginitis
- Decreased size of uterus, ovaries and breast
- Chromosomal abnormalities in cells

Nursing Care
- Provide psychological support
- Genetic counselling

Neurological System
- Decreased brain weight, cerebral blood flow and neurotransmitters
- Increased lipofuscin pigment in neurons
- Alteration in sleep wake cycle
- Decreased baroreflex activity, increased risk of syncope
- Decreased pain, temperature and vibration sensitivity
- Slower DTRs (deep tendon reflex)
- Delirium and dementia seen
- Alzheimer's dementia is commonly seen.

Nursing Care
- Provide assistance
- Assess the symptoms of Alzheimer's disease (wandering away in the late afternoon)
- Administer antidepressants.

Eye and Ear
- Increased rigidity of iris, decreased size of anterior chamber
- Decreased eye sight, reduced lens elasticity
- Retinal deterioration, decreased pupil size
- Increased chance of cataract, glaucoma, presbyopia
- Impaired adaptation to darkness, enophthalmia
- Decreased hearing ability

Nursing care
- Monitor the visual and hearing test
- Provide assistance

Role of a Nurse in Geriatrics

- Act as a liaison for families living at a distance. This includes regular visits, attending physician appointments and notifying families of changes or potential problem.
- Explain and suggest medical and health care options based on expertise in the health care and residential housing field.
- Extend support to client and family members.
- Help the client designate a health care proxy and compose a living will.
- Hire, screen, coordinate, and monitor in home health care and help services.
- Identify problems and services necessary to rectify them.
- Intervene during a crisis.
- Offer a professional, objective point-of-view regarding senior care options.
- Provide community education and client advocacy.
- Recommend resources, support groups, and references for elderly clients and their families.
- Save families time and money by eliminating duplicative and unnecessary service.
- Utilize trusted resources to make physician, mental health, attorney, trust officers, and residential housing referrals.

END-OF-LIFE CARE

Death is the termination of the biological functions that define a living organism. It will eventually afflict all living things.

The important aspects at the end of life care are:

Palliative Care

Today, doctors are able to cure many people diagnosed with cancer. If a cure is not possible, some people receive treatment to manage the symptoms and side effects of cancer and its treatment. This type of treatment is called palliative care, and it helps people with cancer at all stages of their illness live as comfortable as possible.

Preparation at the End of Life

Despite a doctor's best efforts and hard work, disease treatment sometimes stops working and a cure or long-term remission is no longer possible. This stage of illness is called advanced, terminal, or end-stage.

Advanced Directives

Advance directives are legal documents that explain the kind of medical treatment you would want and would not want if you become unable to make these decisions for yourself.

Advance directives protect your rights and preferences for medical treatment and diminish the burden of family members and other caregivers making decisions for you. You can protect your rights and preferences for medical treatment by writing down your wishes in an advance directive and having a witness or witnesses sign the statement.

It is important to talk with your family and doctor about your wishes ahead of time, so they can be aware of your choices. Any adult who is mentally and physically able to understand his or her medical condition and express his or her preferences can make an advance directive.

Hospice Care

Hospice care is programs in local communities to help people with terminal disease who are coping with a limited life expectancy receive care by trained professionals. The emphasis of hospice care is to relieve pain and discomfort to the patient. It is the care of terminally ill patients.

CHAPTER 3

Neurological System

Chapter Objectives

- Keynotes in the neurological system
- Anatomy of the nervous system
- Various diagnostic measures
- Disorders in the nervous system

KEY TERMS

ICP	GCS
MRI	Flaccidity
LP	Tensilon
LOC	Neurons

KEYNOTES

- The deficiency of dopamine leads to parkinsonism.
- Restrict caffeine before the patient going for EEG.
- Provide dim light for a patient with meningitis.
- The common neurotransmitters are dopamine, acetylcholine, serotonin, epinephrine, amino acids, etc.
- Increase dopamine is seen in schizophrenia.
- Elevate the head end of bed in patient with cerebral edema.
- The mode of communication for a patient with CVA and Aphasia is pen and paper or magic slate.
- Normal CSF glucose level 50–70 mg/dl.
- Normal CSF protein 15–45 mg/dl.
- Normal CSF volume is 125–150 ml.
- Normal CSF pressure is 50–175 mm H_2O.
- Presence of RBC in CSF indicates infection.
- Absence of smell is known as anosmia.
- Ataxia is unsteady gait.
- Apraxia is the inability to perform previously learned activity.
- Agnosia is the inability to recognize objects and attach meaning to them.
- Presence of oligoclonal bands in CSF indicates multiple sclerosis.
- Doll's eye test is contraindicated in cervical spinal injury.
- Cryptococcosis is the most common CNS fungal infection.
- Pill rolling movements of hands is the type of tremor in Parkinson's disease and levodopa is the drug of choice.
- Bell's palsy is also known as facial paralysis.
- The priority nursing care of a patient with GBS is monitor for respiratory failure.
- About 750–900 ml of blood is received by the brain in every one minute.

ANATOMY

The nervous system, a network of nerves and fibres helps all the parts of the body to communicate with each other. It also reacts to changes both outside and inside the body. The nervous system uses both electrical and chemical means to send and receive messages (Fig. 1).

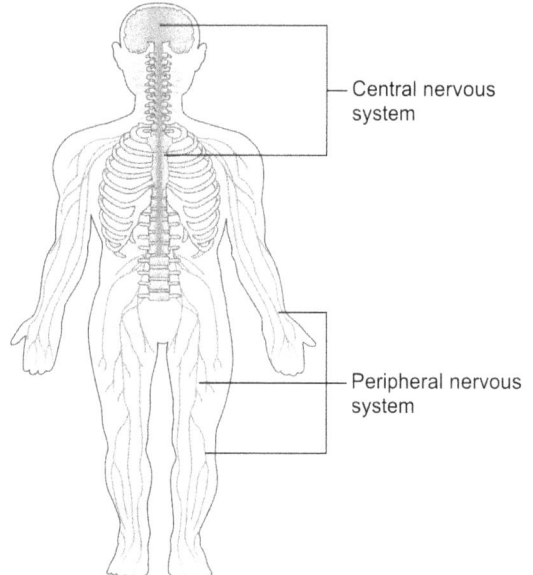

Fig. 1: Structure of nervous system

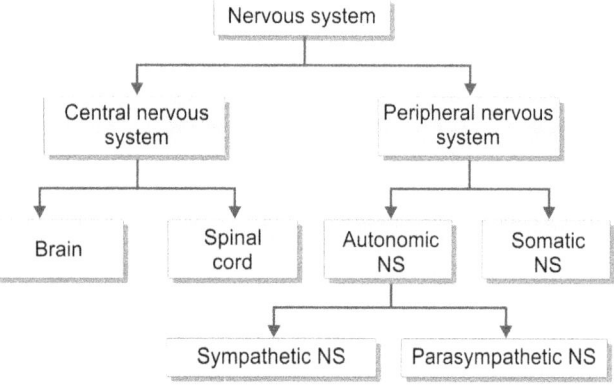

Peripheral Nervous System

The peripheral nervous system (PNS) is the part of the nervous system that is outside the brain and spinal cord consists of nerves and ganglia.

Autonomic Nervous System

The autonomic nervous system (ANS) is a part of peripheral nervous system that controls all the involuntary activities of the body, such as breathing, heartbeat, and digestive processes.

Somatic Nervous System

The somatic nervous system (SoNS) is a part of peripheral nervous system consist of afferent and efferent nerves, such as cranial nerves, spinal nerves, etc. which controls all the voluntary movement of muscles in our body.

Sympathetic Nervous System

The sympathetic nervous system (SNS) is one of two main divisions of the autonomic nervous system controls body's response to perceived threat (arousing) and is responsible for "fight-or-flight" response.

Parasympathetic Nervous System

The parasympathetic nervous system is one of the two main divisions of the autonomic nervous system controls homeostasis and body at rest (calming) and is responsible for body's "rest-and-digest" response.

Central Nervous System

The central nervous system (CNS) is a part of nervous system which consist of brain and spinal cord that controls all the activities of body and mind.

BRAIN

The brain is one of the largest and most complex organs in our body. The weight of brain is 1200 gm.

Functions of Brain

- Thinking or cognition
- Perception or sensing
- Emotion or feeling
- Behavior control
- Physical or somatic control
- Signaling (being responsive and active to stimuli)

Anatomy of Brain (Fig. 2)

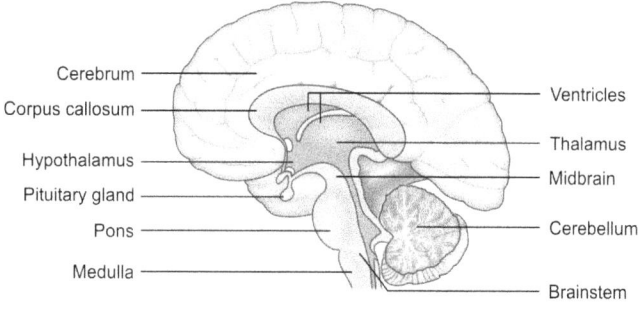

Fig. 2: Structure of brain

Three Parts

1. Cerebrum
2. Cerebellum
3. Brainstem

Cerebrum

It is the largest part of the brain, consisting of two cerebral hemispheres.
- Right hemisphere: Receives the sensory information from the left side of the body.
- Left hemisphere: Receives the sensory information from the right side of the body.

If there is any cessation of blood supply to a part of brain, it may leads to unilateral neglect syndrome.

Cerebellum

It is a part of brain that coordinates all the motor activities of the body.

Brainstem

It consist of mid brain, pons and medulla. Medulla is the respiratory as well as vomiting syndrome.

Limbic system is a part of brain considered as emotional brain.

Cerebral Cortex

It is the outer gray matter which protects the brain from trauma. There are five lobes:
- *Frontal lobe:* Speech sensation, personality and behavior, also known as Broca's area of speech
- *Occipital lobe:* Vision sensation
- *Temporal lobe:* Responsible for hearing, Wernicke's area of speech
- *Parietal lobe:* Responsible for sensory information, taste and smell.

Diencephalon

It is a part of brain that consists of thalamus and hypothalamus.
- Thalamus: Relay station for discrimination of sensory signals, such as pain, temperature, touch, etc.
- Hypothalamus: Play major role in regulation of vital functions, such as blood pressure, sleep, food, etc.

Meninges (Fig. 3)

It is a membrane covering the brain which protects from trauma. There are three layers:
- Dura mater: Outer tough layer
- Arachnoid mater: Middle layer
- Pia mater: Inner layer

The space between the arachnoid mater and pia mater is called subarachnoid space.

There are four ventricles of brain. They are the communicating network of cavities which produce a fluid called as cerebrospinal fluid (CSF).

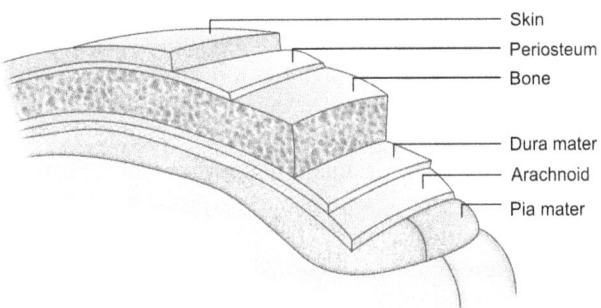

Fig. 3: Layers of meninges

- Normal CSF volume is 125–150 ml
- Normal CSF pressure is 50–175 mm H_2O
- The CSF is produced from the ventricles of the brain and it is drained into the subarachnoid space. It maintains ICP.
- Normal ICP is 5–15 mm Hg

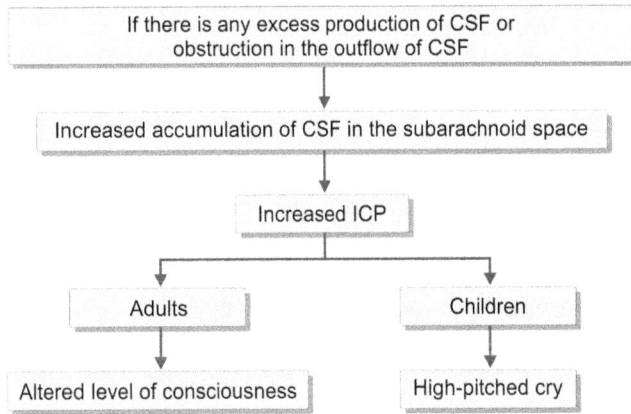

Neurons (Fig. 4)

It is the structural and functional unit of nervous system. It consists of axon, dendrite and cell body.

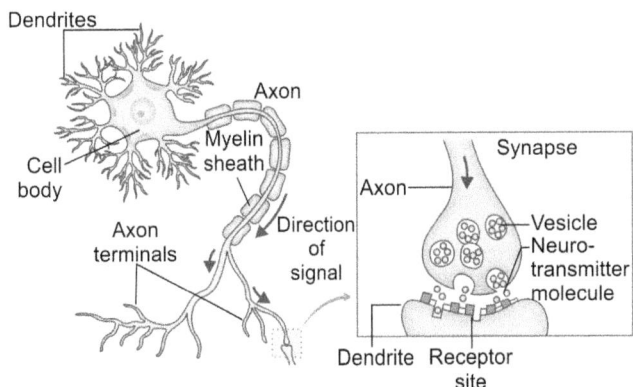

Fig. 4: Structure of neuron

- The transmission of impulse from one neuron to another is called synaptic transmission (i.e. from the presynaptic area to the postsynaptic area). It takes place from the axon of one neuron to the dendrite of another.
- For the easy transmission of impulse, there are a number of neurotransmitters present in the synaptic cleft. They are:
  - Dopamine
  - Serotonin
  - Amino acid
  - Epinephrine
  - Acetylcholine
- From the presynaptic area to the postsynaptic area, if there is any impairment in the transmission of these neurotransmitters will result in certain disorders.
  - Increase dopamine—schizophrenia
  - Decrease dopamine—parkinsonism
  - Increase serotonin—mania
  - Decrease serotonin—depression
  - Increase epinephrine—mania
  - Decrease epinephrine—depression

Spinal Cord (Fig. 5)

Spinal cord is the most important structure between body and brain. It extends from foramen magnum to first or second lumbar vertebrae. The length of spinal cord is 18 inches (45 cm).

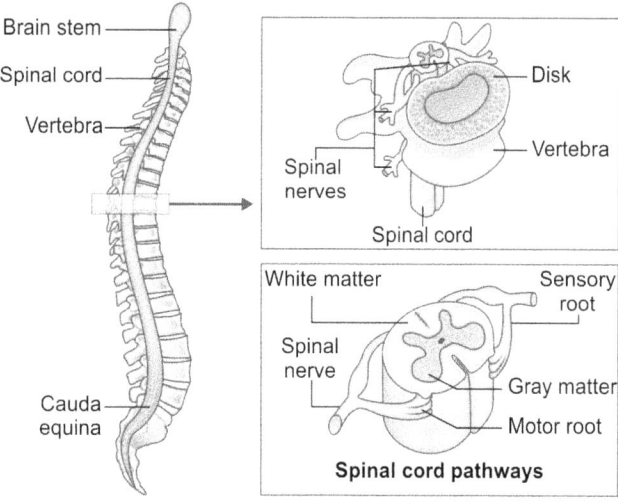

Fig. 5: Structure of spinal cord

- Spinal cord consists of an H-shaped gray mater (cell body) in the center and surrounded by white mater (nerve tract and fibers).
- There are 31 pairs of spinal nerves and 12 pairs of cranial nerves in the peripheral nervous system. The spinal nerves carry impulses to and from the spinal cord and the cranial nerves carry impulses to and from the brain.
- Spinal nerves are divided into 8 cervical, 12 thoracic, 5 lumbar, 5 sacral, and 1 coccygeal nerve. Dorsal and ventral roots enter and leave the vertebral column respectively, through intervertebral foramen at the vertebral segments corresponding to the spinal segment.
- The arterial blood supply to the spinal cord in the upper cervical regions is derived from two branches of the vertebral arteries, the anterior spinal artery and the posterior spinal arteries.

NEUROLOGICAL ASSESSMENT

Assessment of Cranial Nerves

CN I	Olfactory nerve—sense of smell
CN II	Optic nerve—sense of vision
CN III	Oculomotor nerve—responsible for pupillary constriction
CN IV	Trochlear nerve—down ward and inward movement of eye
CN V	Trigeminal nerve—responsible for corneal reflex, largest cranial nerve
CN VI	Abducens nerve—lateral deviation of eye
CN VII	Facial nerve—facial movement
CN VIII	Acoustic nerve or vestibulocochlear nerve—responsible for hearing and balance
CN IX	Glossopharyngeal nerve—movement of pharynx and swallowing
CN X	Vagus nerve—longest cranial nerve, mixed cranial nerve, movement of larynx, pharynx
CN XI	Spinal accessory—movement of sternomastoid muscle and trapezius muscle
CN XII	Hypoglossal nerve—movement of tongue

- **CN I (olfactory):** Ask your patient to identify at least two common substances, such as coffee and cinnamon. Make sure his nostrils are patent before performing this test.
- **CN II (optic):** Test visual acuity with a Snellen chart and the Rosenbaum nearvision card.
- **CN III (oculomotor), CN IV (trochlear), and CN VI (abducens):** Assess these nerves together using the corneal light reflex test, the six cardinal positions of gaze, and the cover-uncover test. Also, inspect the size, shape, and symmetry of your patient's pupils and papillary reactions to light.
- **CN V (trigeminal):** To assess the sensory component of the trigeminal nerve, ask your patient to close his eyes and then touch him with a wisp of cotton on his forehead, cheek, and jaw on each side. Next, test pain perception by touching the tip of a safety pin to the same three areas.

- **CN VII (facial):** To assess the sensory component, test taste by placing items with various tastes on the anterior portion of your patient's tongue, for example, sweet, sour, and bitter. To test motor function, observe his face for symmetry at rest and while he smiles, frowns, and raises his eyebrows.
- **CN VIII (acoustic):** To assess this nerve, use Weber's test—strike a tuning fork lightly against your hand and place the vibrating fork on your patient's forehead at the midline or on the top of his head—and the Rinne test—strike the tuning fork against your hand and place the vibrating fork over his mastoid process.
- **CN IX (glossopharyngeal) and CN X (vagus):** Test these nerves together because their innervation overlaps in the pharynx. Listen to your patient's voice. Then check his gag reflex by touching the tip of a tongue blade against his posterior pharynx and asking him to open wide and say "ah." Watch for symmetrical upward movement of the soft palate and uvula and for the midline position of the uvula.
- **CN XI (spinal accessory):** Assess this nerve by testing the strength of the sternocleidomastoid muscles and the upper portion of the trapezius muscle.
- **CN XII (hypoglossal):** Observe your patient's tongue for symmetry. His tongue should be midline without tremors or muscle twitching. Test tongue strength by asking him to push his tongue against his cheek as you apply resistance.

Assessment of the Level of Consciousness

- Orientation to time, place and person
- Speech of the patient
- Monitor for abnormal posturing
  - **Decorticate posturing:** Also known as flexor, extension of the legs, internal rotation and flexion of arms.
  - **Decerebrate posturing:** Also known as extensor.

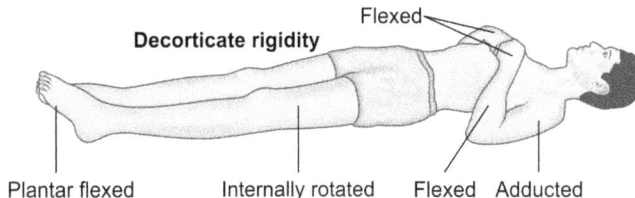

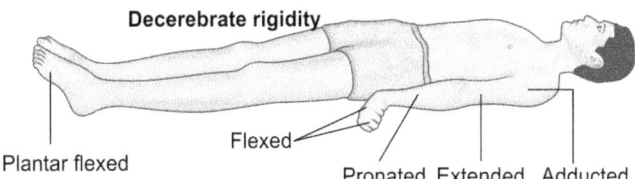

- Pupillary reaction of the patient
- Motor function, movement of extremities
- Glasgow coma scale

Eye opening (4)		Verbal response (5)		Motor response (6)	
Spontaneous	4	Oriented	5	Obeys command	6
To verbal stimuli	3	Confused	4	To painful stimuli	5
To pain	2	Inappropriate words	3	Withdrawal	4
No response	1	Inappropriate sound	2	Flexion	3
		No response	1	Extension	2
				No response	1

- Total score is 15
- Minimum score is 3
- Maximum score is 15
- If the score is less than 7, patient is in coma state

DIAGNOSTIC MEASURES

- **Skull X-ray:** Radiographic examination of the skull to rule out any fracture or deformity. It is contraindicated in pregnant women.
- **CT scan:** Used to detect intracranial space occupying lesion, withhold all metformin preparations because it react with iodine to form metformin induced iodine lactic acidosis.
- **MRI scan:** Magnetic rays are used to detect the intracranial space lesions in brain and spinal cord, contraindicated in pregnant women because it may cause increase in amniotic fluid temperature and cause fetal toxicity.
- **Lumbar puncture:** Insertion of a needle between L3 and L4 to remove CSF for diagnostic and treatment purpose. It is contraindicated in patients with increased ICP because the withdrawal may cause rapid decline in the CSF pressure. While performing LP position the patient in a fetal position (ask the patient to lie in left lateral position and draw the knees toward abdomen and chin towards the trunk).
- **Myelography:** It is used to rule out IVDP (inter vertebral disc prolapse) or tumor. LP is performed, remove a small amount of CSF, mix the dye in the CSF and reinsert again. The dye may be oil based or water based or air based.
  - If water based or oil based dye is used provide flat position with head of bed elevation to prevent

the upward displacement of dye and to prevent meningeal irritation.
- If air based dye is used provide flat position with head lower than the trunk.
- **EEG (electroencephalography):** It is used to rule out the severity of seizure or epilepsy. Withhold all caffeinated beverages and anticonvulsant medications before the test because it may cause false reading.
- **Cerebral angiography:** Used to rule out cerebral vessels and tumors. Injection of radiopaque substance into the cerebral circulation via carotid artery, vertebral artery, femoral artery or brachial artery followed by X-ray. Maintain pressure dressing after the procedure to prevent bleeding.

DISORDERS

Increased ICP

Due to any trauma or RTA, there will be an obstruction in the outflow of CSF which results in the excessive accumulation of CSF in the subarachnoid space results in increased ICP.

Clinical Manifestation

- Altered level of consciousness
- Nuchal rigidity
- Increased systolic pressure
- Widened pulse pressure
- Decreased heart rate
- Vomiting (projectile)
- High pitched cry in children

Nursing Care

- Monitor for increased ICP
- Monitor for Cushing's triad (increased systolic pressure, widened pulse pressure and decreased heart rate)
- Avoid administering morphine sulfate
- Provide mechanical ventilation with slight hyperventilation (to keep the $PaCO_3$ 30-35 mm Hg which results in vasoconstriction and decreases ICP)
- Provide head of bed elevation 30-45 degree
- Administer osmotic diuretics, such as mannitol

Stroke

It is also called as CVA or brain attack. It is the sudden cessation of blood supply to a part of brain. It occurs as a result of ischemia or hemorrhage secondary to thrombi or emboli.

There are two types of stroke:
- Ischemic stroke (83%)
- Hemorrhagic stroke (17%)

Clinical Manifestation

- Headache
- Seizures and disorientation
- Fever
- Aphasia (speech disturbance)
- Apraxia (loss of ability to perform skilled activities)
- Unilateral neglect syndrome (in case of right hemisphere damage, there will be paralysis of the left side of the body and, in case of left hemisphere damage, there is paralysis of the right side of the body).

Nursing Care

- Maintain a patent airway
- Maintain blood pressure of 150/100 mm Hg to proper ensure cerebral perfusion
- Monitor for increased ICP
- Provide head of bed elevation 30-45 degree
- Always approach the patient from the unaffected side
- Reposition the patient every 20 minutes (affected side only for 20 minutes)
- Administer thrombolytic agents, such as streptokinase and urokinase
- Administer anticoagulants, such as heparin and warfarin.
- Administer corticosteroids and osmotic diuretics to decrease cerebral edema.

Myasthenia Gravis

It is a neuromuscular disorder characterized by considerable muscle weakness. It occurs more common among women than men, in women 15-35 years of age and men over 40 years. Thymus gland abnormalities may lead to myasthenia gravis.

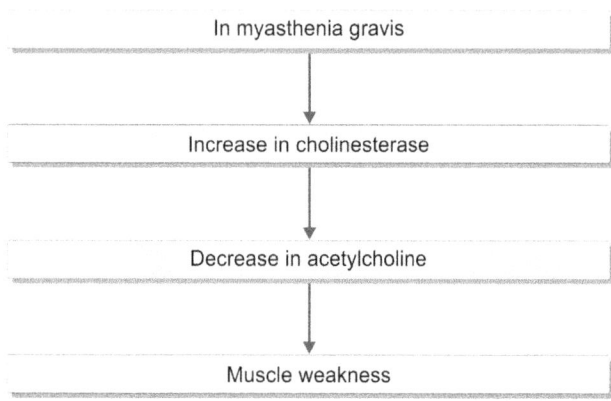

Clinical Manifestation

- Weakness
- Respiratory failure
- Dysphagia
- Diplopia
- Diminished breath sound

Nursing Care

- Monitor the respiratory status
- Encourage the client to sit up while eating
- Check the gag reflex and swallowing reflex
- Administer anticholinesterase medications, such as neostigmine, tilstigmin, physostigmine
- Prepare the patient for tensilon test
- Monitor for myasthenia crisis and cholinergic crisis
- Administer corticosteroids (prednisone)
- Prepare the patient for thymectomy, removal of thymus gland.

Tensilon Test (Fig. 6)

- The other names of tensilon is edrophonium. It is the test used to diagnose myasthenia gravis and to differentiate between myasthenia crisis and cholinergic crisis.
- The priority nursing care of a patient undergoing Tensilon test is keep atropine ready in the emergency tray.

Myasthenic Crisis

- It is the acute exacerbation of myasthenia gravis characterized by weakness, dyspnea, bowel and bladder incontinence, increase respiration and pulse.

Management
- Administer increases dose of anticholinesterase medication.

Cholinergic Crisis

- It occurs as a complication of overmedication of anticholinesterase. It is manifested as blurred vision, hypotension, etc.

Management
- Avoid anticholinesterase medication
- Administer antidote (atropine sulfate)

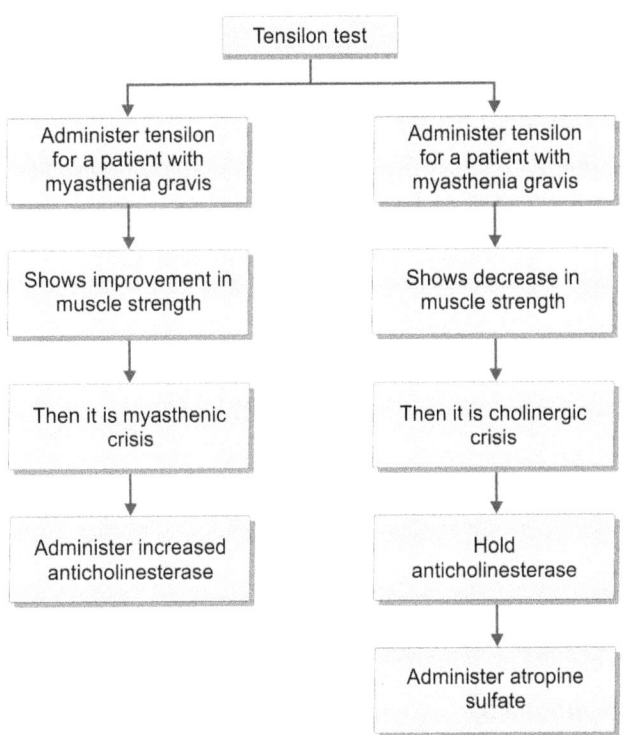

Fig. 6: Tensilon test

Parkinsonism

It is a degenerative disorder characterized by depletion of dopamine in the postsynaptic area leads to inhibition of excitatory muscles (slowing of activities).

Clinical Manifestation

- Bradykinesia and tremor
- Akathisia
- Poor handwriting
- Poor hand-motor coordination

Nursing Care

- Assist with activities of daily living (ADL)
- Provide a safe environment, side rails on bed
- Maintain adequate nutrition
- Assist the patient to improve communication abilities
- Instruct the patient to wear low healed shoes
- Administer anti-Parkinson's drugs (levodopa and carbidopa)
- Avoid administering vitamin B6 along with levodopa and carbidopa

- Avoid administering MAOI along with levodopa and carbidopa, because it may cause hypertensive crisis.

Spinal Cord Injury

A spinal cord injury is an injury to the spinal cord results in loss of function, such as mobility or feeling.

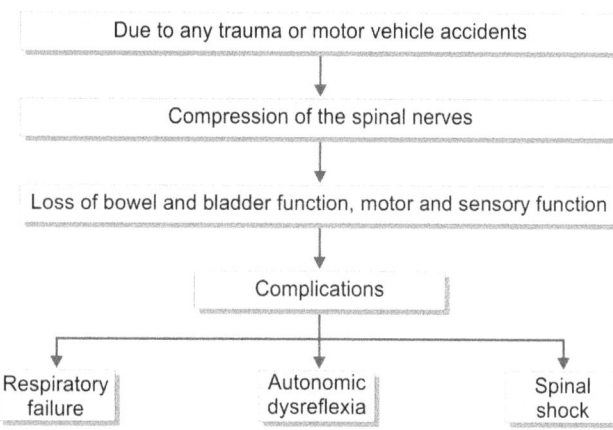

Common Sites
- Cervical—C_5, C_6, C_7
- Thoracic—T_{12}
- Lumbar—L_1

Clinical Manifestation
- Loss of bowel and bladder function
- Loss of motor function
- Loss of sensory function
- Respiratory failure (injury at C_4)
- Bowel and bladder incontinence (injury at S_2 and S_3)
- If the injury between C_1 and C_8, it results in quadriplegia (paralysis of four extremities)
- If the injury between T_1 and L_4, it results in paraplegia (paralysis of lower extremities)
- Absence of sweat in the paralysed area.

Nursing Care
- Assess the injury site, if any patient admitted in the hospital with complaints of RTA always suspect for spinal cord injury (improper handling may results in complete transection of the cord from partial transection)
- Immobilize the patient, place the patient on a spinal backboard
- Provide flat position for the patient except in autonomic dysreflexia
- Place the patient in a skull tongs or halo traction in case of any suspected cervical fracture
- Use log rolling technique while moving the patient
- Monitor for complications.

Autonomic Dysreflexia
It is also known as autonomic hyper-reflexia. It occurs when the injury is above T_6. It is manifested as restlessness, severe hypertension, pupillary dilation, etc.

Management
- Raise the head end of bed 30–45 degree
- Administer antihypertensive medications
- Provide catheterization.

Spinal Shock
It is also called flaccidity or flaccid paralysis or neurogenic shock. It is manifested as hypotension, bradycardia.

Meningitis
- It is the inflammation of the meninges or subarachnoid space (see the Fig. 3, layers of meninges).
- It is the inflammation of the arachnoid mater and pia mater of the brain and spinal cord.
- It is the inflammation of the CSF
- The mode of transmission of meningitis is droplet infection or direct contact.
- It may be viral or bacterial meningitis.

Clinical Manifestation
- Fever and chills
- Headache, photophobia and irritability
- Vomiting and seizures
- Positive Kernig's sign (make the patient to lie down in supine position, flex the legs 90 degree angle to the thigh, suddenly extend the lower leg, there will be pain the hamstring muscle, indicates meningeal irritation)
- Positive Brudzinski's sign (ask the patient to lie in supine position, flex the neck towards the chest, the legs will also flex in case of meningeal irritation).

Nursing Care
- Assess the signs and symptoms of increased ICP
- Provide head of bed elevation 30 degree
- Monitor the CSF (decreased CSF glucose and increased CSF protein in meningitis)
- Provide dark and quiet room
- Provide respiratory isolation for 24 hours after initiation of antibiotic therapy
- Administer prescribed antibiotics
- The drug of choice for meningococcal meningitis is rifampicin.

Seizures
- Seizure is a sudden abnormal electrical discharge in the brain cells.
- Epilepsy is a chronic seizure activity.

- Status epilepticus is a chronic epileptic episodes without interval of consciousness.

Types

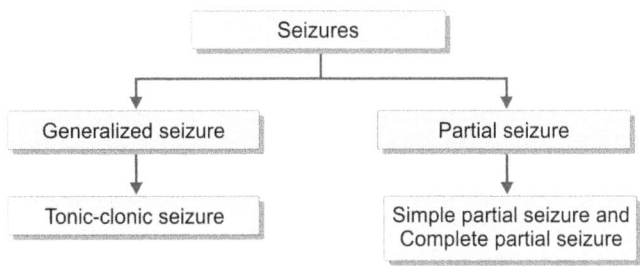

- **Generalized seizure:** Initial onset in both hemispheres, usually involves loss of consciousness and bilateral motor activity.
- **Partial seizure:** Begins in focal area of brain and symptoms are appropriate to a dysfunction of that area.
- **Tonic-clonic seizure:** It consist of a tonic phase and clonic phase. It begins with aura (warning sign). Tonic phase last for 20 seconds and is manifested as sudden stiffness. Clonic phase is manifested as jerky movements. This type of seizure ends with a period of postictal period of confusion and drowsiness.
- **Simple partial seizure:** Seizure confined to one hemisphere of brain.
- **Complex partial seizure:** Seizure begins in one focal area and spread to both hemispheres.

Nursing Care

- Remove all sharp objects near the patient side
- Maintain a patent airway
- Provide side lying position
- Administer anticonvulsant medications, such as Eptoin, carbamazepine
- The nursing care of a patient who is on anticonvulsants is monitor for gingival hypertrophy
- The drug of choice for status epilepticus is IV dilantin.

Head Injury

A head injury is any trauma to the scalp, skull, or brain. It may be a minor injury or major injury.

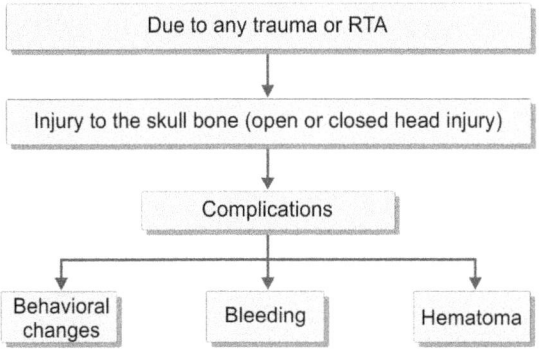

- **Closed head injury:** A head injury in which there is no break in the skull bone.
- **Open head injury:** A head injury in which the skull is open and entered the brain.
- **Contusion:** A bruising type of injury with changes in the level of consciousness.
- **Concussion:** A jarring type of injury with no loss of consciousness (temporary neural dysfunction).
- **Epidural hematoma:** Hematoma which is seen between dura mater and skull bone.
- **Subdural hematoma:** Hematoma which is seen below the dura mater (between dura mater and arachnoid mater).

Clinical Manifestation

- Hematoma and bleeding
- Seizure activity
- Visual disturbances
- Changes in the level of consciousness
- CSF drainage from ear and nose
- Battle sign: Ecchymosis around the mastoid process as a result of head injury

Nursing Care

- Maintain a patent airway
- Monitor the respiratory rate
- Monitor for increased ICP
- Administer morphine sulfate to decrease agitation (do not administer in case of increased ICP)
- Observe for CSF drainage
- Instruct the client to avoid coughing
- Administer mannitol
- Provide psychological support
- Prepare the patient for surgical correction

Surgical Correction (Intracranial Surgeries)
- **Craniotomy:** A surgical procedure that involves opening of the skull bone, an incision is made through the cranium to remove the accumulated blood or tumor.
- **Craniectomy:** Excision of a portion of the skull bone.
- **Cranioplasty:** Repair of a cranial defect with a metal or plastic plate.

Nursing Care (Preoperative)
- Provide emotional support to the patient and relatives
- Perform routine blood investigations
- Administer preoperative medications
- Shave the area, avoid enema because straining increases ICP
- Informed consent.

Nursing Care (Postoperative)
- Maintain a patent airway
- Monitor for increased ICP
- Provide mechanical ventilation with slight hyperventilation for 24–48 hours

- Monitor for the drainage, notify the physician if it is more than 30-50 ml
- Restrict fluid intake 1500 ml per day
- Provide anti-embolism stocking
- Provide proper position, in case of supratentorial surgery elevate the head of bed 15-45 degree, in case of infratentorial surgery keep the head of bed flat or elevate 20-30 degree, in case of bone flap removal turn the patient to nonoperated site, in case of posterior fossa surgery position the client on the side with a pillow under the head.

Cerebral Aneurysm

It is the dilation of the weakened cerebral artery.

Clinical Manifestation

- Headache or head pain
- Diplopia
- Nuchal rigidity

Nursing Care

- Maintain a patent airway
- Provide dark and quiet room
- Provide semi Fowler's position
- Provide seizure precautions
- Limit the number of visitors

Bell's Palsy

It is also known as facial paralysis, damage to the 7th cranial nerve.

Clinical Manifestation

- Inability to raise the eyebrow
- Inability to close the eye lids
- Loss of taste, smile and complete paralysis of one side of face.

Nursing Care

- Administer corticosteroids
- Provide soft diet
- Instruct the client to chew on the unaffected side.

Trigeminal Neuralgia

It is the disorder of 5th cranial nerve (trigeminal nerve).

Clinical Manifestation

- Severe sharp facial pain
- Poor eating and hygiene habits

Nursing Care

- Assess the characteristics of pain
- Provide small and frequent feeding
- Avoid hot or cold fluids

Guillain-Barré Syndrome

Guillain-Barré syndrome (GBS) is a rare disorder in which your body's immune system attacks your nerves (nerve inflammation).

Clinical Manifestation

- Prickling, "pins and needles" sensations in fingers, toes, ankles or wrists
- Weakness in legs that spreads to your upper body
- Unsteady walking or inability to walk or climb stairs
- Difficulty with eye or facial movements, including speaking, chewing or swallowing.

Nursing Care

- Assess the cranial nerve function
- Monitor for respiratory distress
- The priority nursing care of a patient with GBS is monitor for respiratory failure
- Administer corticosteroids.

CHAPTER 4

Respiratory System

Chapter Objectives

- Keynotes in the respiratory system
- Anatomy of the respiratory system
- Oxygen administration
- Various diagnostic measures
- Mechanical ventilation
- Disorders in the respiratory system

KEY TERMS

ABG   Crackles
MRI   Stridor
PFT   Apnoea
COPD   Surfactant

KEYNOTES

- The weight of lungs is 1.09 kg.
- Fine crackles is heard in heart failure and pulmonary edema.
- Coarse crackles is heard in pneumonia.
- Scoline is a muscle relaxant.
- The purpose of Venturi mask is administration of high flow oxygen.
- The purpose of spirometer is expansion of alveoli.
- The first sign of cessation of breathing is hypoxia.
- The first sign of hypoxia is restlessness.
- The confirmation test for TB is sputum AFB (acid-fast bacilli).
- The ABG (arterial blood gas) report for a patient with asthma is respiratory acidosis.
- The complication of morphine is respiratory arrest.
- Hyperventilate the patient before and after suctioning.
- Streptomycin cause ototoxicity.
- Diaphragm is the primary muscle of breathing.
- Barrel chest is seen in emphysema.
- Paradoxical chest movement is most distinctive sign of flail chest.
- Deficiency of alpha antitrypsin will result in emphysema.
- Salbutamol nebulization is the earliest method to decrease serum potassium in patients with CRF associated hyperkalemia.
- Hyperventilation results in respiratory alkalosis.
- Hypoventilation results in respiratory acidosis.
- The side effect of rifampicin is reddish orange urine.
- The side effect of Isoniazid is peripheral neuritis.
- The side effect of ethambutol is optic neuritis.
- Monitor serum uric acid for a patient undergoing pyrazinamide.

INTRODUCTION

The respiratory system plays a vital role in our body. The functions of respiratory system can be classified into two categories.

Primary Functions

- Provide oxygenation for the body
- Removes carbon dioxide along with waste products of metabolism.

Secondary Functions

- Maintain acid base balance
- Maintain heat balance
- Produce and modulate speech

ANATOMY

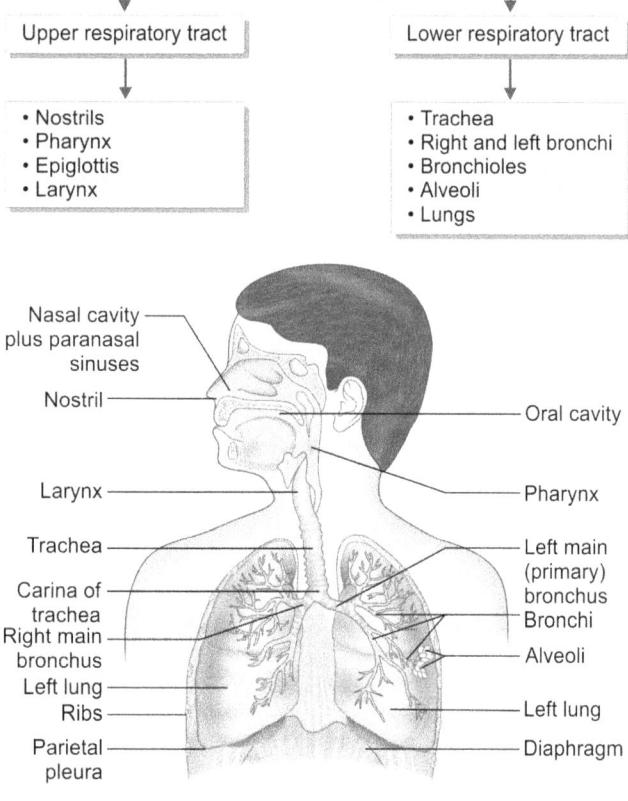

Fig. 1: Anatomy of respiratory system

- **Nostrils:** The nose is the primary opening for the respiratory system, made of bones, muscles and cartilages. From the nostrils, the humidified air enters into the lungs.
- **Pharynx:** It is also known as food pipe, the common passage for food and air. From the pharynx it is turned into two structures, the larynx and esophagus. Larynx is followed by the respiratory tract and esophagus is followed by the digestive tract.
- **Epiglottis:** A leaf-like structure seen at the top of the larynx which prevents the entry of food in to the respiratory tract. Any infection in the epiglottis is called as epiglottitis. The classical manifestation of a child with epiglottitis is diminished cough.
- **Larynx:** It is called as voice box of the human body. It helps in voice modulation.
- **Trachea:** Also known the wind pipe, the trachea is a tube made of cartilage rings that are lined with pseudostratified ciliated columnar epithelium. It is seen in front of esophagus.
- **Right and left bronchi:** The bronchi connect the wind pipe to the lungs, allowing air from external respiratory openings to pass efficiently into the lungs.
- **Bronchioles:** Bronchioles lead to alveolar sacs, which are sacs containing alveoli.
- **Alveoli:** Alveoli are hollow, individual cavities that are found within alveolar sacs which allow the exchange of oxygen and carbon dioxide.
- **Lungs:** There are two lungs, right lung and left lung. Right lung is larger than left lung consist of three lobes. Left lung is little narrower to accommodate heart.

What is Yawning?

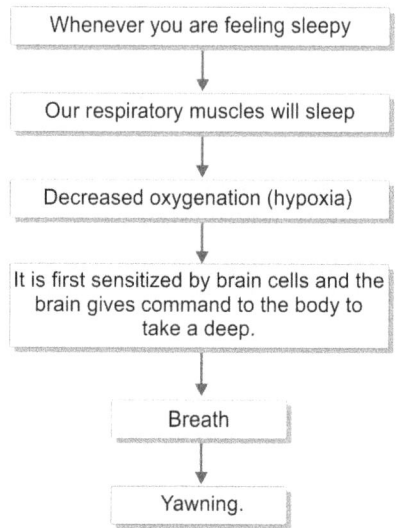

Inspiration and Expiration

Inspiration	Expiration
During inspiration ↓ The diaphragm descends ↓ Increase intrathoracic space ↓ Negative pressure created in the lungs ↓ Air from atmosphere enters to lungs (passage of air from greater concentration to lesser concentration)	During expiration ↓ The diaphragm recoils ↓ Decrease intrathoracic space ↓ Positive pressure created in lungs ↓ Air enters into atmosphere from the lung (passage of air from greater concentration to lesser concentration)

Breath Sounds

Breath sounds can be classified into two categories. These sounds can be heard through stethoscope or auscultation.

Normal Breath Sounds

- **Bronchial:** Bronchial breath sounds consist of a full inspiratory and expiratory phase with the inspiratory phase usually being louder. They are normally heard over the trachea and larynx.

- **Bronchovesicular sounds:** *Bronchovesicular breath sounds consist of a full inspiratory phase with a shortened and softer expiratory phase.*
- **Vesicular sounds:** *Vesicular breath sounds consist of a quiet, wispy inspiratory phase followed by a short, almost silent expiratory phase.*

Abnormal Breath Sounds (Adventitious)

- **Crackles:** *Crackles are discontinuous, explosive, "popping" sounds that originate within the airways like fluid accumulation.*
- **Wheezes:** *A high-pitched whistling sound caused by obstruction of the bronchial tubes*
- **Stridor:** *A harsh, vibratory sound caused by obstruction of the trachea*
- **Rhonchi:** *Snoring sounds.*

Diminished Breath Sounds are heard in:
- Atelectasis (alveolar collapse)
- Emphysema (increased AP diameter)
- Chest injuries (increased AP diameter)
- Road traffic accidents

OXYGEN THERAPY

Oxygen therapy is the administration of oxygen as a medical intervention to prevent excessive carbon dioxide accumulation.
- Normal atmospheric air oxygen concentration is 20.85% or 21%.
- Hyperoxygenation, if the atmospheric air oxygen concentration more than 21%.
- Oxygen toxicity, if the atmospheric air oxygen concentration more than 40%.
- Administer 2 liter oxygen for a patient with COPD (chronic obstructive pulmonary disease), because low arterial oxygen is a thrive to take more oxygen.

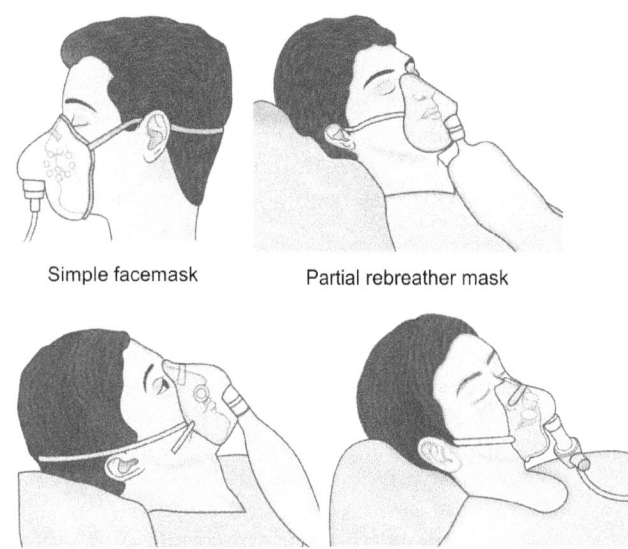

Simple facemask · Partial rebreather mask · Nonrebreather mask · Venturimask

Nasal cannula (nasal prongs) (low flow oxygen)	Facial mask	Partial rebreather mask	Non-rebreather mask	Venturi mask (high flow oxygen delivery)
Amount of oxygen 1–6 liters per minute	Amount of oxygen minimum 5 liters per minute	Amount of oxygen 6–15 liters per minute	Amount of oxygen greater than 15 liters per minute	Amount of oxygen 4–10 liters per minute
Fraction of inspired oxygen (FiO_2) is 24–44%	Fraction of inspired oxygen (FiO_2) is 40–60%	Fraction of inspired oxygen (FiO_2) is 70–90%	Fraction of inspired oxygen (FiO_2) is 60–100%	Fraction of inspired oxygen (FiO_2) is 24–50%

SUCTIONING

Suctioning is a method to remove the mucous from the lungs in order to make airway clear.

Purposes

- To maintain a patent airway
- To promote gas exchange
- To obtain a sample for analysis

Nursing Care

- Hyperventilate the patient before and after suctioning
- Place the patient in semi to high Fowler's position
- Rotate the catheter while applying intermittent suction
- The standard suctioning time is 10 to 15 seconds
- Attach connective tubing to suction regulator/equipment and inlet of suction container. Connect suction machine to vacuum wall outlet. Turn the vacuum on, and occlude tip of connective tubing. If no suction is demonstrated on gauge, tighten all connections. If still no suction occurs increase vacuum. If still no suction occurs, label machine "defective" obtain another suction machine, reassemble and retest.
- Adjust vacuum between 80 and 120 mm Hg for adults or 60 to 80 mm Hg for pediatrics.
- Position the patient by extending the neck slightly to facilitate entrance into the trachea (especially for nasotracheal suctioning).

- Open suction catheter exposing only the connector, attach to connective tubing and maintain sterility of catheter.
- Fill sterile box with sterile water, and place a dab of water-soluble lubricant on sterile envelope if nasotracheal suctioning is to be performed.
- Check heart rate before, during and after procedure. If tachycardia or bradycardia occurs discontinue the procedure until it resolves.
- Hyperoxygenate the intubated patient or request the nonintubated patient to take several deep breaths.
- Auscultate the patient's chest; if secretions can still be heard repeat the suctioning procedure (5–10 ml of normal saline may be used to loosen tenacious secretions). Before re-suctioning, clear catheter with sterile water.
- Monitor for any complications
  - Hypoxia
  - Vagal stimulation: Cardiac arrhythmia
  - Tracheitis
  - Damage to mucous membranes
  - Airway occlusions
  - Sudden death
  - Bleeding disorders

Chest Tube Drainage and Water Seal System

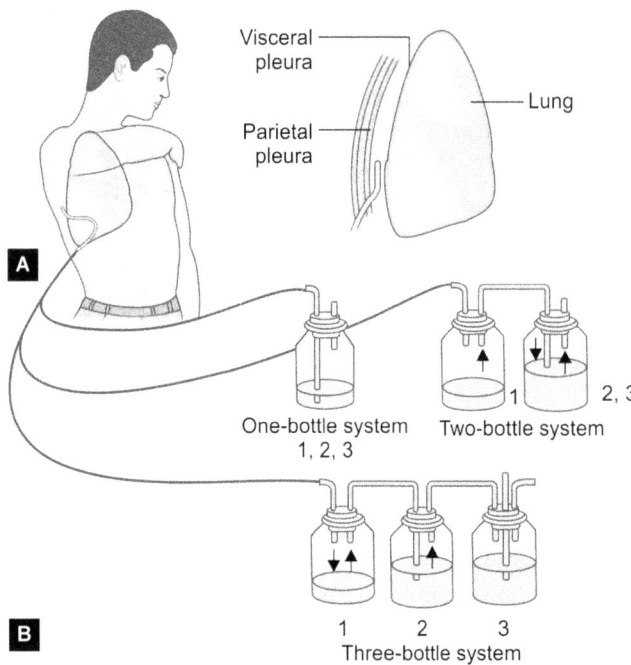

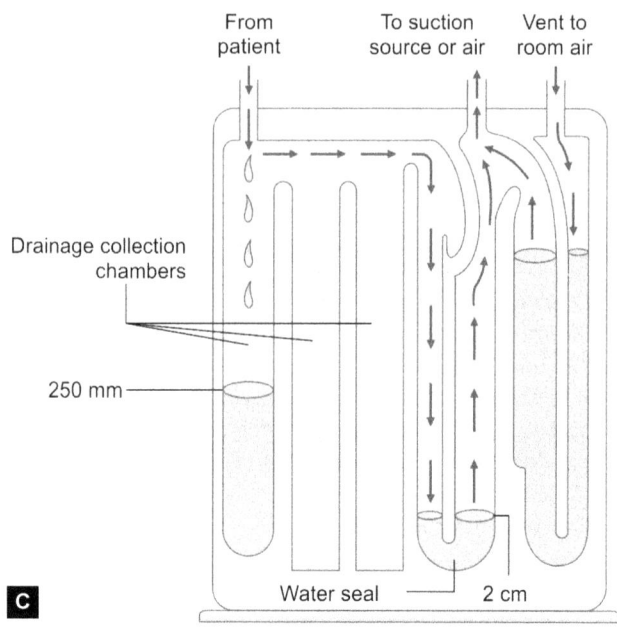

- A chest tube or intercostal drain is a flexible plastic tube that is inserted through the chest wall and into the pleural space or mediastinum to remove air or fluid.
- A chest tube is attached to the water seal drainage system to allow escape of air or fluid and to prevent reflex of air into chest.
- A chest tube is placed in the eighth or ninth intercostal space, midaxillary line for drainage of fluid and second or third for the removal of air.
- Chest tube drainage is connected to the closed gravity drainage system.
- A water seal drainage system suddenly breaks, create an artificial drainage system by dipping the drainage tube in a glass of sterile water.
- A continuous bubbling in the water seal drainage system indicates air leak and an intermittent bubbling in the water seal system indicates normal functioning. No bubbling indicates obstruction or kink in the drainage system or lung is re-expanded.
- Never clamp the chest tube drainage, if a physician instruct the nurse to clamp the chest tube, clamp near the patient side to prevent pneumothorax.
- In case of accidental dislodgment from the body cavity, cover the site with an occlusive dressing (vaseline dressing).
- Do not keep the ICD (intercostal drainage) above the heart level.
- In case of two bottle system, one is suction apparatus and other is water seal drainage (continuous bubbling is seen in the suction apparatus and intermittent bubbling in drainage system).
- In case of three bottle systems, there is a drainage collection, water seal, a suction control bottle. The third bottle controls the amount of pressure in the system. Suction control bottle has three tube inserted in the stopper, two short and one long. Two short tubes, one short tube connected to former air vent of the water seal bottle, second short tube connected to suction. The long tube located between the two short has opened to atmosphere.

- Confirmation of chest tube placement is made by X-ray.
- Bedside equipments needed for a patient with ICD—clamp, bottle of sterile water, vaseline dressing.
- While removing the chest tube drainage, instruct the patient to breath normally or follow valsalva maneuver.

MECHANICAL VENTILATION

Ventilation is performed through a mechanical means is called mechanical ventilation. A mechanical ventilator is a machine that helps a patient breathe (ventilate) when he or she is recovering from surgery or critical illness, or cannot breathe on his or her own for any reason.

- Scoline is a muscle relaxant which is administered before intubation. The particular chest movements after scoline administration are called as fasciculation.
- The antidote of scoline is neostigmine or physostigmine.
- The cuff of ET (endotracheal tube) tube is pilot balloon, to maintain tube in position and to facilitate delivery of air into the lungs.

Indications

- COPD
- Obesity
- Thoracic surgeries
- Cardiac arrest

Types of Mechanical Ventilation

- Positive pressure ventilation (used now)
- Negative pressure ventilation

Types of Positive Pressure Ventilators

- Pressure cycled ventilators: Pushes air into the lungs until a predetermined pressure.
- Volume cycled ventilators: Until a predetermined tidal volume.
- Time cycled ventilators: Until a predetermined or preset time.

Modes of Mechanical Ventilation

1. **CMV mode (continuous mandatory ventilation):** It is also called as control mode. The ventilator is giving full support, the ventilator deliver breath automatically if the client does not trigger it. The same tidal volume is delivered with each breath. Sedate the patient in order to prevent respiratory alkalosis.
2. **SIMV (synchronized intermittent mandatory ventilation):** The client may take breath at own rate and the intermittent mandatory ventilation breaths are delivered under positive pressure in between.
3. **Weaning or spontaneous mode:** Changing of the patient from ventilator to spontaneous breath, the client is taken from the ventilator and T-piece is connected to provide humidified oxygen.

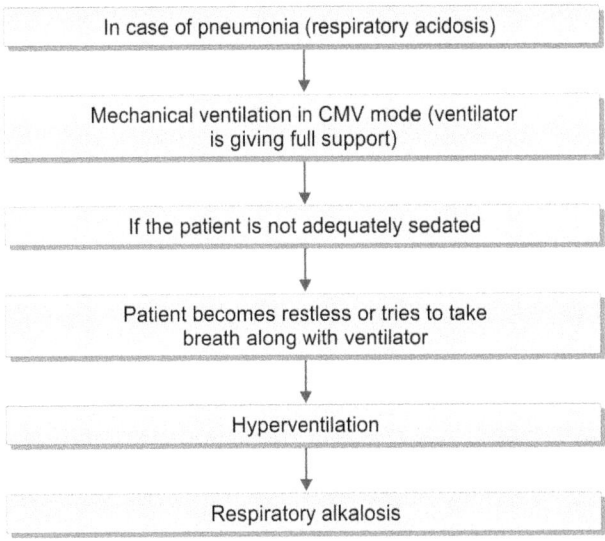

Ventilator Settings

- **PEEP (positive end-expiratory pressure):** A positive pressure is delivered at the end of expiratory phase of ventilation in order to maintain the alveoli open. If the PEEP is more than 15, there is chance to develop barotrauma and tension pneumothorax.
- **CPAP (continuous positive airway pressure):** The application of positive airway pressure throughout the entire respiratory cycle for spontaneous breathing, it keeps the alveoli opened during the inspiration and prevents alveolar collapse. It is primarily used as weaning mode.

Nursing Care

- Assess the cardiac output
- Monitor for peripheral edema
- Monitor barotrauma
- Assess the breath sounds every two hours
- Monitor for any complication
- Monitor for any alarm sound

Alarm System

- **High pressure alarm:** Due to any obstruction or secretion
- **Low pressure alarm:** Due to any disconnection or leakage.

Complications

- Respiratory alkalosis
- Hypotension
- Gastrointestinal bleeding
- VAP (ventilator-assisted pneumonia)
- Pneumothorax

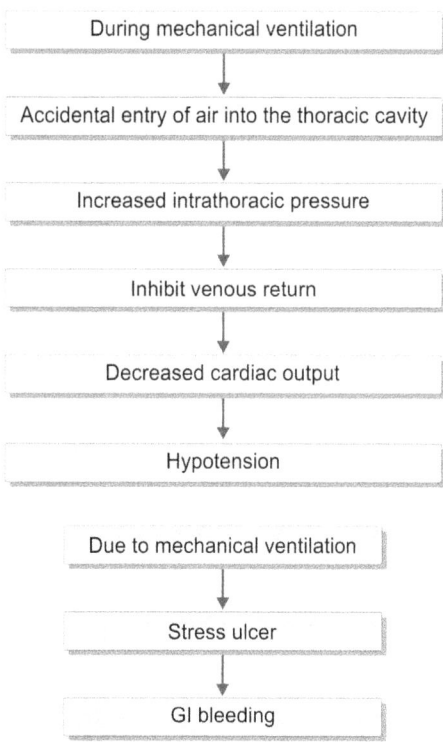

DIAGNOSTIC MEASURES

- **Chest X-ray:** Radiograph of the chest provides information regarding the anatomical location and appearance of lungs. Question the women regarding the possibility of pregnancy before chest radiography.
- **Common X-ray findings**
  - In COPD: Areas of hyperinflation or over inflation
  - In asthma: hyperexpanded lungs, flattened diaphragms, narrowed cardiac shadow
  - In bronchiectasis: Honeycomb appearance in X-ray
  - In pneumonia: Lobar or segmental consolidation
  - In tuberculosis: Multinodular infiltrates with calcification in upper lobes
  - In pleural effusion: Mediastinal shift
- **Sputum examination:** Early morning sterile specimen is obtained either by expectoration or by tracheal suctioning. Obtain sputum before antibiotic therapy.
- **Laryngoscopy:** Direct visualization of larynx, trachea and bronchi with a fiber-optic bronchoscope. Remove all dentures and maintain the client on a semi Fowler's position after Bronchoscopy.
- **Bronchoscopy:** Insertion of a fiberscope into the bronchi for diagnosis, biopsy collection for diagnostic purposes.
- **Pulmonary angiography:** An invasive procedure in which a catheter is inserted via the femoral artery into the pulmonary artery to rule out any abnormalities. Monitor for any allergies for dye before the procedure.
- **Thoracentesis:** Insertion of a needle through the chest wall into the pleural space to remove fluid or air or specimen for diagnostic purposes. Position the patient at the side of bed, sitting upright with arms and shoulder supported on a table. If the patient cannot sit up the client is placed lying in the bed toward the unaffected side with head of bed elevation.
- **Pulmonary function test (PFT):** It is used to evaluate the lung mechanism. A spirometer is used to evaluate the lung volume and capacities. Refrain from smoking or heavy meals for 4–6 hours before the test. Withhold all the bronchodilators before the test. The test is contraindicated in children less than 5 years of age because they cannot follow the instructions.
- **Lung biopsy:** It is used to detect any abnormalities or malignancies. The position used for lung biopsy is prone position or decubitus position.
- **Pulse oximetry:** It is a noninvasive procedure to measure the dissolved oxygen concentration in the blood. Normal saturation 90-100%. A pulse oximetry reading of less than 91% necessitate physician notification, if it is less than 85% oxygen to the body tissue is compromised, if it is less than 70% it is a life-threatening complication.
- **Tuberculin skin test (Mantoux):** It is a test used to determine tuberculosis infection. 0.1 ml solution containing 5 units of tuberculin, purified protein derivative (PPD) is administered intradermally to the client's forearm. The site is monitored for induration between 48 and 72 hours. If the induration is more than 10 mm, the test is positive and if it is between 5 and 10 mm it shows the client is immunocompromised. If it is less than 5, it is negative. Positive Mantoux test indicates body's immunity starts functioning.

Arterial Blood Gas (ABG) Analysis

It measures the dissolved oxygen and carbon dioxide concentration in the arterial blood and to find out the acid-base balance.

Indications of ABG

- Respiratory failure—In acute and chronic states.
- Any severe illness which may lead to a metabolic acidosis-for example:
  - Cardiac failure
  - Liver failure
  - Renal failure
  - Hyperglycemic states
  - Sepsis
  - Burns
  - Poisons/toxins
- Ventilated patients

Nursing Care

- Perform Allen test before drawing blood sample

- Allen's test
  - Elevate the hand and make a fist for approximately 30 seconds.
  - Apply pressure over the ulnar and the radial arteries occluding both (keep the hand elevated).
  - Open the hand which will be blanched.
  - Release pressure on the ulnar artery and look for perfusion of the hand (this takes under eight seconds).
  - If there is any delay then it may not be safe to perform radial artery puncture.
- Avoid suctioning before drawing ABG sample
- After ABG collection, apply pressure over the site for 10 minutes.

Normal ABG Report

- Ph 7.35 to 7.45
- PCO_2—35 to 45 mm Hg
- HCO_3—22 to 28 mEq/L
- PO_2—80 to 100 mm Hg

Acid-Base Imbalances

- Respiratory acidosis
- Respiratory alkalosis
- Metabolic acidosis
- Metabolic alkalosis

RO/ME

Respiratory—opposite direction
Metabolic—equal direction

Respiratory acidosis	Ph ↓	PCO_2 ↑	HCO_3 ↑
Respiratory alkalosis	Ph ↑	PCO_2 ↓	HCO_3 ↓
Metabolic acidosis	Ph ↓	PCO_2 ↓	HCO_3 ↓
Metabolic alkalosis	Ph ↑	PCO_2 ↑	HCO_3 ↑

	Respiratory acidosis	Respiratory alkalosis
Causes	Hypoventilation	Hyperventilation
In which all conditions	Asthma, pneumonia, CNS depressants, brain trauma, pulmonary edema	Fever, hysteria, pain, hypoxia, mechanical ventilation
Manifestations	Increased respiratory rate, hyperkalemia	Decreased respiratory rate, hypokalemia
Management	Administer oxygen	Limit oxygen

RESPIRATORY MEDICATIONS

Bronchodilators		Corticosteroids	
Oral	**Inhaled**	**Oral**	**Inhaled**
Deriphyllin	Albuterol	Methylprednisolone	Fluticasone
Theophy-lline	Salmeterol	Montelukast (Leukotriene modifiers)	Mometasone
Terbutaline	Formoterol		

Nursing Care

- Monitor for peanut allergy in case of administering anticholinergics like ipratropium bromide.
- Monitor serum theophylline (10-20 mcg/ml). If the serum theophylline is more than 20 mcg/ml, it is called theophylline toxicity manifested as tachycardia, nervousness and irritability.
- Monitor the heart rate while administering deriphyllin.

DISORDERS

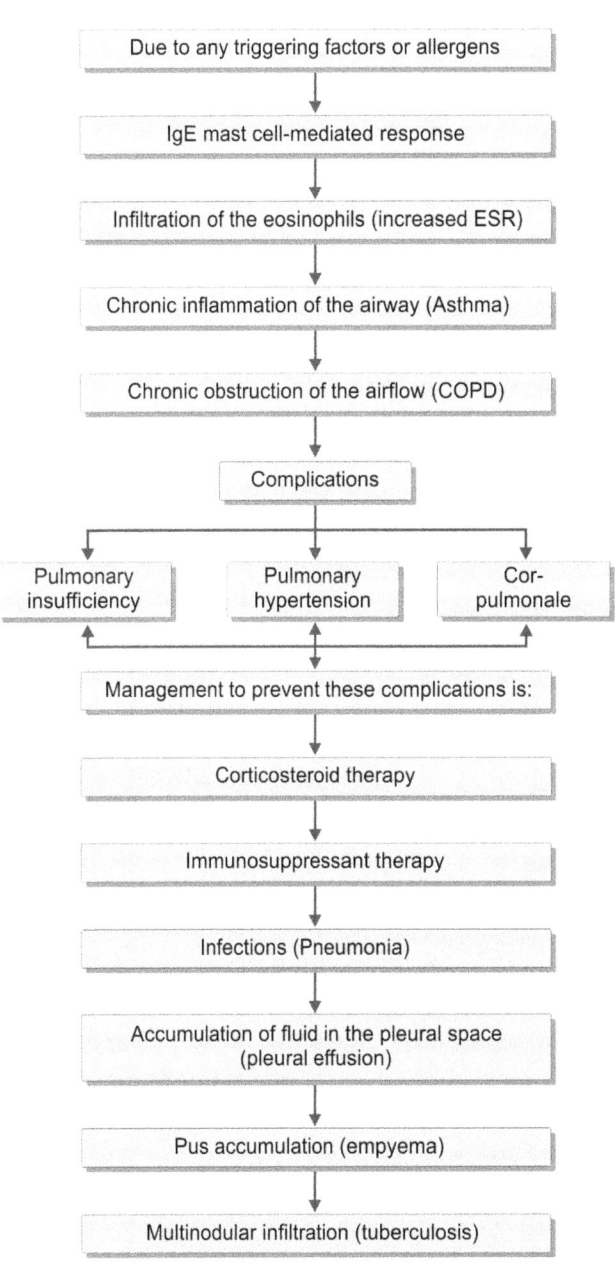

Chronic Obstructive Pulmonary Disease (COPD)

It is also called chronic airway limitation or chronic obstruction of air flow. It consists of 3 disorders. They are:
1. Emphysema: Destruction of the alveolar, bronchial and bronchiolar tissue
2. Bronchitis: Excessive production of mucus in the bronchi with cough
3. Chronic bronchiectasis: Permanent abnormal dilation of the bronchi.

Clinical Manifestations

- Dyspnea
- Barrel chest
- Wheezing and crackles
- Orthopnea (dyspnea in upright position)
- Shortness of breath
- ABG shows respiratory acidosis and hypoxemia
- Chest X-ray shows areas of hyperinflation or over inflation
- PFT shows reduced vital capacity.

Nursing Care

- Monitor vital signs
- Administer low concentration oxygen (2L)
- Teach the patient pursed lip breathing (deep inspiration followed by prolonged expiration I:E = 1:2)
- Provide high calorie high protein diet (low carbohydrate diet for COPD, because the end product of carbohydrate metabolism is carbon dioxide)
- Provide high Fowler's position
- The classical position maintained by COPD patient is tripod position
- Administer mucolites, corticosteroids and bronchodilators
- Monitor for any complications (pulmonary hypertension, pulmonary hypertension and cor-pulmonale).

Asthma

It is a chronic inflammatory disorder of the airway characterized by airway inflammation and hyper-responsiveness to a variety of stimuli. Status asthmaticus is a severe life-threatening asthma episode which may result in pneumothorax, cor-pulmonale and respiratory arrest.

Clinical Manifestations

- Wheezing
- Diminished lung sound or hyper-resonance
- Tachycardia
- Tachypnea
- Diaphoresis
- Chest tightness
- PFT shows decreased airflow rates
- Decreased oxygen saturation

Nursing Care

- Monitor vital signs
- Administer oxygen
- Avoid triggering factors, such as dust or smoke
- Avoid beta-blockers
- Provide comfortable position, sitting upright position.
- Encourage pursed lip-breathing exercise
- Administer bronchodilators
- Administer corticosteroids

Pneumonia

It is the inflammation of the lung parenchyma, interstitial space, alveoli, bronchioles, etc. It may be hospital acquired or community acquired. The main causative organisms are Pneumococci, *E. coli* and *Staphylococcus aureus*.

Clinical Manifestations

- Cough with greenish or rust colored sputum
- High pitch bronchial breath sounds
- Crackles, coarse crackles
- Chest X-ray shows lobar or segmental consolidation
- Increased WBC and ESR

Nursing Care

- Administer oxygen
- Provide high Fowler's position
- Maintain adequate hydration
- Monitor for any pleuritic pain
- Limit the number of visitors
- Provide respiratory isolation
- Teach the patient about proper hand washing and respiratory isolation

Pleural Effusion

Collection of fluid in the pleural space, pleura is a membrane covering the lungs. There are two layers, visceral pleura (inner layer) and parietal pleura (outer layer). The space between these two layers is pleural space and fluid in between is pleural fluid. Normal pleural fluid is 10–20 ml.

Clinical Manifestations

- Pleuritic pain (sharp severe pain)
- Dry and nonproductive cough
- Tachycardia

- Increased temperature
- Chest X-ray shows mediastinal shift, if the amount of fluid is more than 250 ml.

Nursing Care

- Monitor the breath sounds
- Provide Fowler's position
- Prepare the client for thoracentesis
- If there is any recurrent pleural effusion, prepare the patient for pleurodesis or pleurectomy.

Empyema

It is the collection of pus in the pleural space. The fluid becomes thick, opaque and foul smelling.

Clinical Manifestations

- Chest pain
- Dyspnea
- Increased temperature
- Night sweating

Nursing Care

- Provide semi to high Fowler's position
- Encourage coughing and deep breathing exercise
- Administer antibiotics

Tuberculosis (TB)

- It is a highly communicable disease caused by *Mycobacterium tuberculi*, it is a nonmotile acid fast bacteria which secrete niacin which helps in the multiplication of TB pathogen.
- It is primarily affecting the pulmonary system and affect other areas, such as brain, kidney, joints, etc.
- Improper treatment schedules may result in MDR TB (multidrug resistant TB)
- DOTS therapy is related to TB (directly observed treatment short course)
- The mode of transmission of TB is airborne or droplet infection.

Causes

- Drinking unpasteurized milk
- Children less than 5 years of age
- Overcrowded areas
- IV drug abusers
- Nosocomial infections

Clinical Manifestations

- Cough with mucopurulent sputum
- Yellow greenish sputum
- Weight loss
- Low grade fever
- Blood in sputum
- Night sweat
- Chest X-ray shows multinodular infiltrates with calcification in the upper lobe
- Positive Mantoux test
- Sputum AFB (confirmatory test for TB)
- Positive TB gold test

Nursing Care

- Administer Anti-TB drugs
- Provide isolation (reverse isolation)
- Teach about strict handwashing techniques
- Follow standard precautions, like gloves and mask, while handling patient with TB
- Provide proper nutrition
- Monitor weight periodically
- Restrict the number of visitors

Anti-TB Drugs

First line drugs	Second line drugs
1. Rifampicin (Rcin)	Streptomycin
2. Isoniazid (Solonex)	Amikacin
3. Pyrazinamide (PZA)	Levofloxacin
4. Ethambutol (Mycobutol)	

- **Rifampicin (Rcin) 400–500 mg**
  - It is available in capsular form
  - Dose of rifampicin is 10 mg per kg
  - It is taken in empty stomach to prevent gatric irritation
  - It is the drug of choice for meningococcal meningitis
  - The side effect of rifampicin is reddish orange colored body fluids (urine)
- **Isoniazid (Solonex) 300 mg**
  - The dose is 5 mg per kg
  - The side effect is peripheral neuritis
  - Administer along with vitamin B6 or pyridoxine
- **Pyrazinamide (PZA) 500–750 mg**
  - The dose is 15 to 20 mg per kg
  - The side effect of pyrazinamide is nephrotoxicity and gout
  - Administer allopurinol to decrease the serum uric acid level
  - Administer more fluids along with PZA
  - Monitor serum uric acid level
- **Ethambutol (Mycobutol) 300–800 mg**
  - The dose of ethambutol is 25 mg per kg
  - The side effect is optic neuritis
  - Perform periodic visual examination of the patient

- **Streptomycin 1000 mg**
  - The dose of streptomycin is 20 to 40 mg per kg
  - The side effect is ototoxicity (damage to C8 cranial nerve)
  - Monitor for any impairment in hearing and balance

Bronchogenic Carcinoma

The lung cancer is commonly occurs in the right lung, because the blood supply and lymphatic supply is more seen in the right lung. It is associated with cigarette smoking, frequent respiratory infections and asbestos inhalation.

Clinical Manifestations

- Dyspnea
- Persistent cough with bloody sputum
- Chest pain

Nursing Care

- The priority nursing care of a patient with bronchogenic carcinoma is to maintain a patent airway
- Prepare the patient for radiation therapy and chemotherapy
- Provide semi-Fowler's position
- Incase of pneumonectomy same side position is given
- Monitor the ICD (ICD is not performed for a patient undergoing pneumonectomy)
- Prepare the patient for surgical correction, common surgical approaches are:
  - *Exploratory thoracotomy:* Incision through the 3rd, 4th, 5th, 6th, 7th intercostal space to examine the pleura and lung.
  - *Lobectomy:* Removal of a lobe
  - *Segmentectomy:* Removal of a segment
  - *Wedge resection:* Removal of the lesion
  - *Pneumonectomy:* Removal of a part of lung

Laryngeal Cancer

It is one of the most common upper respiratory malignancies. The larynx contains the vocal cords, which vibrate and make sound when air is directed against them. Laryngeal cancer is a disease in which malignant (cancer) cells form in the tissues of the larynx. The main causative factors are smoking, alcoholism and vocal abuse.

Clinical Manifestations

- Progressive hoarseness of voice
- Burning sensation while drinking hot liquids or orange juice.

Nursing Care

- Maintain a patent airway
- Prepare the patient for radiation therapy and chemotherapy
- Prepare the patient for surgery
- The priority nursing care of a patient undergoing surgical correction of laryngeal cancer is make the patient to accept the body image (the surgical correction of laryngeal cancer is laryngectomy, after laryngectomy we will keep an artificial larynx, it does not have the ability to vibrate and the patient exhibits monotonous sound. So, instruct the patient to accept the body image).

Flail Chest

It occurs from blunt trauma.

Clinical Manifestations

- Paradoxical chest movement
- Diminished breath sounds
- Hypotension
- Dyspnea

Nursing Care

- Monitor for any respiratory difficulty
- Administer oxygen
- Monitor for the signs of shock

Pneumothorax

It is a condition characterized by air in the thoracic cavity, it may be:
- Open pneumothorax: Due to any trauma
- Tension pneumothorax: Due to any complication of PEEP
- Spontaneous pneumothorax: Due to damage to the pulmonary bleb or tissue
- Hemothorax: Blood in the thoracic cavity

Clinical Manifestations

- Hypotension
- Chest pain, sharp pain
- Tachycardia
- Tachypnea
- Absence of breath sound in the affected area

Nursing Care

- Monitor for any bleeding from nose, mouth
- Maintain an ICD and closed gravity drainage system
- Provide high Fowler's position

CHAPTER 5

Cardiovascular System

Chapter Objectives

- Keynotes in the cardiovascular system
- Anatomy of heart
- Various diagnostic measures
- ECG
- Disorders in cardiovascular system
- Vascular disorders

KEY TERMS

Stokes-Adams syndrome
NTG
Angina
Raynaud's syndrome
Swan-Ganz catheter
PCWP
Pacemaker
Emboli

KEYNOTES

- The weight of heart is 315 gm.
- Heart is located in the left mediastinum.
- Normal amount of pericardial fluid is 5–20 ml.
- Accumulation of more amount of pericardial fluid in the pericardial space is called as cardiac tamponade.
- The classical manifestation of cardiac tamponade is Beck's triad.
- Normal capillary refill time is 2–3 seconds.
- Normal PCWP (pulmonary capillary wedge pressure) is 4–12 mm Hg.
- The catheter which is used to measure pulmonary artery pressure and pulmonary capillary wedge pressure is Swan-Ganz catheter.
- Golden rule of management of CAD is diet-exercise-medication
- The classical manifestations of heart failure are fine crackles and air hunger (left ventricular failure) and Jugular vein distention (right ventricular failure).
- Normal coagulation time 5–15 minutes
- Normal prothrombin time (PT) 9.8–11.6 seconds (9.5–12 seconds)
- Normal activated partial thromboplastin time (APTT) 20–45 seconds
- Left anterior descending artery is also known as widow maker artery.
- The hormones produced by the heart are atrial natriuretic peptide (ANP) a hormone of 28 amino acids released from stretched atria. Brain natriuretic peptide (BNP) hormone of 32 amino acids which is released from the ventricles, increased BNP is seen in heart failure.
- The first step of CPR is assessing the response of the patient.
- The causative organism of endocarditis is group A beta hemolytic streptococci.
- Virchow's triad is seen in thrombophlebitis.
- The symptoms of cardiology or clogged arteries are chest pain combined with the following symptoms:
  - Sweating, cool clammy skin, and paleness
  - Shortness of breath
  - Nausea or vomiting
  - Dizziness or fainting
  - Unexplained weakness or fatigue
  - Rapid or irregular pulse

INTRODUCTION

Heart is a hollow muscular organ which is located in the left mediastinum. There are two lungs, the right lung and left lung: Right lung is little larger than the left lung consists of three lobes. The left lung appears little narrower in order to accommodate the heart. The weight of heart is 315 gm (9–11 oz). In males 300–350 gm, in females 250–300 gm.

The main function of the cardiovascular system is to transport nutrients and oxygen to the entire body. The human heart is a four-chambered muscular organ, shaped and sized roughly like a man's closed fist.

CHAMBERS OF HEART

1. Right atrium
2. Right ventricle
3. Left atrium
4. Left ventricle

The deoxygenated blood from different parts of the body reaches the right atrium through the inferior and superior vena cava (venous return). From the right atrium through the Tricuspid valve it enters into the right ventricle, from the right ventricle with the help of pulmonary artery it enters to the lungs for purification. This circulation we can call **pulmonary circulation**. The purified blood (oxygenated blood) from the lungs reaches the left atrium with the help of pulmonary veins. From the left atrium it enters to the left ventricle through the Bicuspid valve (mitral valve). With the help of Aorta the purified blood reaches to all body part and this circulation we can call it as **systemic circulation (Fig. 1)**.

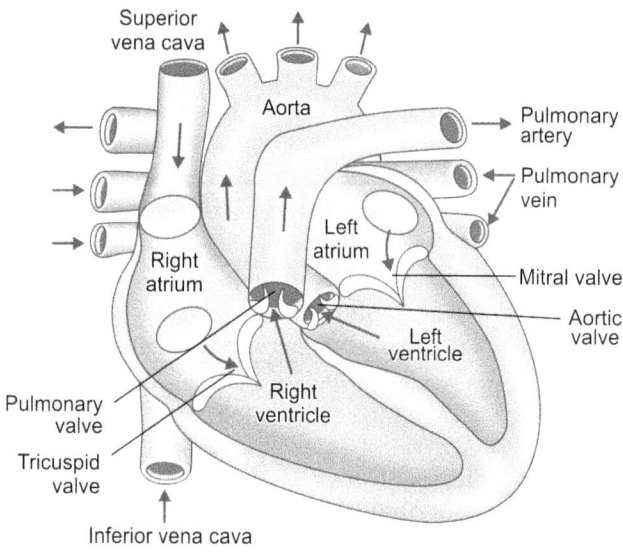

Fig. 1: Structure of heart

The heart uses a series of valves to ensure that blood flows in one direction into an out of the heart. Heart valves are made of tough, flexible tissue that is oriented in such a way that blood can only go through the valve in one direction. Blood flows in the direction of the arrows.

A valve only opens when the blood exerts enough pressure on it, forcing it open for blood to flow through. When this pressure drops, the valve returns to its originally closed position, preventing blood from flowing in the wrong direction. A pressure gradient is developed as blood flows through the body, and blood only flows from a high pressure to a lower one.

Layers of Heart

Heart is covered with three layers:
- Epicardium (outer layer)
- Myocardium (middle layer)
- Endocardium (inner layer)

Pericardial Sac

It protect the heart from trauma, there are two layers:
- Parietal pericardium (outer tough layer)
- Visceral pericardium (inner serous layer)

The space between the two pericardium is pericardial space, the fluid seen in the pericardial space is called as pericardial fluid, and normal amount of pericardial fluid is 5–20 ml.

Accumulation of more amount of pericardial fluid in the pericardial space is called as cardiac tamponade.

The classical manifestation of a patient with cardiac tamponade is Beck's triad.
- Hypotension due to decreased ventricular contraction
- Jugular vein distention
- Distant heart sound

CONDUCTION SYSTEM OF THE HEART

The heart has its own built-in electrical system, called the conduction system. The conduction system sends electrical signals throughout the heart that determine the timing of the heartbeat and cause the heart to beat in a coordinated, rhythmic pattern.

The electrical signals, or impulses, of the heart are generated by a clump of specialized tissue called the sinus node. Each time the sinus node generates a new electrical impulse, that impulse spreads out through the heart's upper chambers, called the right atrium and the left atrium. This electrical impulse, as it spreads across the two atria, stimulates them to contract, pumping blood into the right and left ventricles.

The electrical impulse then spreads to the atrioventricular (AV) node, which is another clump of specialized tissue located between the atria and the ventricles. The AV node momentarily slows down the spread of the electrical impulse, to allow the left and right atria to finish contracting. From the AV node, the impulse spreads into a system of specialized fibers called the His bundle and the right and left bundle branches. These fibers distribute the electrical impulse rapidly to all areas of the right and left ventricles, stimulating them to contract in a coordinated way. With this contraction, blood is pumped from the right ventricle to the lungs, and from the left ventricle throughout the body (Fig. 2).

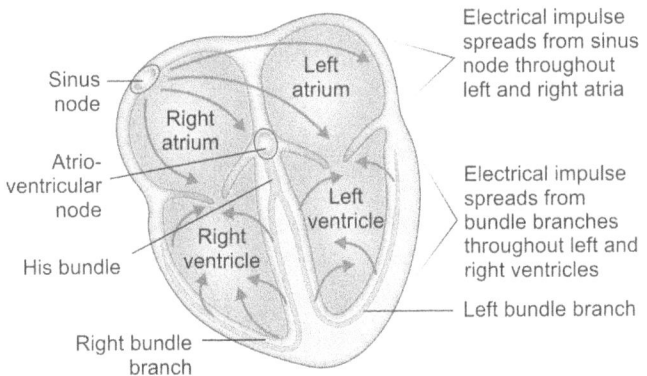

Fig. 2: Conduction system of heart

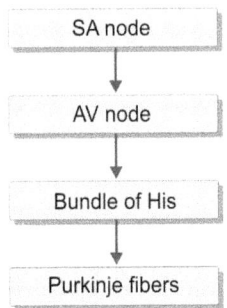

SA Node

- It is called as the pacemaker of heart.
- It is located at the junction of superior vena cava and right atrium.
- It stimulate at a rate of 60–100 beats/minute.

AV Node

- It is located at the base of right atrium.
- It stimulate at a rate of 40–60 beats/minute.

From the AV node the impulse travels through the bundle branches and through the Purkinje fibers to the ventricular myocardium, causing ventricular depolarization and ventricular contraction.

Heart Block

Any impairment in the conduction system of the heart leads to slowing the pumping system of the heart and causes heart block. Based on the severity of the block, it is classified into three categories.

First-Degree Heart Block (1st Degree)

Any delay in the transmission of impulse from SA to AV is called as first degree heart block. The management of first degree heart block is temporary pacemaker.

Second-Degree Heart Block (2nd Degree)

Not all impulse is generated to AV node from SA node is called as second degree heart block. The management of second degree heart block is temporary pacemaker.

Third-Degree Heart Block (3rd Degree)

No impulse is generated from SA to AV node is called as third degree heart block. The management of third degree heart block is permanent pacemaker.

What is Stokes-Adams Syndrome?

Sudden collapse into unconsciousness due to a disorder of heart rhythm in which there is a slow or absent pulse resulting in syncope (fainting) with or without convulsions. It is also called cardiovascular syncope.

It is the temporary loss of consciousness that occurs when the blood flow stops to the brain cells as a result of ventricular fibrillation or ventricular asystole. The management of Stokes-Adams syndrome is permanent pacemaker.

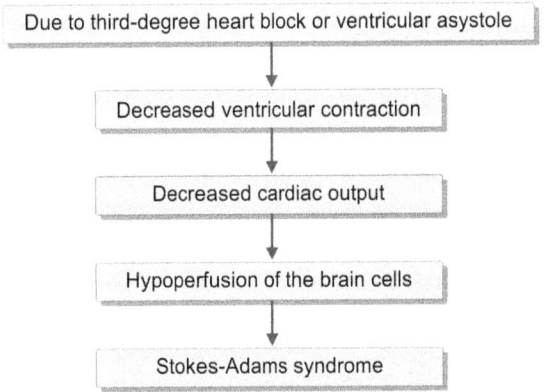

BLOOD SUPPLY TO HEART

The heart receives its own supply of blood from the coronary arteries (Figs 3 and 4).

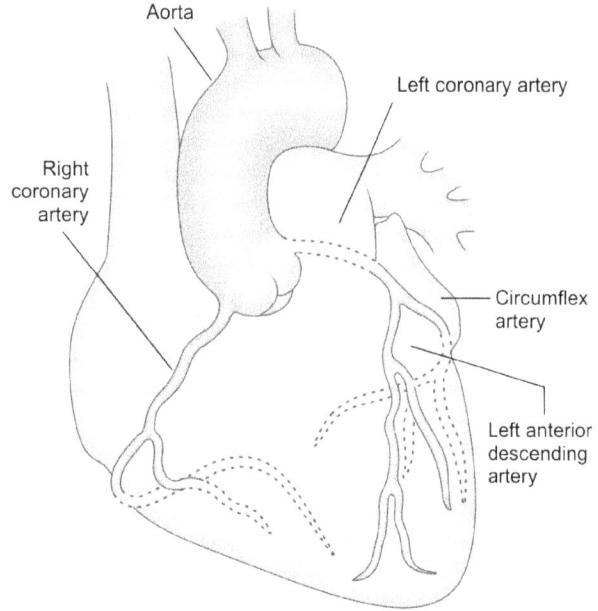

Fig. 3: Blood supply to the Heart

the aortic valve is approximately 7.5 cm. The pulmonic valve cusps are termed *right anterior* (right), *left anterior* (anterior), and *posterior* (left); the positions of the cusps in the fetus are indicated parenthetically. It prevents backflow of blood into the ventricles when the ventricles relax.

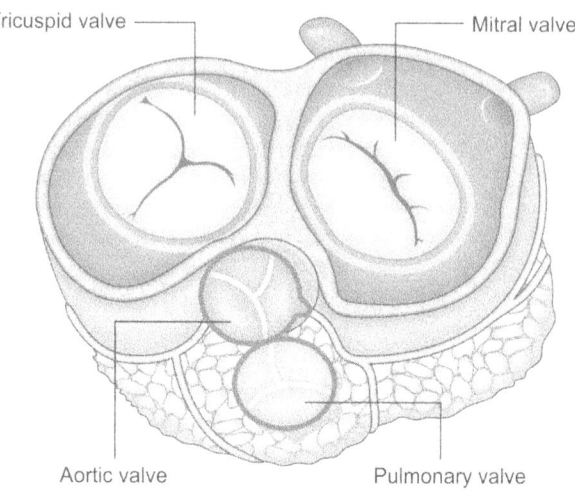

Fig. 4: Heart valves

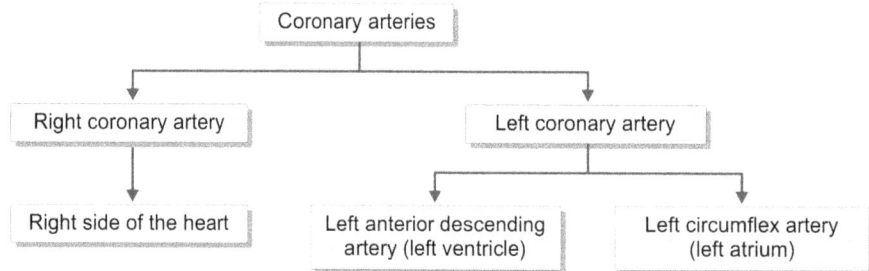

Left anterior descending artery (LAD) is also called as "Widow Maker Artery".

HEART VALVES

The four heart valves are:
- The tricuspid valve, located between the right atrium and the right ventricle.
- The bicuspid valve or mitral valve, between the left atrium and left ventricle.
- The pulmonary (pulmonic) valve, between the right ventricle and the pulmonary artery.
- The aortic valve, between the left ventricle and the aorta.

Each valve has a set of flaps, which are also known as leaflets or cusps. The mitral valve normally has only two flaps while the others all have three flaps. The pulmonary valve orifice is approximately 8.5 cm in circumference, and

HEART SOUNDS

S1 and S2 are the normal heart sounds. S3 and S4 are the abnormal heart sounds heard in heart failure, mitral stenosis, etc.
- **S1 due to AV valve closure:** The first heart sound (lub) can be heard the loudest at the mitral area, at the apex. However, if you want to listen specifically for the tricuspid valve, it is heard best at the left lower sternal border in the 4th intercostal space. This sound represents the closure of the mitral and tricuspid valves and is a low pitched, dull sound at the beginning of ventricular systole.
- **S2 due to semilunar valve closure:** The second heart sound ("dub") is produced by the closure of the aortic and pulmonic valves. It is also a high frequency

sound. Pulmonic closure is best heard in the 2nd/3rd intercostal space left sternal border and aortic closure is best heard in the 2nd/3rd intercostal space right sternal border.

- **S3 ventricular gallop:** This is an abnormal heart sound that occurs at the end of the passive filling phase of either ventricle during early to mid diastole. It can best be heard as a dull, low pitched noise immediately following S2 due to tensing of the chordae tendineae during rapid filling and expansion of the ventricle. S3 can best be heard with the bell of the stethoscope with the patient in a supine or left lateral decubitus position. If it is heard at the tricuspid area then the right ventricle is faulty. If the sound occurs at the mitral area then the left ventricle is faulty. A pathological S3 can be referred to as a "ventricular gallop". You can think of it in terms of a horse gallop which can be sounded out as: "Lub-Dub-By".
- **S4 presystolic gallop:** This is another abnormal heart sound known as the "presystolic gallop" precedes S1 of the next cardiac cycle. It can be heard in late diastole and is caused by the vibration of the ventricular wall during atrial contraction characterized by the acceleration and deceleration of blood entering a chamber that resists additional filling. In other words, this sound is produced by the atrium forcefully contracting against a stiffened ventricle. It is also a dull, low pitched sound. You can sound it out as "Le-Lub-Dub" and can best be heard with the patient in supine position. Depending on which ventricle is faulty, you will have to listen for this sound in the tricuspid valve which would represent the right ventricle, and the mitral valve representing the left ventricle.

Notes

Normal BP 120/80 mm Hg
Systolic BP 120 mm Hg
Diastolic BP 80 mm Hg
Pulse pressure = systolic BP–diastolic BP = (120 − 80) = 40 mm Hg
MAP (mean arterial pressure) = [systolic BP + (2 × diastolic BP)] ÷ 3
= [120 + (2 × 80)] ÷ 3
  (120 + 160) ÷ 3
   280 ÷ 3
= 93.3
Cerebral perfusion pressure (CPP) = MAP−ICP

BARORECEPTOR MECHANISMS IN CONTROLLING BLOOD PRESSURE

There are two baroreceptor mechanisms:
- Renin angiotensin mechanism
- ADH mechanism

Renin Angiotensin Mechanism

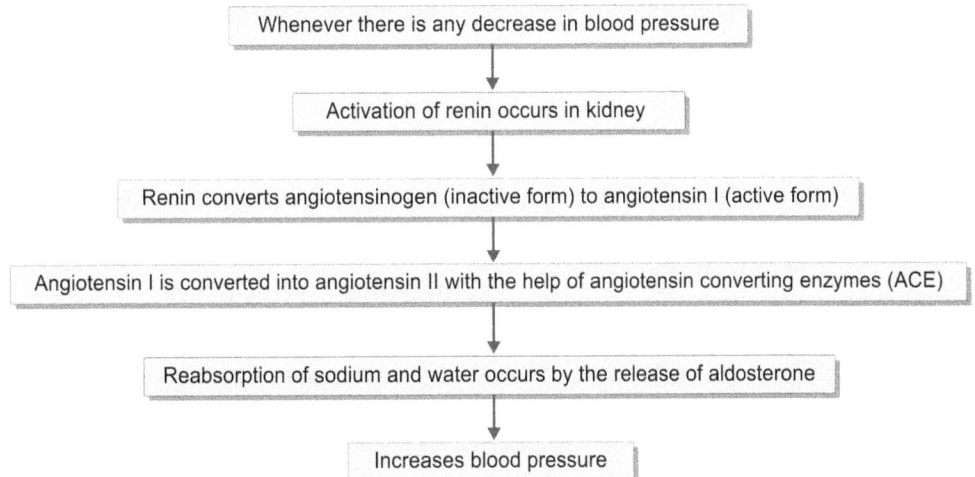

ADH Mechanism (Antidiuretic Hormone)

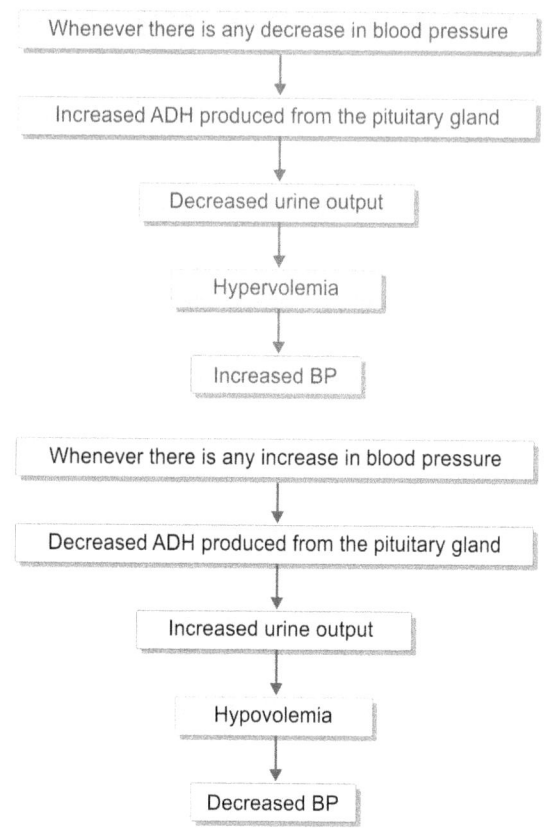

DIAGNOSTIC MEASURES

Cardiac Enzymes

- CPK-MB (Creatine kinase myocardial muscle)
  - A muscle enzyme found in the heart and muscles.
  - Increased CK-MB is seen with heart muscle damage.
  - Increased CPK-MB indicates myocardial infarction
  - A peak elevation is seen in first 18 hours
  - Normal value = 0 – 5% of total, total = 26–174 U/L.
- LDH (lactate dehydrogenase)
  - LDH is an enzyme released in the blood with cell injury. It is often used as a late marker to detect a heart attack.
  - It is also elevated with liver and kidney disease, pernicious and megaloblastic anemias, malignancy, progressive muscular dystrophy, and pulmonary emboli.
  - Elevation of LDH occurs in first 24 hours and peak elevation seen in 48-72 hours.
  - Normal value = 140–280 U/L.
- Cardiac troponin
  - It composed of three proteins. Troponin I, Troponin T and Troponin C.
  - Troponin T is a protein found in the blood and is related to contraction of the heart muscle. Troponin T is valuable for detecting heart muscle damage and risk.
  - Normal Troponin I: Less than 10 μg/L. Troponin T: 0–0.1 μg/L.
- Aspartate Aminotransferase (AST)
  - A liver enzyme that is released into the bloodstream following injury or death of cells. Increased AST is seen with liver disease, myocardial infarction (MI) and some medications. May increase when using cholesterol-lowering medications. It is also called as serum glutamic oxalacetate.
  - Normal value = 7–40 U/L.

Homocysteine

- It is a chemical in the blood that is produced when an amino acid (a building block of protein) called methionine is broken down in the body. We all have some homocysteine in our blood. Elevated homocysteine levels (also called hyperhomocysteinemia) may cause irritation of the blood vessels.
- Increased homocysteine indicates cardiovascular disorders.
- Normal homocysteine < 14 micromoles/liter.
- Administer vitamins B6 and B12 to clear homocysteine from the blood.

CRP (C-reactive Protein)

- C-reactive protein (CRP) is a marker of inflammation in the body. Therefore, its level in the blood increases if there is any inflammation in the body.
- Normal value, if CRP level is lower than 1.0 mg/L there is low risk of developing cardiovascular disease, at average risk of developing cardiovascular disease if levels are between 1.0 and 3.0 mg/L and high risk for cardiovascular disease if CRP level is higher than 3.0 mg/L.

Electrolytes Monitoring

- Sodium (Na) 135–145 mEq/L
  - In hyponatremia, there will be symptoms of confusion, convulsion and coma
  - In hypernatremia, there will be symptoms of hypovolemia, tachycardia and coma.
- Potassium (K) 3.5–5.5 mEq/L
  - In hypokalemia, there will be ST depression, T-wave inversion and presence of U-wave in ECG.
  - In hyperkalemia, there will be prolonged PR interval, widened QRS complex and tall T-wave and flat P-wave in ECG.

- **Calcium (ca) 4.5–5.3 mEq/L**
  - In hypocalcemia prolonged QT and ST interval in ECG.
  - In hypercalcemia short ST and widened T wave in ECG
- **Magnesium (Mg) 1.3–2.1 mEq/L**
  - In hypomagnesemia there will be tall T wave and ST segment depression in ECG.
  - In hypermagnesemia, there will be prolonged PR interval and widened QRS complex.

Serum Lipids (Cholesterol)

- Total cholesterol: 150–200 mg/dL (< 200)
- HDL (High density lipids): 30–85 mg/dL
- LDL (Low density lipids): 50–140 mg/dL (< 130)
- Triglycerides: 10–150 mg/dL (< 200)
- Increased LDL and decreased HDL levels predispose to cardiovascular disease.
- Increased triglycerides leads to atherosclerotic heart disease.
- Administer fenofibrate medications to decrease triglycerides.

Blood Studies

- CBC
- Coagulation time: 5–15 minutes. Increased level indicates bleeding. Used to monitor heparin therapy.
- Bleeding time (BT): 3–10 minutes and clotting time (CT): 2–6 mins.
- Prothrombin time (PT): 9.5–12 seconds. Used to monitor warfarin therapy.
- INR (International normalized ratio): 1–2. The INR is a test of blood clotting, which is primarily used to monitor warfarin therapy, where the aim is to maintain an elevated INR in a certain range, e.g. 2.0 to 3.0.
- Activated partial thromboplastin time (APTT): 20–45 seconds. Increased levels indicate bleeding.
- Erythrocyte sedimentation rate (ESR) < 20 mm/hr.
- ANP or BNP (atrial and brain natriuretic peptides): Brain natriuretic peptide, uretic peptide or ventricular natriuretic peptide (still BNP), is a 32 amino acid polypeptide secreted by the ventricles of the heart in response to excessive stretching of heart muscle cells (cardiomyocytes). The release of BNP is modulated by calcium ions. Increased BNP indicates heart failure. Normal BNP less than 100 pg per milliliter.
- Myoglobin: It is a heme protein released from all damaged tissues. Increases normal: < 92 ng/ml (men), < 72 ng/ml (women).

Cardiac Catheterization

- It is an invasive procedure in which a catheter is inserted into the right or left side of the heart for diagnostic procedures.
- **Purpose:**
  - To measure intracardiac pressures and oxygen levels.
  - Injection of dye
  - Visualization of heart chambers and blood vessels
  - To rule out any obstruction in the blood flow
- In right side, catheterization a catheter is inserted through the antecubital vein or femoral vein and advanced into the vena cava, right atrium, right ventricle and to the pulmonary artery as seen in Figure 5.
- In left side catheterization a catheter is inserted through brachial artery or femoral artery and advanced into the aorta and left ventricle as seen in Figure 6.
- In pediatrics select only femoral vein for cardiac catheterization.

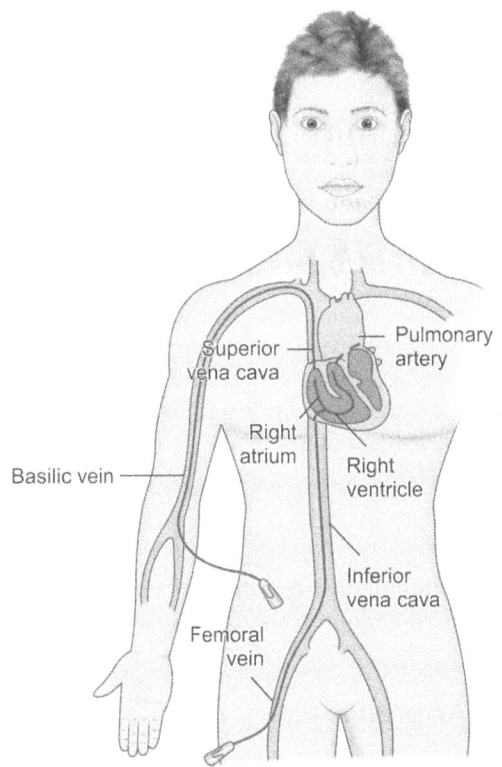

Fig. 5: Right heart catheterization

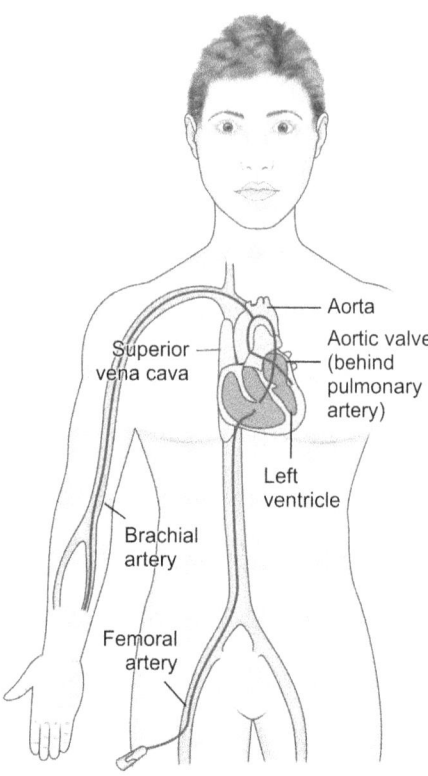

Fig. 6: Left heart catheterization

Nursing Care (Preoperative)

- Informed consent
- Check for any allergies to iodine
- NPO for 8-12 hours
- Explain the procedure to the patient

Nursing Care (Postoperative)

- Assess the circulation to the extremity
- Check the peripheral pulses, color, sensation, coolness of the affected extremity every 15 minutes for 4 hours.
- Observe the catheter insertion site for redness, swelling.
- Apply pressure dressing.
- Assess the vitals.

Aortography

Insertion of a radiopaque dye into the aorta to visualize the aorta and major blood vessels and to detect any abnormalities.

Coronary Arteriography

Visualization of coronary arteries by injection of radiopaque dye for ruling out any lesions or evidences of coronary artery diseases.

Echocardiogram

A noninvasive procedure to record the cardiac structures using an ultrasound.

Electrocardiogram (ECG)

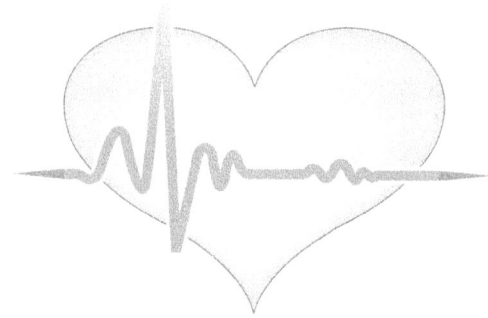

- It is a noninvasive procedure which measures the electrical contractility of the heart at a rate of 25 mm/sec.
- It is used to determine the cardiac rhythms and reveal dysrhythmias and block of right and left bundle branch.
- ECG consists of horizontal and vertical lines, horizontal lines represent time and vertical lines represent the voltage.
- In the ECG, there are small squares and large squares. Each small sqaure represent 0.04 second and large square represent 0.20 second.
- For example, how much time is required to complete the QRS interval? (QRS consists of 6 small squares)
  $6 \times 0.04 = 0.24$ second
- Holter monitoring provides continuous recording of ECG for up to 24 hours.

P wave	First wave indicates atrial depolarization or atrial contraction
QRS	Second wave indicates ventricular depolarization or contraction. Consist of three deflections Q wave is the first negative deflection, R wave is the first positive deflection and S wave is the first negative deflection after R wave. **Normal QRS interval: 0.04–0.1 second**
T wave	Indicates ventricular repolarization
PR interval	Distance between the beginning of P wave and beginning of QRS complex. It measures the time during which a depolarization wave travels from the atria to the ventricle **Normal PR interval: 0.12–0.2 second**
ST interval	Distance between S wave and the beginning of T wave. Measures time between ventricular depolarization and beginning of repolarization. **Normal ST interval: 0.080 to 0.120 sec**

Contd...

Contd...

QT interval	Measured from the beginning of QRS to the T wave represents total ventricular activity. **Normal QT interval: 0.32–0.4 second**
U wave	A small round wave following T wave represents the repolarization of purkinje fibers

Normal ECG

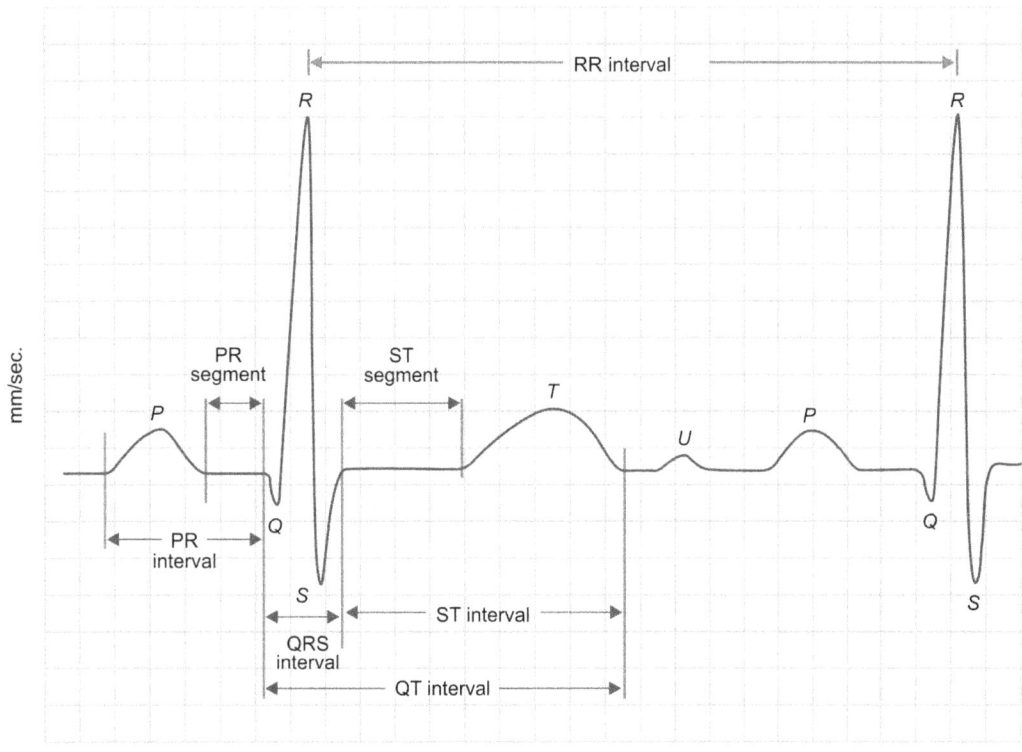

mm/mV   1 square = 0.04 sec/0.1 mV

Method I

Regular rhythms can be quickly determined by counting the number of large graph boxes between two R waves. To calculate the rate 300 divided by number of large squares.

Examples: The number of large squares between two R interval is 5

So, heart rate = 300/5 = 60 beats/minute

Method II

Sometimes, it is necessary to count the number of small boxes between two R waves for fast heart rates. To calculate the rate 1500 divided by number of small boxes between two R intervals.

Calculation of Heart Rate

Heart rate is calculated as the number of times the heart beats per minute. It usually measures ventricular rate (the number of QRS complexes) but can refer to atrial rate (the number of P waves). There are two common methods.

Examples: If there are ten small boxes between two R waves—1500/10 = 150 beats/minute.

CARDIAC ARRHYTHMIAS (DYSRHYTHMIAS)

Sinus Tachycardia

Heart rate > 100 beats/min

Causes

- Fever
- Increased physical activity
- Anemia
- Deriphyllin toxicity or theophylline toxicity
- Stimulants, such as caffeine, alcohol, coffee, etc.
- Hyperthyroidism

Signs and Symptoms (Fig. 7)

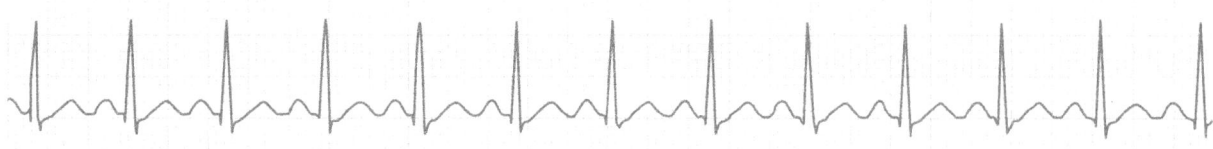

Fig. 7: Sinus tachycardia

- Heart rate = 300/number of large squares = 300/2 = 150 = sinus tachycardia
- Rhythm is regular
- P waves normal, PR interval normal and QRS complex normal

Management

- The drug of choice for sinus tachycardia is propranolol (inderal), beta blockers.
- Treat the underlying cause.

Sinus Bradycardia

Heart rate < 60 beats/minute

Causes

- Increased vagus nerve stimulation
- Increased ICP
- Hypothyroidism
- Well-trained athletes

Signs and Symptoms (Fig. 8)

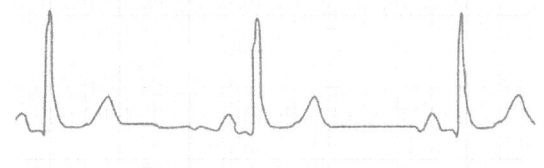

Fig. 8: Sinus bradycardia

- Heart rate = 300/number of large squares = 300/6 = 50 = sinus bradycardia
- Rhythm is regular
- P waves normal, PR interval normal and QRS complex normal
- Severe bradycardia may cause dizziness, fatigue, palpitation, even syncope.

Management

- The drug of choice for sinus bradycardia is atropine sulphate
- Administer glycopyrrolate or scopolamine (anticholinergics)
- If medical therapies are unsuccessful apply pacemaker.

Atrial Fibrillation

Irregular contractions of the atria

Causes

- Mitral valve stenosis
- CAD
- Left ventricular hypertrophy
- Heart failure

Signs and Symptoms (Fig. 9)

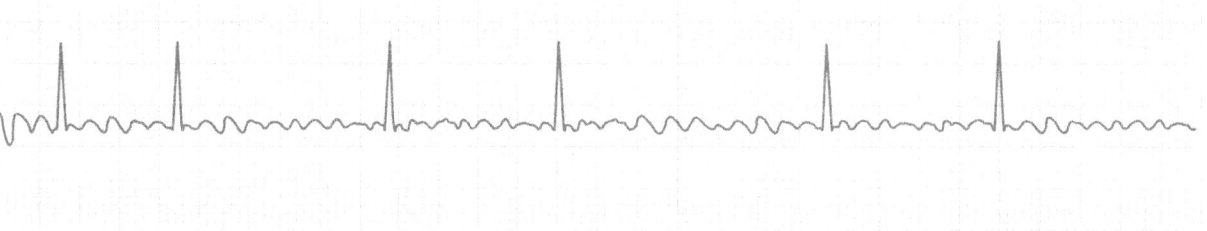

Fig. 9: Atrial fibrillation

- No definite P wave
- Normal QRS complex
- Atrial rate is 300–600 beats/minute
- Manifestations of syncope due to decreased blood supply to the brain and decreased ventricular filling.

Management

- Administer digoxin
- Administer verapamil (calcium channel blocker)
- Prepare the patient for cardioversion or defibrillation.

Premature Ventricular Contraction (PVC)

- A premature ventricular contraction (PVC), also known as a premature ventricular complex, ventricular premature contraction (VPC), ventricular premature beat (VPB), or ventricular extrasystole (VES), is a relatively common event where the heartbeat is initiated by Purkinje fibers in the ventricles rather than by the sinoatrial node, the normal heartbeat initiator.
- Irritable impulse originating from the ventricles.
- We can see ectopics in the ECG

Causes

- Hypokalemia
- Drug toxicity (digoxin toxicity, quinidine and anti-anxiety drug)
- Cardiac failure

Signs and Symptoms

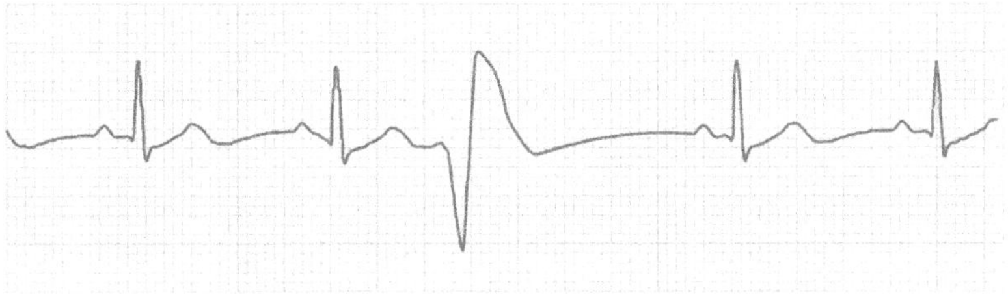

- Presence of ectopics in the ECG as seen in Figure 10
- Palpitation, dizziness and syncope
- Loss of second heart sound

Management

- Treat the underlying cause
- Administer electrolytes such as potassium to prevent VT
- IV push of lidocaine followed by IV infusion of the same

Ventricular Tachycardia

- Ventricular tachycardia (VT) is a rapid heartbeat that starts in the lower chambers of the heart (ventricles).
- Repetitive firing of the ventricles of the heart

Types of Ventricular Tachycardia

- Monomorphic ventricular tachycardia means that the appearance of all the beats match each other in each lead of a surface electrocardiogram (ECG).
- Polymorphic ventricular tachycardia, on the other hand, has beat-to-beat variations in morphology. This may appear as a cyclical progressive change in cardiac axis, previously referred to by its French name torsades de pointe (twisting of the spikes). However, at the current time, the term torsades is reserved for polymorphic VT occurring in the context of a prolonged resting QT interval.

Fig. 10: Premature ventricular contraction

Causes

- Digoxin toxicity
- Hypokalemia
- Myocardial infarction
- Myocarditis

Signs and Symptoms

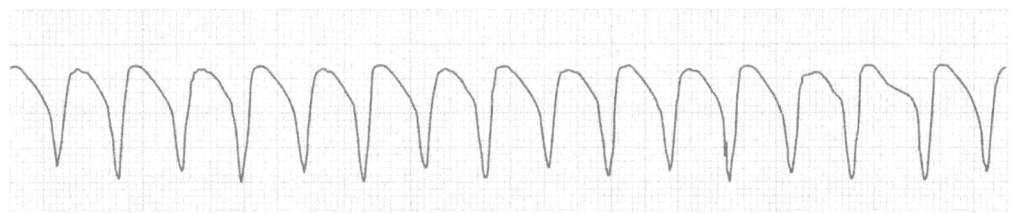

Fig. 11: Ventricular tachycardia

- No definite P wave as seen in Figure 11
- Ventricular rate 110–250 beats/minute

Management

- Treat the underlying cause
- If it is a pulseless VT same as cardiac arrest (defibrillation)
- If the VT with pulse administer Cordarone or amiodarone.
- In case of supraventricular tachycardia (SVT) administer adenosine.

Signs and Symptoms

Ventricular Fibrillation

- If the ventricular tachycardia is in an irregular or haphazard manner as seen in figure 12, it is called as ventricular fibrillation.
- Ventricular fibrillation is an abnormal and irregular heart rhythm in which there are rapid uncoordinated fluttering contractions of the lower chambers (ventricles) of the heart. Ventricular fibrillation disrupts the synchrony between the heartbeat and the pulse beat. Ventricular fibrillation is commonly associated with heart attacks and scarring of the heart muscle from previous heart attacks. Ventricular fibrillation is life-threatening.
- Ventricular fibrillation is a cause of cardiac arrest and sudden cardiac death.

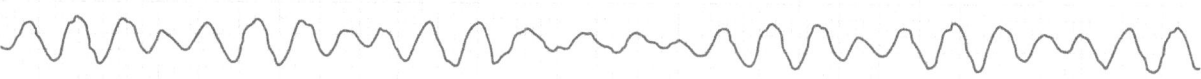

Fig. 12: Ventricular fibrillation

- Shortness of breath
- Loss of consciousness

Management

- Defibrillation
- Antiarrhythmic agents, such as amiodarone or lidocaine

DEFIBRILLATION AND CARDIOVERSION

Defibrillation	Cardioversion
Emergency procedure	Elective procedure
No need for consent	Consent required
It is non synchronized, delivery of energy to any phase of the cardiac cycle	It is synchronized, delivery of energy to the large R wave or QRS complex. If the synchronized mode is off the current discharges to T wave and produce ventricular fibrillation
Energy 200–360 joules	Energy 50–150 joules

PACEMAKER

Pacemaker is an electronic device that produce repeated electric stimulation to the heart muscles.

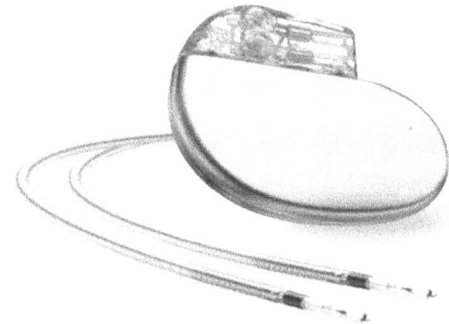

- A pacemaker is a small device that is placed in the chest or abdomen to control abnormal heart rhythms. This device uses low-energy electrical pulses to prompt the heart to beat at a normal rate. Pacemakers are used to treat arrhythmias.

Types of Pacemaker

- **Temporary pacemaker**
  - It is used in emergency situations and is kept at the bedside (e.g. in CABG).
- **Permanent pacemaker**
  - It is a subcutaneous implantation of the pulse generator into the right or left subclavian area.

Modes of Pacemaker

There are two common modes of pacemaker. They are:
- **Demand mode:** Pacemaker produce electrical stimulation only when the client's heart rate drops below the preset rate (when demand, it is also called as synchronous mode).
- **Fixed mode:** It is used in patients with profound bradycardia (in a preset rate, it is also called as asynchronous mode).

Nursing Care

- Assess the pacemaker function
- Monitor the pacemaker spikes on ECG. In atrial pacemaker, we can see a spike before the P wave (spikes followed by a P wave).
- In ventricular pacemaker, we can see a spike before the QRS complex (spikes followed by a QRS complex).

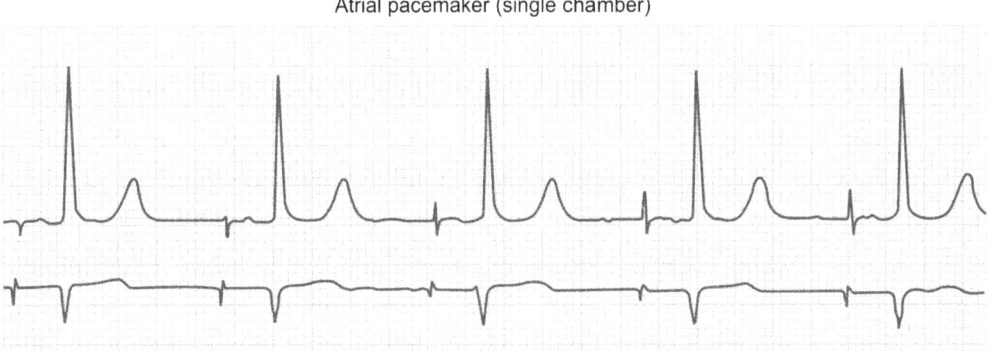

Atrial pacemaker (single chamber)

One spike producing an abnormal P wave (atrial capture) followed by a normal QRS

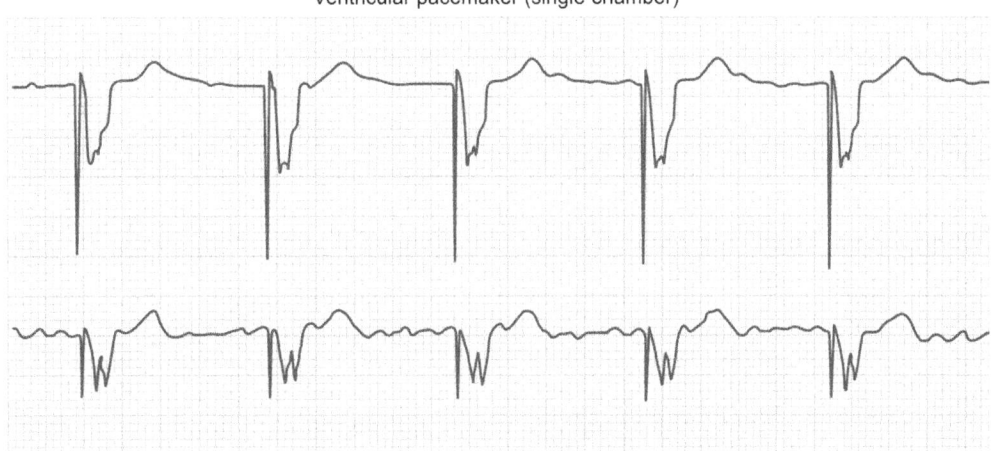

Ventricular pacemaker (single chamber)

One spike producing a wide QRS (ventricular capture)

- Monitor the pulse for one full minute.
- Monitor the signs and symptoms of pacemaker malfunction like weakness, fainting, hypotension, etc.
- Ensure that the catheter terminals are connected or properly attached to the pulse generator (in case of temporary pacemaker).
- Monitor the serum potassium level.
- Instruct the patient to wear loose fitting cloths.
- Instruct the patient to avoid heavy activities.
- Instruct the patient to undergo a hand scanner.
- Monitor the modes of pacemaker (e.g. AVI or VVI or DDD mode)

Paced	Sensed	Response
O–none	O–none	I–inhibition
A—Atrial	A—Atrial	T–triggering
V–ventricular	V–ventricular	D–dual
D–dual	D–dual	

For example, AVI (atrial pacing, ventricular sensing, inhibition)

DISORDERS

Coronary Artery Disease

Coronary artery disease (CAD) is the most common type of heart disease. It is the leading cause of death in the United States in both men and women.

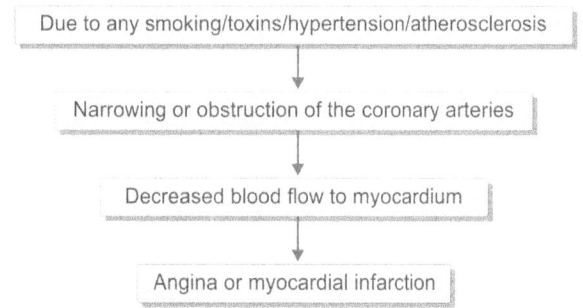

Causes

- Smoking
- High blood pressure
- Increased cholesterol level
- Toxins

Signs and Symptoms

- Chest pain, substernal radiating to the left side of the body
- Dyspnea
- ECG shows ST depression and T wave inversion
- Increased serum cholesterol level

Nursing Care

- Provide rest (semi to high fowlers position).
- The golden rule of management of CAD is rest + nitrates
- The priority nursing care of a patient with CAD is **Diet → Exercise → Medication**
- Administer NTG (nitroglycerin) is a coronary vasodilator.
- Provide low fat and low cholesterol diet.

ANGINA

Angina is a term used for chest pain caused by reduced blood flow to the heart muscle. Angina is a symptom of coronary artery disease. Angina is typically described as squeezing, pressure, heaviness, tightness or pain in your chest.

Angina, also called angina pectoris, can be a recurring problem or a sudden, acute health concern.

A transient paroxysmal chest pain produced by insufficient blood flow to the myocardium resulting in myocardial ischemia.

Causes

- Decreased blood supply to the myocardium
- Obstruction of coronary arteries

Risk Factors

- Tobacco use
- Diabetes
- High blood pressure
- High blood cholesterol or triglyceride levels.
- History of heart disease
- Older age. Men older than 45 and women older than 55 have a greater risk than do younger adults.
- Lack of exercise
- Obesity: Obesity raises the risk of angina and heart disease because it's associated with high blood cholesterol levels, high blood pressure and diabetes
- Stress: Stress can increase your risk of angina and heart attacks. Too much stress, as well as anger, can also raise your blood pressure. Surges of hormones produced during stress can narrow your arteries and worsen angina.

Signs and Symptoms

- Chest pain, substernal radiating to the neck, jaw, back and arms relieved by rest
- Palpitation
- Fatigue
- Shortness of breath
- Sweating or diaphoresis
- ECG shows ST depression and T-wave inversion

Types of Angina

- **Stable angina:** It is also called as exertional angina. Stable angina is usually triggered by physical exertion. When you climb stairs, exercise or walk, your heart demands more blood, but it's harder for the muscle to get enough blood when your arteries are narrowed. Besides physical activity, other factors, such as emotional stress, cold temperatures, heavy meals and smoking, also can narrow arteries and trigger angina.

- **Unstable angina:** It is also called as pre infarction angina. Unstable angina worsens and is not relieved by rest or your usual medications. If the blood flow doesn't improve, heart muscle deprived of oxygen and leads to heart attack. Unstable angina is dangerous and requires emergency treatment.
- **Variant angina:** Variant angina, also called Prinzmetal's angina or vasospastic angina. This occurs in same time each day. The classical manifestation of variant angina is ST elevation in ECG. It is caused by a spasm in a coronary artery in which the artery temporarily narrows. This narrowing reduces blood flow to your heart, causing chest pain. Variant angina can occur even when you're at rest, and is often severe. It can be relieved with medications.

Nursing Care

- Administer oxygen (3 liters/minute)
- Monitor vitals and ECG
- Provide semi to high Fowler's position
- Provide emotional support
- Avoid smoking and extremes of temperature.
- Avoid large meals.
- Avoiding stress is easier said than done, but try to find ways to relax. Talk with your doctor about stress reduction techniques.
- Eat a healthy diet with lots of whole grains, many fruits and vegetables, and limited amounts of saturated fat.
- Administer medications, such as nitrates, aspirin, clopidogrels, beta blockers, calcium channel blockers, ranolazine, etc.
- Prepare the patient for angioplasty and stenting if the medical therapies become unsuccessful.

MYOCARDIAL INFARCTION

Death of a segment of myocardium due to inadequate oxygenation caused by blockage of coronary arteries.

Myocardial infarction (MI) or acute myocardial infarction (AMI), commonly known as a heart attack, occurs when blood flow stops to the heart causing damage to the heart muscle. The most common symptom is chest pain or discomfort which may travel into the shoulder, arm, back, neck, or jaw.

- Usually MI is confined to the anterior wall of left ventricle.
- The emergency medication of MI is IV morphine.
- The classical manifestation of acute MI is increased CKMB.
- Dressler's syndrome is one of the late complication of MI.

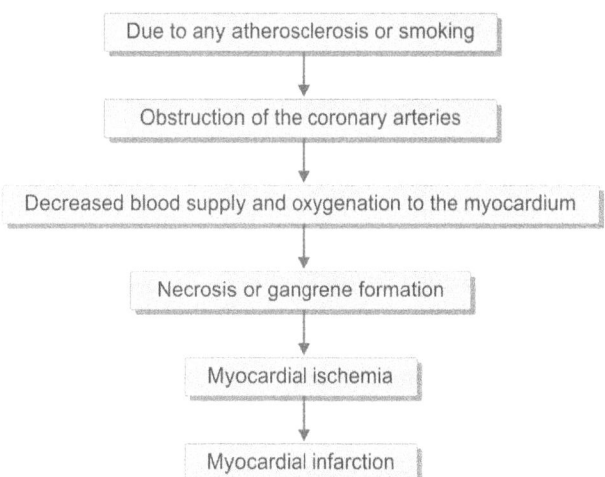

Causes

- Atherosclerosis
- Coronary vasospasm

Risk Factors

- Tobacco use
- Diabetes
- High blood pressure
- High blood cholesterol or triglyceride levels.
- Lack of exercise
- Obesity

Signs and Symptoms

- Severe crushing chest pain radiating to neck, jaw and left arm
- Presence of S3 heart sound
- Presence of pericardial friction rub and split S_1 and S_2
- Restlessness and dyspnea
- Palpitation
- Cool and clammy skin
- Nausea and vomiting

Diagnosis

- Increased CKMB, peak elevation in the first 18 hours and normal in 48–72 hours
- ECG shows ST elevation and T-wave inversion
- Increased serum cholesterol level
- Increased troponin levels
- Increased LDH
- Increased ESR and WBC count
- Echocardiogram
- Coronary angiogram

Nursing Care

- Administer morphine sulfate IV for pain relief.
- Administer oxygen as ordered
- Provide bed rest with semi Fowler's position to decrease cardiac workload.
- Monitor the urinary output and inform if it is less than 30 ml/hour, it indicates decreased cardiac output.
- Maintain a quiet environment
- Provide full liquid diet and slowly increase to soft with low sodium.
- Administer aspirin 325 mg as a loading dose
- Administer anticoagulants (heparin).

Classification of Heparin

Unfractionated heparin	Low molecular weight heparin	Hirudin derivative	Coumadin derivative
e.g. heparin sodium or beparine	e.g. clexane or enoxaparin	e.g. lepirudin	e.g. warfarin sodium
Route IV	Route subcutaneous	Route oral/IV/Sc	Route oral
Therapeutic effect is monitored by APTT	Therapeutic effect is monitored by CBC	Therapeutic effect is monitored by APTT	Therapeutic effect is monitored by PT INR
Antidote of heparin is protamine sulfate			Antidote of warfarin is vitamin K

Client Teaching

- Teach the dietary restrictions, low sodium and low cholesterol diet
- Avoid caffeine
- Teach the use of NTG patches.
- In case of NTG patch application shave the area and do not cut the NTG patch
- Teach the patient to avoid cranberry juice if he is on warfarin therapy (cranberry is an antioxidant and it may alter PT INR).
- Teach the importance of participation in a progressive activity program.

Complications

- Heart failure
- Pulmonary edema
- Cardiac arrest

Surgical Management

Coronary Angiography and Percutaneous Transluminal Coronary Angioplasty

Coronary angiography and percutaneous transluminal coronary angioplasty (PTCA) is the most direct method of opening a blocked coronary artery. The procedures are performed in the catheterization laboratory in a hospital. Under X-ray guidance, a tiny plastic catheter with a balloon on its end is advanced over a guide wire from a vein in the groin or the arm and into the blocked coronary artery. Once the balloon reaches the blockage, it is inflated, pushing the clot and plaque out of the way to open the artery. PTCA can be effective in opening up to 95% of arteries. In addition, the angiogram (X-ray pictures taken of the coronary arteries) allows evaluation of the status of the other coronary arteries so that long-term treatment plans may be formulated.

Percutaneous transluminal coronary angioplasty can be performed instead of coronary artery bypass graft surgery in various clients with single vessel coronary disease.

The aim of PTCA is to revascularize the myocardium, decrease angina and increase survival.

The most serious complication of PTCA is an abrupt closure of the coronary artery within the first few hours after PTCA. Abrupt coronary artery closure (that can lead to further heart damage) occurs in some patients after simple balloon angioplasty (without stenting). The risk of abrupt closure of the coronary arteries can be reduced by aspirins, anticoagulants, nitrates and the application of coronary artery stents.

Nursing Care (Preoperative)

- Informed consent.
- Check for any allergies to iodine.
- NPO for 8–12 hours.
- Explain the procedure to the patient.

Nursing Care (Postoperative)

- Assess vitals and monitor the circulation to the extremity.
- Check the peripheral pulses, color, sensation, coolness of the affected extremity every 15 minutes for 4 hours.
- Observe the catheter insertion site for redness, swelling.
- Apply pressure dressing.

Coronary Artery Bypass Grafting

A coronary artery bypass graft is the surgery of choice for clients with severe CAD. The procedure requires a heart lung machine (cardiopulmonary bypass) or extra heart lung machine or extracorporeal circulation. That is why it is also known as open heart surgery.

Coronary artery bypass graft (CABG) surgery reestablishes sufficient blood flow to deliver oxygen and nutrients to the heart muscle. The bypass graft for a CABG can be a vein from the leg or an inner chest wall artery.

The common grafts are left internal mammary artery, radial artery or saphenous vein graft.

Nursing Care (Preoperative)

- Explain the anatomy and physiology of the heart.
- Explain the time required for surgery and length of surgery.
- Explain the equipments used for surgery.
- Teach breathing and coughing exercises.

Nursing Care (Postoperative)

- Maintain a patent airway.
- Monitor the drainage from the chest tube. Intercostal chest tube drainage (ICD) is present in all thoracic surgeries except in pneumonectomy.
- Monitor the cardiac status.
- Administer pain relief medications, such as narcotics.
- Maintain fluid electrolyte balance by monitoring the lab values particularly BUN, creatine, sodium and potassium levels.
- Monitor the urine output and inform if it is less than 30 ml/hour. It reflects renal perfusion.
- Monitor cerebral functions.
- Monitor frequent neurovascular assessment.
- Monitor for complications (DVT, pulmonary embolism, cardiac tamponade, pneumonia, heart failure, arrhythmia, etc.)
- Monitor nasogastric drainage and maintain patency of the system to prevent abdominal distension.

Client Teaching

- Encourage walking and gradual increase the distance
- Avoid heavy lifting
- Avoid sexual activities until physician allows
- Low sodium and low cholesterol diet
- Report the following symptoms, such as fever, dyspnea, chest pain.

HEART FAILURE (CONGESTIVE HEART FAILURE)

Heart failure is the inability of the heart to pump blood for meeting the metabolic demands of the body.

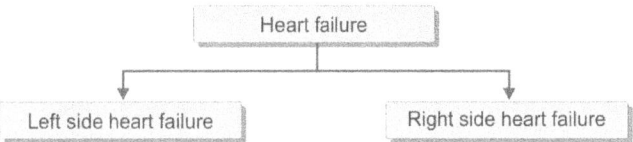

Left ventricular failure is evident in pulmonary circulation and right ventricular failure is evident in systemic circulation.

Left Side Heart Failure

It is the inability of the left ventricle to pump blood through the aorta. It may cause back flow of blood to the left atrium and pulmonary veins.

Causes

- Left ventricular damage
- Mitral stenosis
- Ischemic heart disease

Signs and Symptoms

- Air hunger (dyspnea and orthopnea)
- Fine crackles (coarse crackles in pneumonia)
- PMI displaced (point of maximum impulse will be displaced. PMI is 5th intercostal area)
- PND (paroxysmal nocturnal dyspnea)
- Tachycardia
- Decreased PO_2 and increased PCO_2

Right Side Heart Failure

It may occur as a complication of left ventricular failure (LVF leads to RVF).

Causes

- Left side heart failure
- Pulmonary embolism
- Pulmonic stenosis
- COPD

Signs and Symptoms

- JVD (jugular venous distension)
- Oliguria
- Edema
- Increased CVP (normal central venous pressure is 2–8 cm H_2O or **2–6** mm Hg)
- Bounding pulse

Why the doctor instruct the nurse to monitor hepatojugular reflex for a patient with mitral stenosis or left ventricular failure?

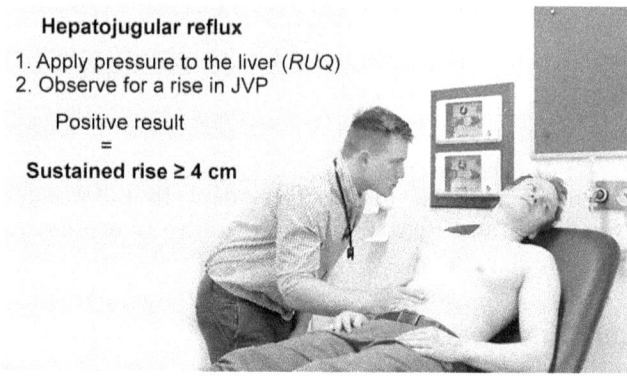

Hepatojugular reflux
1. Apply pressure to the liver (*RUQ*)
2. Observe for a rise in JVP

Positive result
=
Sustained rise ≥ 4 cm

To assess the presence of JVD, you can perform hepatojugular assessment. Make the patient to lie down in semi Fowler's position and press the examiner's finger on the hepatic margin, there will be distension of the jugular veins.

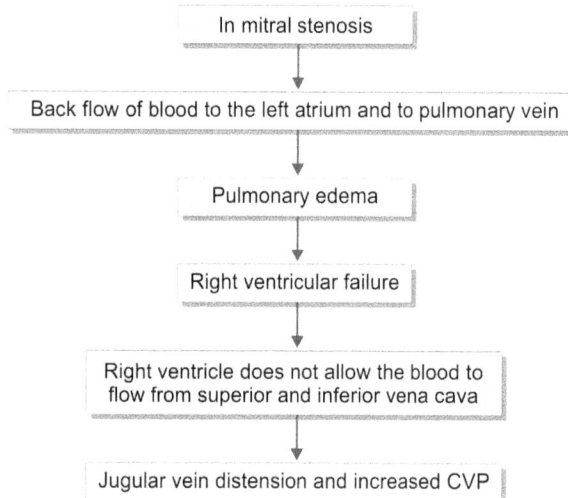

Diagnosis

- Chest X-ray reveals cardiac hypertrophy
- Echocardiography
- Coronary angiogram
- Increased BNP

Management of Heart Failure

1. Medical management
2. Mechanical management
3. Surgical management
4. Nursing management

Medical Management

4Ds of management
- D: Digoxin
- D: Dilators
- D: Diuretics
- D: Diet

Digoxin

- It is called cardiac glycoside.
- It is indicated for a patient with heart failure.
- Monitor serum digoxin level for a patient udergoing digoxin therapy.
- Normal serum digoxin level is 0.5–2 nanogram/milliliter.
- The side effects of digoxin are bradycardia, nausea, vomiting.
- The complications of digoxin are digoxin toxicity, yellowish vision, hypokalemia.
- The antidote of digoxin is digibind or digoxin immune fab.

Dilators

- NTG or nitroglycerin is called as coronary vasodilator.
- It is also available as NTG patches, instruct the patient to shave the area before applying.
- The common side effect of NTG is throbbing headache
- The complication of NTG is hypotension

Diet

- Administer low sodium and low fat diet.

Diuretics

Classification of diuretics:

Loop diuretics	Thiazide diuretics	Osmotic diuretics	Potassium sparing diuretics
Lasix or frusemide	Hydrochlorothiazide or diuril	Mannitol	Spironolactone or lasilactone
Side effect	**Side effect**	**Side effect**	**Side effect**
Hypokalemia, hyponatremia, hyperglycemia, ototoxicity	Hypokalemia, hyponatremia, hyperglycemia	Hypokalemia, hyponatremia	Hyperkalemia
Administer potassium rich diet and monitor potassium daily	Administer potassium rich diet and monitor potassium daily	Administer via an inline filter and shake before administering. Monitor potassium daily	Avoid potassium rich diet

Mechanical Management

IABP (Intra-aortic Balloon Pump)

The balloon is designed to sit in the proximal descending aorta. It comes in various lengths according to body height, with balloon volumes of about 30–50 mL. The balloon is usually filled with helium gas, and when inflated should fill up 80-90% of the aortic diameter.

The IABP works by inflating and deflating at different phases of the cardiac cycle. Balloon **inflation** augments diastolic blood pressure and balloon **deflation** decreases afterload during systole.

The position of balloon is 1-2 cm below the left subclavian artery. IABPs are usually inserted using the Seldinger technique via the femoral artery so that the tip of the catheter is advanced proximally into the aorta.

Surgical Management

Heart Transplantation

A heart transplant is a surgery to remove a damaged or diseased heart and replace it with a healthy donor heart. Finding a donor heart can be difficult. The heart must be donated by someone who is brain-dead but is still on life support. The donor heart must be matched as closely as possible to your tissue type to reduce the chance that your body will reject it.

After transplantation there will be two p waves in ECG because the new heart is connected to the right atrium of the old one.

Nursing Management

- Maintain respiration and adequate ventilation
- Administer oxygen
- Provide semi to high Fowler's position
- Administer digoxin
- Administer diuretics
- Provide physical and emotional rest
- Monitor the signs and symptoms of heart failure (e.g. pedal edema and weight gain of 1-2 kg in a 2 days period)

PULMONARY EDEMA

Pulmonary edema is a condition caused by excess fluid in the lungs. This fluid collects in the numerous air sacs in the lungs, making it difficult to breathe. It occurs as a complication of left ventricular failure.

Causes

- Left ventricular failure
- Rapid administration of IV fluids in children

Signs and Symptoms

- Dyspnea
- A feeling of suffocating or drowning
- Frothy secretion
- Cough with blood tinged sputum
- Jugular vein distention (JVD)
- Crackles

Management

- Administer oxygen
- Administer morphine sulphate (it may increase smooth muscle constriction and leads to the compression of saphenous vein and thereby leads to decrease venous return. This reduces the severity of pulmonary edema)
- Administer aminophylline
- Prepare the patient for phlebotomy (removal of 300-500 ml of blood).

CARDIAC ARREST

Cardiac arrest, also known as cardiopulmonary arrest or circulatory arrest, a sudden or unexpected cessation of breathing and circulation.

A cardiac arrest is different from a myocardial infarction (also known as a heart attack), where blood flow to the muscle of the heart is impaired. It is different from congestive heart failure, where circulation is substandard, but the heart is still pumping sufficient blood to sustain life.

Signs and Symptoms

- Unresponsiveness
- Cessation of respiration
- Pallor and cyanosis
- Absence of pulse
- Dilation of pupil

Management of Cardiac Arrest

Cardiopulmonary Resuscitation (CPR)

- Management of cardiac arrest is CPR
- Assess the response is the first step of CPR (call the victim by his or her name or shake victim's shoulder).
- If there is no response call for help
- Place the patient on a firm surface
- Check the carotid pulse in case of adult and brachial pulse in infants. (In infants its very difficult to palpate carotid pulse due to the short structure and fat)
- Start CPR
- Ratio of compression is 30:2 or 15:2 in case of two rescuers.
- Depth of compression is 1½ to 2 inch (5 cm) in adults and ½ to 1 inch in infants.
- Position of the hand is on the center of the chest on the nipple line.

- Proper hand placement is very important to prevent rib fracture.
- While giving CPR check the pupillary response because it is the excellent method to know whether the oxygen reaches the brain.
- It the CPR is not given with in 4–6 minutes, it may leads to brain death.
- While applying pressure on the xyphoid process, there is chance to get liver damage.
- While giving CPR, open the airway by head tilt and chin lift method (in case of spinal cord injury use jaw thrust method).
- Based on AHA, connect the patient to an AED (automated external defibrillator) in case of ventricular fibrillation.

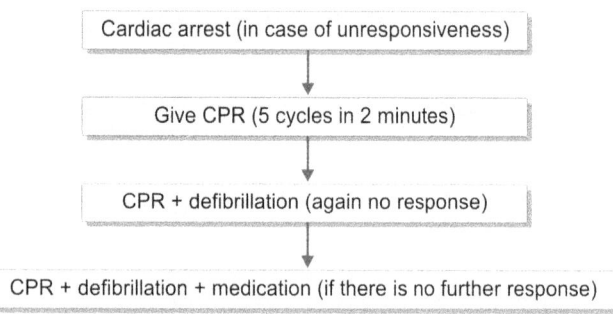

- Administer adrenaline or epinephrine to enhance the force of myocardial contractility.

Drug Therapy

- Antiarrhythmic agents, such as amiodarone (cordarone).
- Adrenaline or epinephrine to enhance force of myocardial contractility
- Atropine sulphate to control heart rate by reducing vagus nerve stimulation
- Sodium bicarbonate to correct respiratory and metabolic acidosis.

INFLAMMATORY DISORDERS OF HEART

Endocarditis

Endocarditis is an infection of the inner lining of the heart (endocardium). Inflammation of endocardium caused by bacteria (e.g. Group A beta hemolytic streptococci).

Endocarditis generally occurs when bacteria or other germs from another part of your body, such as your mouth, spread through your bloodstream and attach to damaged areas in your heart. Left untreated, endocarditis can damage or destroy your heart valves and can lead to life-threatening complications.

Causes

- Certain dental procedures
- Any obstetrical procedures
- Any open heart surgery
- Rheumatic heart disease
- Common among IV drug abusers

Signs and Symptoms

- Fever and chills
- Dyspnea
- Night sweats
- Persistent cough
- Swelling and joint pain
- Increased ESR and WBC count
- Tenderness in your spleen—an infection-fighting abdominal organ on your left side, just below your rib cage
- Osler's nodes—red, tender spots under the skin of your fingers
- Petechiae (puh-TEE-key-ee)—tiny purple or red spots on the skin, whites of your eyes or inside your mouth

Management

- Administer antibiotics (Penicillin)
- Avoid personal contacts with infectious patients.

Pericarditis

Inflammation of pericardium caused by bacteria, virus and fungi. It is also seen as a complication of antitumor antibiotics (adriamycin).

Signs and Symptoms

- Sharp piercing chest pain with deep inspiration and relieved by sitting up position.
- Pericardial friction rub
- Jugular vein distention
- Increased WBC and ESR
- ECG shows ST elevation in all leads

Management

- Control the underlying cause
- Administer corticosteroids and colchicine to reduce inflammation.
- Provide semi to high Fowler's position.
- Administer antibiotics.

Cardiac Tamponade

Accumulation of blood or fluids in the pericardial space, resulting in decreased ventricular filling.

Causes

- Gunshot or stab wounds
- Blunt trauma to the chest from a car or industrial accident
- Accidental perforation after cardiac catheterization, angiography, or insertion of a pacemaker
- Punctures during placement of central lines, a type of catheter used to administer fluids or medications
- Invasion of the sac by breast, lung, or other cancers
- A ruptured aortic aneurysm

Signs and Symptoms

- Chest pain
- Increase CVP
- Trouble breathing or taking deep breaths
- Rapid breathing
- Discomfort that is relieved by sitting or leaning forward
- Fainting, dizziness, and loss of consciousness
- Pericardial friction rub
- Cardiac tamponade has three classical sign called as **Beck's triad**, which includes
  - Hypotension
  - Jugular vein distention (JVD)
  - Distant or muffled heart sound

Management

- Administer oxygen
- Position the patient supine with head of bed elevation 30–40 degree.
- Assist with pericardiocentesis (insertion of a needle into the pericardial sac to remove the excess blood or fluid and to reduce the pressure on the heart).
- After pericardiocentesis, the blood pressure will be normalized.

VASCULAR DISORDERS

Vascular disease includes any condition that affects the circulatory system. As the heart beats, it pumps blood through a system of blood vessels called the circulatory system. The vessels are elastic tubes that carry blood to every part of the body. Arteries carry blood away from the heart while veins return it (arteries carry blood from the proximal to the distal area where as veins carry blood from the distal to proximal).

The common vascular disorders are:
1. Hypertension
2. Arteriosclerosis obliterans
3. Thromboangiitis obliterans (TAO or Buerger's disease)
4. Raynaud's phenomena
5. Aneurysms
6. Pulmonary embolism
7. Varicose vein
8. Venous stasis ulcer
9. Thrombophlebitis
10. Deep vein thrombosis
11. Amputation

Hypertension

Hypertension is also known as high blood pressure, a chronic medical condition in which the blood pressure in the arteries is persistently elevated (systolic BP above 140 mm Hg and diastolic BP above 90 mm Hg).

Blood pressure is determined both by the amount of blood your heart pumps and the amount of resistance to blood flow in your arteries. The more blood your heart pumps and the narrower your arteries, the higher your blood pressure.

Types of Hypertension

- **Primary hypertension:** It is also called as essential hypertension or idiopathic hypertension. About 95% hypertension is primary hypertension. It occurs between 30 and 50 years of age.
- **Secondary hypertension:** Hypertension due to some other medical conditions, such as Cushing syndrome, renal artery occlusion, adrenal gland tumors, etc.

Signs and Symptoms

- Chest pain similar to anginal pain
- Intermittent claudication (pain in the calf muscle after ambulation or exercise)
- Retinal damage
- Epistaxis
- Edema in the lower extremities
- Rise in systolic BP from supine to standing position is the classical symptom of essential hypertension.
- Increased serum cholesterol
- Increased blood sodium and uric acid levels

Management

- Administer antihypertensives
- Restrict sodium and cholesterol
- Monitor BP in all position
- Instruct the patient to stop smoking
- Alcohol moderation
- Avoid abrupt discontinuation of medication because it result in rebound hypertension.
- Avoid hot bath or alcohol or vigorous exercise at least three hours after antihypertensive medication because it may result in severe vasodilation and hypotension.

Classification of Antihypertensives

ACE inhibitors	ACE II inhibitors	Alpha blockers	Beta blockers	Calcium channel blocker	Direct acting vasodilator
Pril	**Sartan**	**Zin**	**Lol**		
Lisinopril	Losartan	Terazosin	Propranolol	Verapamil	Apresoline
Captopril	Telmisartan	Prazosin	Metoprolol	Nifedipine	Hydralazine
Enalapril	Losar, revas	Minipress	Atenolol	Diltiazem	
Side effect					
Hyperkalemia Edema Pruritis	Hyperkalemia	Syncope	Smooth muscle constriction	Constipation Palpitation	Weight gain Edema
Nursing care					
Monitor potassium level	Monitor potassium level	Administer at night time	Contraindicated in COPD, HF asthma, DM,	Administer more fluids, fiber rich diet	Monitor for weight gain

Arteriosclerosis Obliterans

Arteriosclerosis obliterans is an occlusive arterial disease most prominently affecting the abdominal aorta and the small- and medium-sized arteries of the lower extremities, which may lead to absent dorsalis pedis, posterior tibial, and/or popliteal artery pulses.

Cigarette smoking is the major cause.

Signs and Symptoms

- Pain in the calf muscle
- Diminished or absent pulse in the lower extremities
- Hair loss in the lower extremity
- Dizziness
- Doppler study shows decreased blood flow to the lower extremity
- Elevated serum triglyceride levels

Management

- Administer vasodilators, such as papaverine hydrochloride or nylidrin hydrochloride
- Administer lipid lowering agents
- Provide low fat diet
- Teach Buerger-Allen Exercise

Buerger exercise is an active exercise of the feet. These exercises consist of flexion, extension, and circumduction of the ankles and are done during the phase of dependency of the legs, as suggested in 1931 by Arthur W. Allen (1887–1958).

A specific exercises intended to improve circulation to the feet and legs. The lower extremities are elevated to a 45 to 90 degree angle and supported in this position until the skin blanches (appears dead white). The feet and legs are then lowered below the level of the rest of the body until redness appears (care should be taken that there is no pressure against the back of the knees); finally, the legs are placed flat on the bed for a few minutes. The length of time for each position varies with the patient's tolerance and the speed with which color change occurs. Usually, the exercises are prescribed so that the legs are elevated for 2 to 3 minutes, down 5 to 10 minutes, and then flat on the bed for 10 minutes.

Thromboangiitis Obliterans (Buerger's Disease)

Buerger's disease, also called thromboangiitis obliterans, is a disease that causes blockages in the blood vessels of your feet and hands. The blood vessels become inflamed, which reduces blood flow. Its an inflammatory disease affecting the arteries and veins of the lower extremities.

Cigarette smoking is the major cause.

Signs and Symptoms

- Intermittent claudication
- Decreased or absent pulse in the lower extremity
- Pain in the hands and feet of legs and arms (this pain may come and go)
- Open sores on the toes or fingers
- Inflamed veins
- Pale toes or fingers when in cold temperatures

Management

- Administer vasodilators
- Maintain warmth in cold weather
- Instruct the patient to stop smoking

Raynaud's Phenomenon

Arterial spasm of the fingers and toes resulting in decreased blood flow.

Women are more likely than men to have Raynaud's disease, also known as Raynaud or Raynaud's phenomenon or syndrome. It appears to be more common in people who live in colder climates.

Signs and Symptoms

- Coolness
- Numbness and tingling sensation

Management

- Administer vasodilators
- Maintain a warm environment
- Instruct the patient to stop smoking
- Instruct the patient to use gloves while handling cold objects

Aneurysms

An aneurysm is an abnormal swelling or bulge in the wall of a blood vessel, such as an artery. It is also called as dilatation in the weakened arterial wall.

Classification

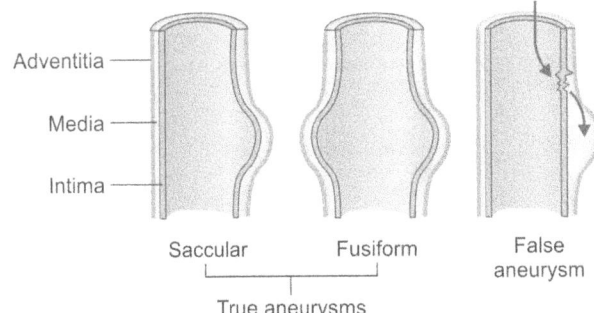

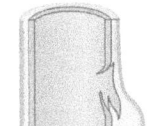

Dissecting aneurysm

- **True aneurysm:** A true aneurysm is one that involves all three layers of the wall of an artery (intima, media and adventitia).
- **False aneurysm:** A false aneurysm, or pseudo-aneurysm, is a collection of blood leaking completely out of an artery or vein, but confined next to the vessel by the surrounding tissue.
- **Saccular aneurysm:** A saccular aneurysm is spherical in shape and involve only a portion of the vessel wall; they vary in size from 5 to 20 cm (8 in) in diameter, and are often filled, either partially or fully, by a thrombus.
- **Fusiform aneurysm:** A fusiform aneurysm is a uniform spindle-shaped involves the entire circumference of the artery.
- **Dissecting aneurysm:** A dissecting aneurysm is a type of aneurysm in which there is separation of the arterial wall layer to form a cavity that fills with blood.

Types of Aneurysm

Common types of aneurysms are:
- Thoracic aortic aneurysm
- Abdominal aortic aneurysm

Thoracic aortic aneurysm: Aneurysm occurs at the descending, ascending and transverse section of the thoracic aorta.

Causes

- Arteriosclerosis
- Infection
- Hypertension

Signs and Symptoms

- Diffuse chest pain
- Dyspnea
- Distended neck vein
- Edema of the hands and extremities

Management

- Treat the underlying cause
- Surgical repair of aneurysm with teflon or Dacron graft

Abdominal aortic aneurysm: Aneurysm in the abdominal aorta just below the renal arteries.

Signs and Symptoms

- Mid to low abdominal pain
- Low back pain
- A pulsating periumbilical mass
- Diminished or absent pulse in the lower extremity.

Management

- Monitor CVP (central venous pressure) and PCWP (pulmonary capillary wedge pressure)

- Monitor serum Creatinine and BUN
- Monitor urine output and Instruct the patient to report if the urine output is less than 30 ml per hour (this indicates renal impairment due to the clamping of aorta during the surgical repair of abdominal aortic aneurysm).
- Monitor for any back pain (it indicates retroperitoneal hemorrhage).
- Assess for the signs of DVT (deep vein thrombosis).
- Provide flat position to avoid hip or knee contractures
- Monitor for any complication (spinal cord ischemia is tend to occur if abdominal aneurysm ruptures).

Pulmonary Embolism

Emboli which is seen in the pulmonary system resulting in the blockage of pulmonary artery is called as pulmonary embolism.

Causes

- Thrombosis
- Fat emboli
- Fracture or trauma
- Pregnancy
- Pre and postoperative stages
- Immobility

Signs and Symptoms

- Chest pain
- Dyspnea
- Tachypnea
- Tachycardia

Management

- Administer thrombolytic agents (streptokinase or urokinase)
- Administer anticoagulants
- Provide Fowler's position
- Prepare the patient for embolectomy
- Treat the underlying cause

How Fracture leads to Pulmonary Embolism

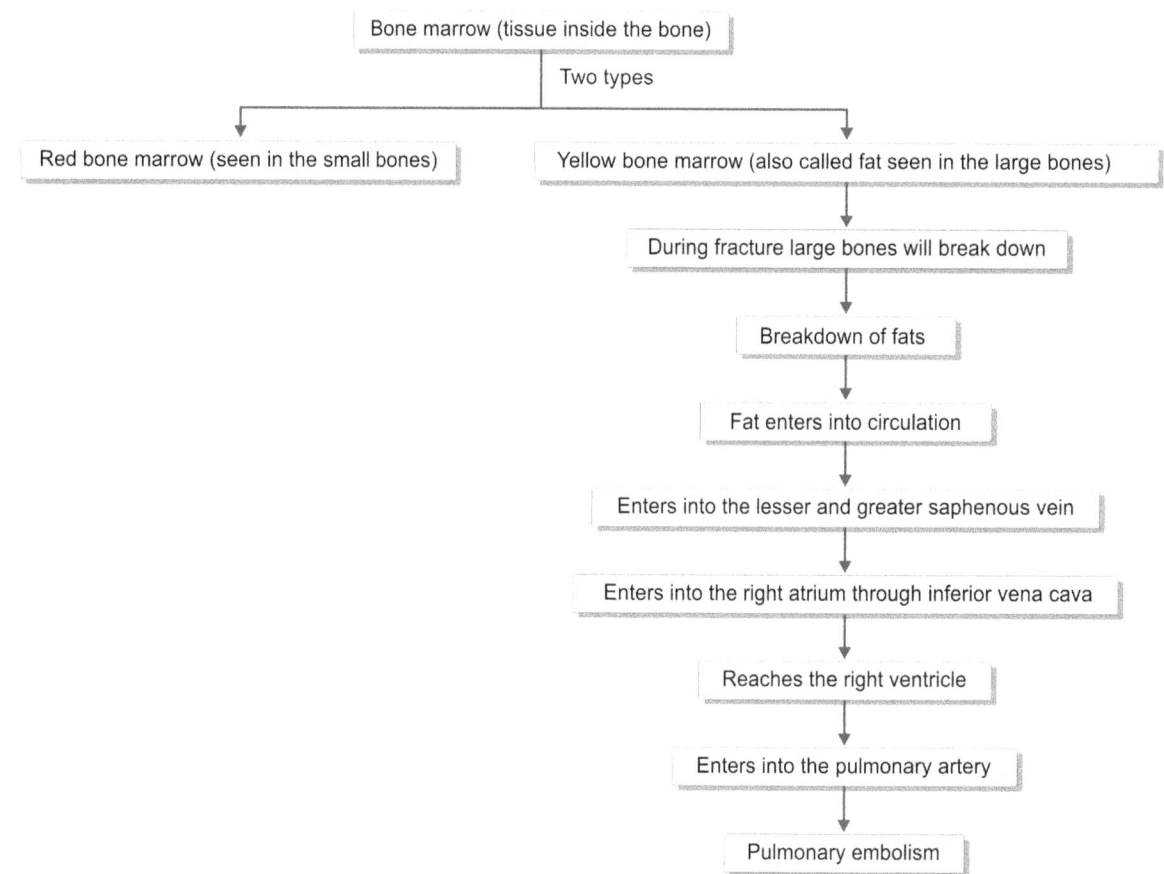

Varicose Vein

It is the abnormal dilation of the veins in the lower extremities. It is the permanently distended veins due to valvular incompetence.

Common Sites

- Greater and lesser saphenous veins
- Perforated veins in the angles

Risk Factors

- Prolonged standing
- Thrombophlebitis
- Pregnancy
- Obesity
- Heart diseases

Signs and Symptoms

- Swollen and dilated veins
- Pain after prolonged standing and relieved by elevation of extremities.
- Veins that are dark purple or blue in color
- Veins that appear twisted and bulging; often like cords on your legs
- Doppler ultrasound shows right or left femoral saphenous valvular incompetence.

Management

- Perform trendelenburg test. Ask the patient to lie down, elevate the affected extremity above the heart level for 2 minutes, ask the patient to stand up soon after the elevation, if the veins distend very quickly (less than 35 seconds), it indicates faulty valvular mechanism. In veins the blood flow from the distal to the proximal but in varicose vein the blood flow from the proximal to distal).
- Administer medications, such as vasodilators
- Apply varicose vein stocking or compression stocking
- Instruct the patient to wear the stocking before getting up from the bed.
- Teach the patient to wear the stocking throughout the day, remove after 8 hours for a short period of time and reapply.

Thrombophlebitis

Inflammation of the vessel wall due to any thrombi or clot formation.

Signs and Symptoms

- Redness and swelling
- Virchow's triad (venous stasis, hypercoagulability and injury to the vessel wall)
- Positive Homans' sign (dorsiflexion of the feet may cause pain in the calf muscle)
- Increased WBC and ESR

Management

- Administer anticoagulants
- Assess for any bleeding
- Avoid aspirin or aspirin contained drugs
- Monitor for chest pain
- Provide antiembolism stocking
- Prepare the patient for placation of inferior vena cava (insertion of an umbrella like prosthesis into the lumen of inferior vena cava to filter the incoming clots)

Deep Vein Thrombosis

Deep vein thrombosis, or deep venous thrombosis (DVT) is the formation of a blood clot (thrombus) within a deep vein predominantly in the legs.

Signs and Symptoms

- Pain and swelling
- Redness
- Distention of surface veins
- Positive Homans' sign

Venous Stasis Ulcer

It is an end stage complication of thrombophlebitis, ulcer resulting from incompetent valves in the vein.

Signs and Symptoms

- Pain
- Edema
- Skin is lathery and brownish

Management

- Administer antibiotics
- Prepare the patient for wound debridement
- Elevate the extremity above the heart level

Amputation

Amputation is the removal of a limb by trauma, medical illness, or surgery. As a surgical measure, it is used to control pain or a disease process in the affected limb, such as malignancy or gangrene. In some cases, it is carried out on individuals as a preventative surgery for such problems. A surgical treatment for the peripheral vascular disorders.

Nursing Care (Preoperative)

- Provide routine investigations
- Provide support and encouragement to accept the client's feeling
- Discuss the use of prosthesis.

Nursing Care (Postoperative)

- Describe about phantom limb sensation
- Prevent hip or knee contractures by providing prone position several times in a day
- Avoid elevation of the stump after 24 hours; elevate the stump for the first 24 hours
- Observe the stump dressing for any bleeding
- Administer pain medication

CHAPTER 6

Endocrine System

Chapter Objectives

- Key notes in the endocrine system
- Endocrine and exocrine glands
- Diagnostic measures
- Endocrine disorders
- Diabetes mellitus
- Pancreatitis

KEY TERMS

SIADH   Cystic fibrosis
ADH   SPGC
VMA   RAIU
DKA   HHNS

KEYNOTES

- Pancreas is the only one gland that has both exocrine and endocrine function.
- Urine acetone is positive in diabetic ketoacidosis.
- Cystic fibrosis is an inflammation of exocrine gland.
- Sweat test is performed for a patient with cystic fibrosis
- Classical manifestation of cystic fibrosis is presence of more amount of salt in the sweat.
- Night sweat is seen in cystic fibrosis.
- Leptin is a hormone produced by the adipose tissues.
- Hashimoto disease is an autoimmune disease associated with thyroid gland.
- The priority nursing care of a patient undergoing thyroidectomy is monitor for any numbness or tingling in the lower extremities due to the accidental removal of parathyroid gland.
- Parathyroid gland maintain calcium metabolism.
- The classical manifestation of SIADH is hyponatremia and hypervolemia.
- The classical manifestation of a patient who develops complication of management of diabetes Insipidus is hypervolemia (symptoms of SIADH).
- Biguanides (metformin) is a category of OHA also indicated for PCOD.
- Withhold metformin preparations before CT scan because iodine which is used for these procedures will react with metformin and cause metformin induced iodine lactic acidosis.
- Meglitinides (Repaglinide) is also used as an OHA.
- Papillary carcinoma is associated with thyroid disorder.
- Addison's disease ADD salt.
- Cushing's disease CUT salt.

INTRODUCTION

The endocrine system is the collection of glands that produce hormones that regulate metabolism, growth and development, tissue function, sexual function, reproduction, sleep, and mood, and so on.

GLANDS

These are organs or structures that secrete hormone or milk in our body. Glands can be classified into two:
1. Endocrine glands
2. Exocrine glands

Endocrine Glands

These are ductless glands which secrete hormones directly into the blood stream. The common endocrine glands are:
- Pituitary glands
- Pineal glands
- Thyroid gland
- Parathyroid gland
- Adrenal glands
- Pancreas
- Ovaries and testes

Exocrine Glands

These are glands with duct which secrete hormones into the body cavities. The common exocrine glands are:
- Salivary glands
- Sweat glands
- Sebaceous glands
- The pancreas

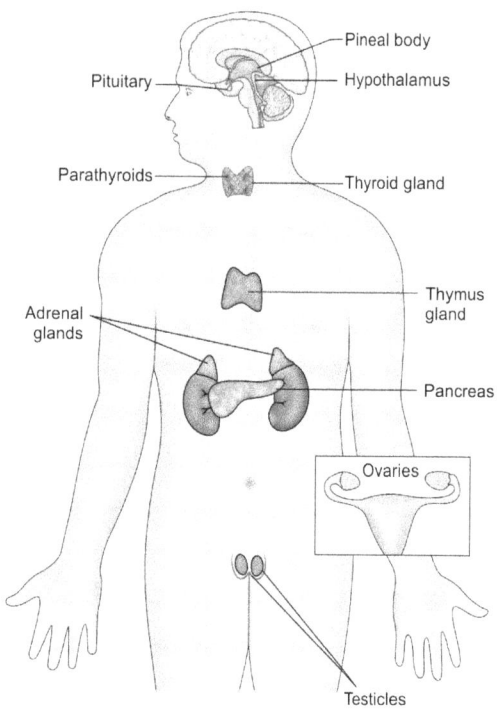

Fig. 1: Endocrine system

PITUITARY GLAND

It is called the master gland of endocrine system because it controls all the endocrine glands. The weight of pituitary gland is 0.5 gm and is located at the base of the brain as seen in Figure 1. In the base of the brain there is a cavity called as sella turcica, inside the sella turcica pituitary gland is located. So it is also known as hypophysis.

Hormones

The pituitary gland is divided into three lobes:

Anterior lobe	Posterior lobe	Intermediate lobe
TSH	ADH	MSH
ACTH	Oxytocin or Pitocin	
FSH & LH		
GH		
Prolactin		

Anterior lobe: The hormones are:
- **TSH (Thyroid stimulating hormone)**
  It stimulate the thyroid gland to produce thyroid hormones.
- **ACTH (Adrenocorticotropic hormones)**
  It stimulate the adrenal gland to produce adrenal hormones.
- **FSH & LH (Follicle-stimulating hormone and luteinizing hormone)**
  It stimulate the growth and function of secondary sexual organs.
- **GH (growth hormone)**
  It stimulates the growth of bones and tissues.
- **Prolactin**
  It stimulates the mammary glands and helps in the ejection of milk during lactation.

Posterior lobe: The hormones are:
- **ADH (Antidiuretic hormone)**
  It maintains water metabolism.
- **Pitocin or oxytocin**
  It stimulate uterine contraction during delivery and release of milk during lactation.

Intermediate lobe: The hormones are:
- **MSH (Melanocyte-stimulating hormone)**
  It helps in skin pigmentation.

DISORDERS OF PITUITARY GLAND

Hypopituitarism

Hypofunction of the anterior lobe of pituitary gland results in deficiency of pituitary hormones (growth hormones).

Causes
- Tumor
- Trauma
- Irradiation of pituitary gland

Clinical Manifestation
- Dwarfism in children (due to decrease in the growth hormone).

- Bitemporal hemianopsia or peripheral vision loss (due to any tumor).

Nursing Care

- Administer hormone replacement therapy as ordered.
- If the cause is due to tumor prepare the patient for hypophysectomy.

Hyperpituitarism

Hyperfunction of the anterior lobe of pituitary gland results in the increased production of pituitary hormones (growth hormones).

Causes

- Tumor
- Trauma
- Irradiation of the gland

Clinical Manifestation

- Gigantism in children (due to increased growth hormone).
- Acromegaly in adults (due to increased growth hormone).
- Enlargement of the bones especially scapular and pelvic bones in acromegaly.

Nursing Care

- Monitor for any hyperglycemia due to hormonal imbalance.
- Prepare the patient for hypophysectomy (removal of pituitary gland).

Hypophysectomy

Partial or complete removal of the pituitary gland, there are two approaches:
- *Craniotomy: Through open skull*
- *Transphenoidal hypophysectomy: An incision is made between upper lip and gingiva and a catheter is passed to remove the pituitary gland.*

Nursing care of patient after hypophysectomy
- *Monitor the urine output, report the physician if the urine output is greater than 800 ml per 2 hour and urine specific gravity is less than 1.004 (Indicates Diabetes Insipidus).*
- *Elevate the head end of bed in case of transphenoidal hypophysectomy is performed (to decrease ICP).*
- *Observe for any CSF leakage through nose or mouth.*
- *No tooth brushing for 10 days.*
- *Monitor the CSF glucose level (decreased CSF glucose indicates meningitis.*

Diabetes Insipidus

Hypofunction of the posterior lobe of pituitary gland results in deficiency of ADH leads to increased urine output (Polyuria).

Causes

- Surgery of the pituitary gland
- Due to any tumor
- Trauma

Clinical Manifestation

- Polyuria
- Decreased urine specific gravity
- Polydipsia
- Muscle weakness
- Dehydration
- Tachycardia

Nursing Care

- Administer antidiuretic hormone (Vasopressin)
- Maintain fluid electrolyte balance
- Monitor urine specific gravity
- Monitor intake output chart
- Monitor weight daily

SIADH (Syndrome of Inappropriate Antidiuretic Hormone Secretion)

Hyperfunction of the posterior lobe of pituitary gland results in the increased ADH production leads to decreased urine output (Oliguria).

Causes

- Due to any tumor
- Trauma

Clinical Manifestation

- Oliguria
- Edema
- Hypervolemia
- Hyponatremia (due to hormonal imbalance)

Nursing Care

- Administer diuretics
- Adequate salt diet
- Monitor for any confusion and disorientation due to hyponatremia.

THYROID GLAND

Thyroid gland is a butterfly like gland which is located on the either side of Adam's apple as seen in Figure 1. The weight of thyroid gland is 15-35 gm. The TSH (thyroid stimulating hormone) is produced from the anterior pituitary gland activate the thyroid gland to produce thyroid hormones. The thyroid gland maintains carbohydrate, protein and fat metabolism of our body.

Thyroid Hormones

- T_3 (Tri-iodothyronine)
- T_4 (Thyroxine)
- Calcitonin

Thyroid Medications

They are classified into two:

Thyroid hormones	Antithyroid medications
Given for hypothyroidism	Given for hyperthyroidism
Levothyroxine (Eltroxin, Thyronorm, Thyrox)	Levimazole, Carbimazole, Neomercazole, PTU or Propylthiouracil

Administer Thyroid Medications throughout the Pregnancy

In case of hypothyroidism in pregnant women, there is decreased T_3 and T_4 and this will leads to MR (Mental Retardation) in the fetus. So in order to prevent MR in the fetus administer thyroid hormones throughout the pregnancy.

In case of hyperthyroidism in pregnant women, there is increased T_3 and T_4 and this will not cross the placental barrier, but the iodine may cross the placental barrier and in the fetus it turns to thyroxine and leads to MR. In order to prevent iodine conversion administer antithyroid medications in pregnancy.

Diagnostic Measures

Thyroid Function Test (No Need for Fasting)

- T_3 : 80-230 ng/dL
- T_4 : 5-12 mcg/dL
- TSH : 0.2-5.4 mu/mL

Radioactive Iodine Uptake Test (RAIU)

- Administer iodine 123 or iodine 131 orally or IV and perform thyroid function test.
- Increased uptake of iodine indicates hyperthyroidism.
- Decreased uptake of iodine indicates hypothyroidism.

Thyroid Scan

- It is used to visualize any thyroid malignancies.

DIOSRDERS OF THYROID GLAND

Goiter

A simple enlargement of thyroid gland not due to any inflammation or neoplasm.

Causes

Due to excess production of TSH from the pituitary gland, it stimulate the thyroid gland to produce more thyroid hormones.

Types

- *Endemic goiter:* Due to iodine deficiency areas where the soil and water are deficient in iodine, common in adolescents and pregnancy.
- *Sporadic goiter*: Due to some goiterogenic substances such as cabbage, soyabean, spinach, radish, due to some drugs such as large dose of lithium, etc.

Diagnosis

- Thyroid hormones are normal (T_3 and T_4)
- TSH is increased.

Nursing Care

- Administer thyroid hormones such as eltroxin or levothyroxine.
- Administer iodine solution (Lugol's iodine)
- In case of administration of lugol's iodine solution administer with as straw to prevent staining of the teeth
- Prepare the patient for thyroidectomy.

Hypothyroidism

Hypofunction of the thyroid gland leads to decrease in the production of thyroid hormones which results in slowing the metabolism of carbohydrate and fat. It causes myxedema in adults and cretinism in children.

Causes

- Due to any atrophy of the thyroid gland.
- Surgical removal of thyroid gland (after thyroidectomy).

Clinical Manifestation

- Weight gain
- Cold intolerance
- Anorexia
- Constipation
- Dry scaly skin

- Brittle nails
- Menstrual irregularities (increased menstrual blood flow)
- Increased sensitivity to cold and narcotics.

Diagnosis

- Decreased T_3 and T_4 level
- RAIU shows decreased uptake of iodine.

Nursing Care

- Administer more fluids and high fiber diet.
- Avoid sedatives and narcotics.
- Provide comfortable warm environment.
- Administer thyroid hormones for life long (Levothyroxine).
- Instruct the patient to take medications in empty stomach in order to prevent insomnia.
- Provide low calorie diet.

Myxedema Coma

It is a medical emergency characterized by exaggerated hypothyroidism and leads to coma.

Causes

- Failure to take prescribed medications
- Any infections
- Trauma
- Exposure to cold

Clinical Manifestation

- Subnormal body temperature
- Hypertension

Nursing Care

- Administer IV thyroid hormones
- Provide warm environment
- Provide low calorie diet.

Hyperthyroidism (Grave's Disease)

Hyperfunction of the thyroid gland leads to increased production of thyroid hormones result in increased metabolism of carbohydrate and fat.

Causes

- Due to any autoimmune diseases
- Idiopathic

Clinical Manifestation

- Weight loss
- Heat intolerance
- Increased temperature
- Tremor
- Diaphoresis
- Exophthalmos
- Menstrual irregularities (decreased menstrual blood flow)
- Diarrhea

Diagnosis

- Increased T_3 and T_4
- RAIU shows increased uptake of iodine.

Nursing Care

- Administer antithyroid medications (PTU or Propylthiouracil).
- Administer beta blockers in case of tachycardia.
- Provide high calorie diet.
- Reduce stress in the environment.
- Provide proper rest.
- Prepare the patient for thyroidectomy.

Thyroid Storm

It is the sudden or uncontrolled life threatening hyperthyroidism caused by excessive release of thyroid hormones in to the blood stream.

Causes

- Severe stress
- Unprepared thyroid surgery

Clinical Manifestation

- High temperature up to 106 degree F
- Tachycardia
- Respiratory distress
- Coma

Nursing Care

- Maintain a patent airway
- Administer oxygen
- Administer antithyroid medications
- Prepare the patient for thyroidectomy.

THYROIDECTOMY

Partial or complete removal of the thyroid gland.

Nursing Care (Pre-operative)

- Maintain a stable cardiac status.
- Maintain normal weight.
- Perform all the routine laboratory investigations.
- Administer antithyroid medications so as to decrease the secretion of thyroid hormones.
- Administer lugol's iodine solution to reduce the size and vascularity of thyroid gland and to prevent bleeding.

Nursing Care (Post-operative)

- Monitor vital signs.
- Monitor for any signs of bleeding, redness around the neck.
- Provide semi-fowler's position.
- Monitor for any respiratory distress due to any damage to laryngeal nerve or edema in the glottis.
- Monitor for any signs and symptoms of tetany (numbness and tingling of the extremity).
- Provide voice rest, report if there is any extreme hoarseness of voice.
- Administer medications to get relief from sore throat.
- Administer thyroid hormones after thyroidectomy (hormone replacement therapy for lifelong).
- Keep the tracheostomy set, oxygen and suctioning ready after thyroidectomy.

PARATHYROID GLAND

It is a gland which is located just above the thyroid gland as seen in figure 1. Parathyroid gland secretes parathyroid hormone or parathormone which helps in calcium metabolism.

DISORDERS OF PARATHYROID GLAND

Hypoparathyroidism

Hypofunction of the parathyroid gland leads to decrease in the parathormone which results in hypocalcemia (decreased serum calcium and increased serum phosphorus).

Causes

- Idiopathic
- Accidental removal of parathyroid gland during thyroidectomy.

Clinical Manifestation

- Hypocalcemia
- Chvostek's sign (sharp tapping over the facial nerve may cause twitching around the mouth, nose and eyes)
- Trousseau's sign (severe carpopedal spasm while inflating a BP cuff for 2-3 minutes)
- Symptoms of rickets and tetany (muscle spasm, cardiac arrhythmias, numbness, seizure).

Diagnosis

- Decreased serum calcium
- Increased serum phosphorus.

Nursing Care

- Administer calcium supplements.
- In case of chronic hypocalcemia administer calcium gluconate IV slowly.
- Administer vitamin D_3 (cholecalciferol) for helping calcium absorption.
- Administer calcium rich diet such as milk, milk products, yogurt, cheese etc.
- Administer amphogel to decrease serum phosphorus.

Hyperparathyroidism

Hyperfunction of the parathyroid gland leads to increased production of parathormone results in hypercalcemia (increased calcium and decreased phosphorus).

Causes

- Any tumor
- Hyperplasia of the parathyroid gland.

Clinical Manifestation

- Hypercalcemia
- Renal calculi (renal calcium calculi)
- Cardiac arrhythmias (Short QT interval)
- Bone demineralization.

Diagnosis

- Increased serum calcium
- Decreased serum phosphorus.

Nursing Care

- Administer IV fluids (Forcing fluids)
- Administer diuretics
- Administer acid-ash diet
- Provide low calcium diet.

ADRENAL GLAND

These are called as supra-renal gland, located above each kidney as seen in figure 1. The weight of adrenal gland is 7-10 gm. It maintains overall kidney functions.

Hormones produced by the Adrenal Gland

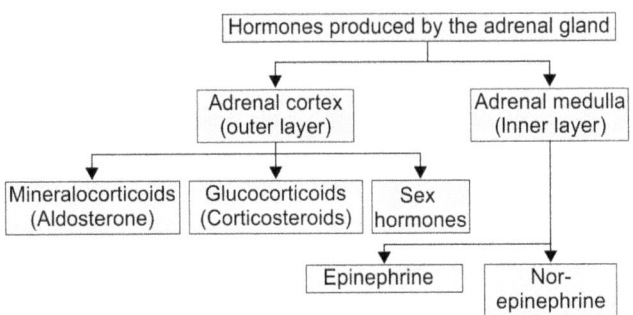

- Mineralocorticoids or aldosterone maintains the water metabolism.
- Glucocorticoids or corticosteroids maintains carbohydrate metabolism.
- Epinephrine and Nor-epinephrine functions in acute stress.

DISORDERS OF ADRENAL GLAND

Addison's Disease

Hypofunction of the adrenal gland (adrenal cortex) leads to decreased production of mineralocorticoids, glucocorticoids and sex hormones.

Causes

- Idiopathic atrophy of the adrenal gland
- Autoimmune
- Destruction of gland through TB or HIV infections.

Clinical Manifestation

- Bronze like pigmentation over the skin
- Hyponatremia
- Hypotension, Hyperkalemia, Hypoglycemia, Hypercalcemia.

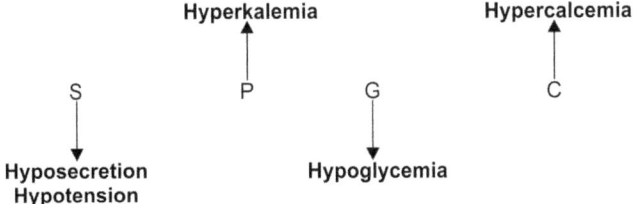

Nursing Care

- Administer salt rich diet (Addison's disease = ADD salt)
- Monitor vital signs especially BP
- Restrict potassium rich diet
- Provide high calorie, high carbohydrate diet
- Provide more fluids to wash out renal calculi
- Administer hormones.

Addisonian Crisis

It is also called as acute adrenal failure. Severe exacerbation of Addison's disease.

Causes

- Sudden withdrawal of hormones
- Surgery of the pituitary gland
- Severe infection or stress.

Clinical Manifestation

- Same as Addison's disease
- Hypovolemia
- Muscle weakness
- Hyperkalemia and hyponatremia
- Shock
- Loss of consciousness

Nursing Care

- Administer IV fluids (Dextrose)
- Administer IV hormones
- Correct the underlying cause (treat infection with antibiotics and provide stress management methods).

Cushing's Syndrome

Hyperfunction of the adrenal gland (adrenal cortex) leads to increased secretion of mineralocorticoids, glucocorticoids and sex hormones.

Causes

- Prolonged use of corticosteroids
- Tumor of the adrenal gland
- Increased production of ACTH from pituitary
- Tumor elsewhere in the body that produce more ACTH.

Clinical Manifestation

- Decreased resistance to infection
- Menstrual dysfunction
- Osteoporosis
- Cushing triad (Moon-like face, buffalo hump and pendulous abdomen)
- Hypertension, Hypokalemia, Hyperglycemia, Hypocalcemia.

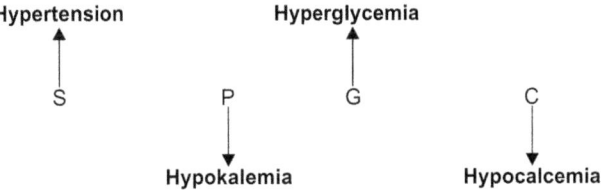

Nursing Care

- Avoid administering salt (Cushing's syndrome = CUT salt)
- Administer fresh fruits for a patient with Cushing's syndrome
- Maintain skin integrity
- Administer high potassium diet
- Administer insulin as per order
- Monitor blood glucose level (when the patient is undergoing treatment for Cushing's syndrome there will be fluctuations in blood sugar level)
- Provide high calcium diet
- Provide psychological support.

Primary Aldosteronism (Conn's Syndrome)

Excessive production of aldosterone from the adrenal cortex resulting in decreased renin levels.

Causes

- Hyperfunction of adrenal gland
- Tumor of adrenal gland.

Clinical Manifestation

- High blood pressure
- Muscle weakness
- Polyuria
- Hypokalemia
- Metabolic alkalosis
- Cardiac arrhythmias

Nursing Care

- Monitor vitals especially BP.
- Administer potassium sparing diuretics (aldactone, the side of aldactone is hyperkalemia so it will cope with hypokalemia).
- Provide salt restriction.
- Prepare the client for adrenalectomy.

Pheochromocytoma

A pheochromocytoma is a rare non-cancerous tumor of the adrenal medulla.

Causes

- Excessive secretion of adrenaline and nor-adrenaline.

Clinical Manifestation

- Severe hypertension
- Severe headache
- Severe hyperglycemia
- Rapid or forceful heart beat
- Tremor
- Shortness of breath
- Dilation of pupil
- Profound sweating

Nursing Care

- Perform VMA test (Vanillylmandelic acid test), elevated catecholamine while collecting 24 hour urine or blood examination, normal level of catecholamine is 14–110 mcg/24 hours), three days prior to the test patient must avoid vanilla, chocolate banana, etc.
- Monitor vitals especially BP.
- Administer medications to control hypertension.
- Monitor urine and blood sugar.
- Provide bed rest.
- Prepare the patient for adrenalectomy.

ADRENALECTOMY

Surgical removal of one or both adrenal glands.

Indications

- Cushing's syndrome
- Addison's disease
- Pheochromocytoma

Nursing Care (Pre-operative)

- Correct the metabolic and cardiovascular problems.
- In pheochromocytoma correct hypertension and hyperglycemia.
- In Addison's disease correct hyperkalemia.
- In Cushing's syndrome correct hypokalemia.
- Administer glucocorticoids in the morning of surgery to prevent acute adrenal insufficiency.

Nursing Care (Post-operative)

- Monitor vital signs.
- Monitor for any hemorrhage and symptoms of shock.
- Maintain intake output chart.
- Administer IV fluids.
- Administer hormones as per order.
- In case of unilateral adrenalectomy hormone replacement therapy (HRT) for 1 year and in case of bilateral adrenalectomy HRT for lifelong.

PANCREAS

The weight of pancreas is 98 gram. It is a leaf like structure which is located on the right side of the duodenum as seen in Figure 2. It has both exocrine and endocrine function.

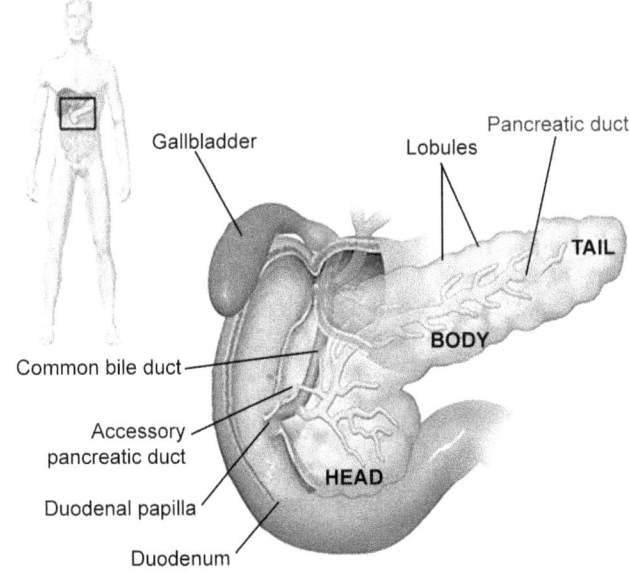

Fig. 2: Structure of pancreas

Hormones produced by the pancreas

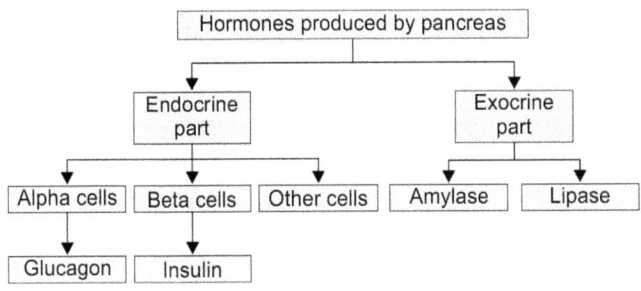

Why diabetes mellitus is called sweet urine disorder

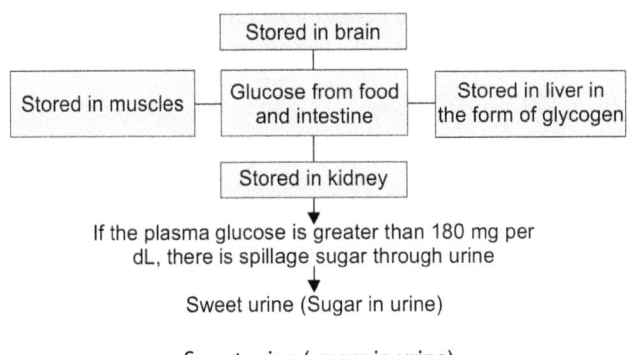

How blood sugar is normalized in individuals

In hyperglycemia	In hypoglycemia
Whenever we are taking more sweet ↓	Whenever we are fasting ↓
Increases blood sugar level ↓	Decreases blood sugar level ↓
Activate the beta cells of pancreas ↓	Activate the alpha cells of pancreas ↓
To produce more insulin ↓	Alpha cells will give command to the liver to use stored glycogen ↓
Which will cope with the sugar level	Which will cope with decreased sugar level

What is the difference between diabetic coma and insulin coma?

Diabetic Coma	Insulin Coma
Seen in severe hyperglycemia	Seen in severe hypoglycemia
In severe hyperglycemia ↓ Polyuria, polyphagia and Polydipsia ↓ To meet the energy demand stored glycogen is used ↓ End product of glucose metabolism is ketones or acetone ↓ Cross the blood brain barrier ↓ Coma	In severe hypoglycemia or insulin overload ↓ The plasma glucose level is less than 20 mg per dL ↓ Coma
Administer IV fluids and regular insulin	Administer dextrose solution

DIABETES MELLITUS (DM)

It is a metabolic disorder characterized by disturbance in carbohydrate, protein and fat metabolism and results in increased blood sugar level.

Types

Type I DM

- It is also called as insulin dependent diabetes or juvenile diabetes.
- It is seen at birth.
- No insulin is produced from the pancreas.
- The management is insulin therapy.

Type II DM

- It is also called as non-insulin dependent diabetes mellitus.
- It is seen in adult period.
- A small amount of insulin is produced from the pancreas.
- The management is oral hypoglycemic agents (OHA).

Gestational Diabetes Mellitus (GDM)

- Newly detected diabetes at the time of gestation.
- Seen between 20-28 weeks of gestation.
- The nutrients are transferred from mother to fetus through the placenta, during the transmission so many hormones are developed in the placenta, among those hormones HPL (Human placental lactogen) is a hormone having an anti insulin effect, so there is increased blood sugar level in mother.
- The management is insulin therapy.

Secondary Diabetes Mellitus

- Diabetes due to any disease conditions such as Cushing's syndrome or steroid therapy.
- The management is treatment of underlying causes.

Causes
- Insufficient production of insulin by the body
- Inability of the body to use insulin properly by the body
- Obesity
- Sedentary life style habits
- Smoking
- Pregnancy

Clinical Manifestation
- Polyuria, Polyphagia, Polydipsia
- Weight loss
- Anorexia
- Weakness

Diagnostic Measures

FBS & PPBS

- Fasting blood sugar examination (FBS), Normal FBS = 60-110 mg/dL.
- Post Prandial blood sugar (PPBS), Normal PPBS = less than 140 mg/dL.
- *DM = impaired blood glucose + associated symptoms.*
- *Impaired blood glucose = FBS ≥ 126 and RBS ≥ 200 mg/dL*
- *DM = FBS ≥ 126 and RBS ≥ 200 mg/dL + Polyuria, polyphagia, Polydipsia.*

Glycosylated Hemoglobin Count (HbA$_1$c)

- Excellent method to detect DM.
- A blood test can measure the amount of glycosylated hemoglobin in the blood. The glycosylated hemoglobin test shows what a person's average blood glucose level was for the 2 to 3 months before the test. This can help determine how well a person's diabetes is being controlled over time.
- It reflect the blood glucose of past 120 days.
- No need for fasting.
- *Normal HbA$_1$c = 4-5.9%*
- *Well controlled DM = less than 6%*
- *Poor controlled DM = less than 7 %*
- *Uncontrolled DM = greater than 7%*

Oral Glucose Tolerance Test (OGTT)

- Step I—monitor the blood glucose in fasting.
- Step II—ingest 50-100 gram of glucose.
- Step III—monitor blood glucose in the 30th and 60th minute up to 5 hours.

Management

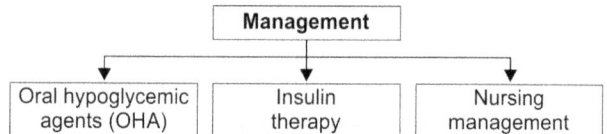

Oral Hypoglycemic Agents (OHA)

- It is given for a patient with Type II DM.
- It will activate the beta cells of pancreas to produce more insulin.
- Sulfonylureas is a category of OHA shows disulfiram like reaction when ingested along with alcohol.

Classification of OHA

Sulfonylureas	Biguanides	Alpha glucosidase inhibitor	Thiazolidinedione	Gliptins
Glimepiride	Metformin	Acarbose	Pioglitazone	Sitagliptin
Glipizide	Glyciphage	Glucobay	Rosiglitazone	Januvia
Glimulin	Glucophage	Precose	Pioglit	Vildagliptin
Amaryl	Melmet		Piomed	Jalra
diapride	Obimet		Pioz	Janumet
Glide	Glucored		Avandia	
1–5 mg	500–1000 gm	50–100 mg	15–30 mg	50–100 mg

Endocrine System

Insulin Therapy
- It is given for a patient with Type I DM.
- Regular insulin is the only one type of insulin we can give IV.
- We can keep an insulin bottle in room temperature for 30 days when it is left open.
- If you want to mix insulin in a same syringe, first withdraw the regular or clear insulin then cloudy or intermediate acting insulin.
- Insulin glargine or Lantus should not be mixed with any other insulin.

Classification of Insulin

Rapid acting	Short acting	Intermediate acting	Long acting
Insulin Lispro Insulin aspart	**(Regular insulin)** Human actrapid Huminsulin R Insugen R	**(Cloudy insulin)** Human mixtard Huminsulin N Huminsulin 30/70	Lantus Glargine
Peak action 1–2 hours	Peak action 2–4 hours	Peak action 4–12 hours	Peak action more than 12 hours

Complications of Insulin Therapy
- **Local allergic reaction:** Redness or itching at the site of administration of insulin.
- **Insulin lipodystrophy:** Damage to the lipid cells as a result of prolonged insulin administration. In order to prevent insulin lipodystrophy gently rotate the site in one anatomical direction.
- **Somogyi phenomenon:** Normal or elevated blood sugar level at bed time and hypoglycemia occurs at 2-3 am. The treatment is decrease the evening dose of insulin or increase the bed time snacks.
- **Dawn phenomenon:** It is also called as pre-breakfast hyperglycemia. Hyperglycemia between 5-8 am. The treatment is administer an evening dose of intermediate acting insulin at 10 pm.

Complications of Diabetes Mellitus

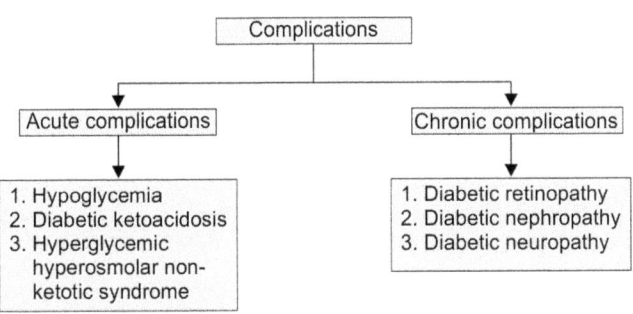

Acute Complications

Hypoglycemia
- If the plasma glucose level is less than 70 mg/dL, it is called as hypoglycemia.
- Mild hypoglycemia: Plasma glucose level less than 60 mg/dL.
- Moderate hypoglycemia: Plasma glucose level less than 40 mg/dL.
- Severe hypoglycemia: Plasma glucose level less than 20 mg/dL.

Nursing Care
- In mild hypoglycemia, administer 10-15 gram of simple carbohydrate orally.
- In moderate hypoglycemia, administer 15-25 gram of simple carbohydrate orally.
- In severe hypoglycemia, donot administer anything orally because the patient is in a state of coma, so administer 25-50 mL of dextrose in water IV.

Diabetic Ketoacidosis (DKA)

It is a life threatening complication of Type I DM.

Clinical Manifestation
- Serum glucose greater than 300 mg/dL.
- Kussmaul's respiration (fruity or acetone breath).
- Ph less than 7.35.
- Serum bicarbonate less than 15 mEq/L.

Nursing Care
- The priority nursing care is to administer IV fluids, normal saline to treat dehydration.
- Administer regular insulin IV (Dextrose with insulin).
- Monitor serum potassium level.
- Monitor for increased ICP (Intracranial pressure) (in severe DKA the fluid is pulled into CSF and causes cerebral edema and increased ICP).

HHNS (Hyperglycemic Hyperosmolar Non-ketotic Syndrome)

It is a complication of Type II DM.

Clinical Manifestation
- Serum glucose greater than 600 mg/dL
- Ph greater than 7.35
- Serum bicarbonate greater than 20 mEq/L
- Serum osmolarity greater than 350 mOsm/L.

Nursing Care

- Administer IV fluids (normal saline)
- Administer regular insulin IV.

Chronic Complications of Diabetes

- **Diabetic retinopathy:** Diabetic retinopathy is a diabetes complication that affects eyes. It is caused by damage to the blood vessels of the light-sensitive tissue at the back of the eye (retina). At first, diabetic retinopathy may cause no symptoms or only mild vision problems. Eventually, it can cause blindness.
- **Diabetic nephropathy:** Diabetic kidney disease, or diabetic nephropathy, is a complication of type 1 or type 2 diabetes caused by damage to the kidneys' delicate filtering system. Diabetic nephropathy is a clinical syndrome characterized by the following: Persistent albuminuria (>300 mg/d or >200 µg/min) that is confirmed on at least 2 occasions 3-6 months apart. Progressive decline in the glomerular filtration rate and after (GFR) and elevated arterial blood pressure.
- **Diabetic neuropathy:** Diabetic neuropathy is a type of nerve damage that can occur if you have diabetes. High blood sugar can injure nerve fibers throughout your body, but diabetic neuropathy most often damages nerves in your legs and feet.

Nursing Care of Diabetes Mellitus

- Administer insulin or OHA as per order.
- Monitor blood sugar and urine sugar.
- Provide emotional support.
- Instruct the client never skip the meal.
- Perform finger strip method to monitor blood glucose level.
- During stress or infection the OHA should be replaced by insulin.
- In case of urine testing perform the test before the meal and at bed time.
- During cold or flu do not omit the insulin because infection may cause increased blood sugar.
- Exercise is best performed after meals when the blood sugar level is rising.
- Teach the patient proper foot care.
  - Wash the legs with mild soap and water.
  - Cut the toe nails straight.
  - Purchase properly fitting shoes.
  - Apply some emollients to prevent dryness of the foot.
  - Corns should be treated under a podiatrist.

PANCREATITIS

It is the inflammation of the pancreas due to any viral infections, alcoholism or due to any metabolic disorders such as diabetes mellitus and hyperparathyoidism.

Clinical Manifestation

- Pain in the left upper quadrant
- Tachycardia
- Positive grey turner spot (Ecchymosis or bluish discoloration in the flank region)
- Cullen's sign (Bluish discoloration in the periumbilical area).

Diagnosis

- Increased serum amylase and lipase (5 times than normal)
- Normal serum amylase = 40-140U/L
- Normal serum lipase = 0-160 U/L
- Decreased serum calcium levels.

Nursing Care

- Administer analgesics as ordered, Demerol or meperidine
- Withhold food and fluids
- Eliminate the odor and site of food
- Provide knee-chest or fetal position for comfort
- Provide high calorie, high protein and low fat diet
- Avoid caffeine and alcohol.

CYSTIC FIBROSIS

It is an inflammation of the exocrine gland, commonly affecting the lungs, pancreas, liver and reproductive system.

Causes

- Unknown
- Genetic

Clinical Manifestation

- Cough
- Muscle cramps
- Night sweat
- Presence of more amount of salt in sweat.

Nursing Care

- Administer antibiotics as ordered.
- Perform sweat test, more amount of sodium chloride in the sweat.
- Provide high calorie, high protein diet and high fat diet.

CHAPTER 7

Gastrointestinal System

Chapter Objectives

- Keynotes in the gastrointestinal system
- Anatomy of gastrointestinal system
- Various diagnostic measures
- Disorders in the gastrointestinal system

KEY TERMS

SGOT   Dyspepsia
SGPT   Acidosis
CEA   Alkalosis
COL   Pylorus

KEYNOTES

- Sengstaken-Blakemore tube is used for esophageal varices.
- Pain after meals and relieved by food intake in duodenal ulcer.
- In upper GI bleeding the color of stool is black.
- The stool occult blood positive in patient with GI bleeding.
- Signs and symptoms of gastric ulcer is pain occurs 1-2 hours after meal.
- How to prevent dumping syndrome—avoid fluids during meal.
- Clay or grey colored stool is the manifestation of Cholelithiasis.
- Aluminium based antacid is used in constipation.
- Position used in liver biopsy is right lateral position or supine with hand flexed behind the head.
- Position used after nasogastric tube feeding Fowler's position.
- Color of stool and urine in hepatitis is light colored stool (stercobilinogen) dark colored urine (urobilinogen).
- Tender and rigid abdomen is seen in patient with Perforated peptic ulcer.
- Nursing care of a patient with abdominal paracentesis, ask the patient to empty the bladder before paracentesis.
- The 1st priority in post endoscopy—check gag reflex.
- Carbonated beverage cause gastritis.
- Morphine is contraindicated in pancreatitis and demerol is the drug of choice.
- Dimercaprol should not given to patient has peanut allergy.
- Provide fatty meal before ERCP (Endoscopic Retrograde Cholangio-Pancreatography) to drain bile from gallbladder.
- Ribbon shaped stool is seen in colorectal cancer.
- The acid base imbalance in vomiting is metabolic alkalosis.
- The acid base imbalance in diarrhea is metabolic acidosis.
- The acid base imbalance in hyperemesis gravidarum is metabolic acidosis.
- The pH of gastric juice is 1.5–3.5.
- The pH of saliva is same as that of pH of blood and pH of spinal fluid and it is 7.4.
- In case of colostomy application temporary colostomy is created on the ascending colon or transverse colon and permanent colostomy is created on the descending or sigmoid colon (To prevent fluid electrolyte imbalance).

- In case of intestinal obstruction there will be hyperactive bowel sound or high pitched bowel sound.
- In case of paralytic ileus we can hear low pitched bowel sound.
- Dyspepsia is also known as indigestion.
- Heart burn is also known as pyrosis.
- Brunner's gland which is seen in submucosa of duodenum secretes mucus.
- Normal flora (bacteria of intestinal tract) produce vitamin K helps to prevent bleeding disorders.
- "Kissing ulcers" are seen in first part of duodenum.
- Caput medusa is the dilated veins around the umbilicus seen in liver cirrhosis.
- Icterus is a sign of hepatic coma.
- Organ of the body which has greater width than length is caecum.
- Roving's sign is seen in acute appendicitis.
- "Rat tail" appearance on barium swallow examination is seen in carcinoma of esophagus.
- "Pseudo kidney sign" on USG is seen in Ca stomach.
- Administer vitamin K for a newborn soon after the delivery in order to prevent bleeding disorders because the intestinal tract of newborn are sterile, so there is no normal floras.
- Rapid loading of the small intestinal content with hyper-osmolar stomach content can lead to rapid entry of water into the intestine results in osmotic diarrhea, hypovolemia and cramping.
- Do not give pancreatic enzymes in an empty stomach.
- Administer pancreatic supplements with apple sauce. (Better absorbed with carbohydrate).
- Do not dilute dopamine and dobutamine with dextrose containing solutions.
- Normal color of stoma is pink to bright red, shining and slight swelling. Pale pink indicate low hemoglobin and low hematocrit. Black purple color indicate necrosis—notify it immediately to physician.
- While inserting the NG tube, patient becomes cyanosed, what will be the nurse's next action? Remove the tube and observe the patient.
- After cholecystectomy, why do we put NG tube? To relieve gastric compression.

ANATOMY

The food passes through a long tube inside the body known as the alimentary canal or the gastrointestinal tract (GI tract). The digestive system is a group of organs working together to convert food into energy and basic nutrients to feed the entire body. The alimentary canal is made up of the oral cavity, pharynx, esophagus, stomach, small intestines, and large intestines.

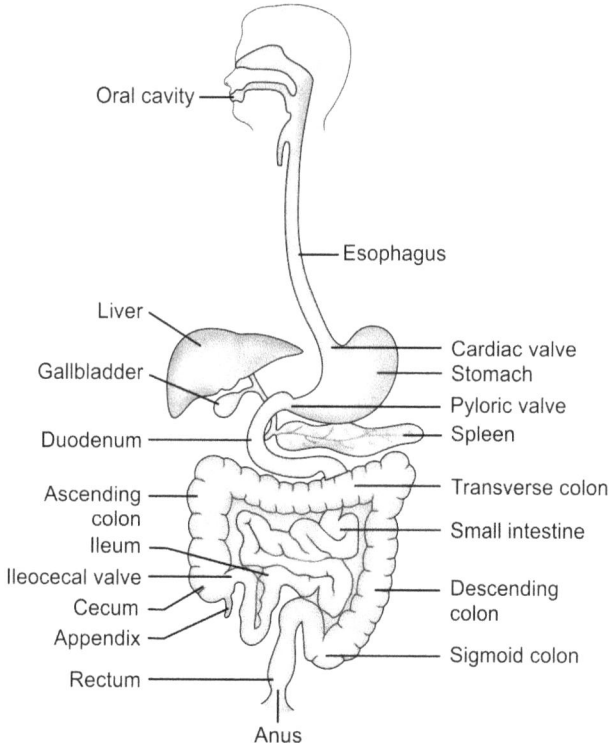

Fig. 1: Anatomy of gastrointestinal system

Mouth (Oral Cavity)

With the help of lips and oral cavity the food enters in to the digestive tract as seen in Figure 1.

Pharynx

It is the common passage for food and air, from the pharynx it is divided into two structures. The larynx and esophagus, the larynx is followed by the respiratory tract and esophagus is followed by the digestive tract.

Esophagus

It is called as the food pipe. The length of esophagus is 23–25 cm. There are two sphincters or valves, cardiac sphincter or lower esophgeal sphincter and the pyloric sphincter or valve. The cardiac sphincter is located between esophagus and stomach and the pyloric sphincter located between esophagus and duodenum as seen in Figure 1.

Stomach

Stomach is divided into three parts, the fundus, body and antrum as seen in Figure 2. Fundus is a portion of stomach which lies above the cardiac notch. The body is the main and central portion and the antrum is the lower part. The pylorus is considered as having two parts, the pyloric antrum (opening to the body of the stomach) and the pyloric canal (opening to the duodenum). The pyloric canal ends as the pyloric orifice, which marks the junction between the stomach and the duodenum.

Gastric juice is commonly seen at the antrum of the stomach and it is acidic in nature. The ph of gastric juice is 1.5 to 3.5. The commonest site of occurrence of peptic ulcer is the antrum of the stomach.

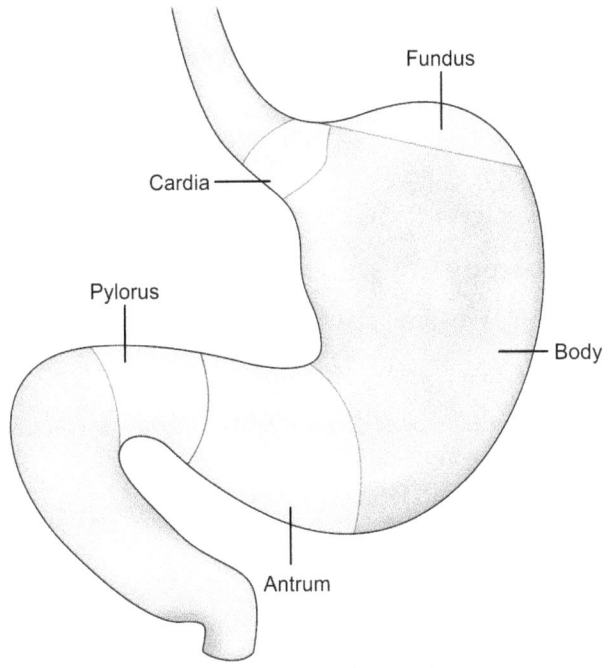

Fig. 2: Structure of stomach

Small Intestine

Small intestine or small bowel is the largest part (6 meters) of gastrointestinal tract which is seen between stomach and large intestine. The main functions of small intestine are digestion and absorption of nutrients. Villi are specialized structure which is seen in the small intestine helps in the absorption of nutrients. Small intestine is divided into three parts as seen in Figure 1.

- **Duodenum:** It is located at the junction of the stomach and the small intestine, the duodenum is the first part of the small intestine. It is C-shaped and about 25 cm long.
- **Jejunum:** It is the middle section of the small intestine that serves as the primary site of nutrient absorption. It measures around 3 feet in length.
- **Ileum:** The ileum is the final portion of the small intestine, which leads into the large intestine. The ileum measures 2–4 m in length.

Large Intestine

Large intestine or large bowel is the final part of gastrointestinal tract where the waste products from the food you eat are collected and processed into feces. It is 1.5 m long. It consists of caecum, colon and rectum as seen in Figure 1.

- **Caecum:** The caecum is the first part of the large intestine. Shaped like a small pouch and located in the right lower abdomen, it is the connection between the small intestine (ileum) and the colon. Between the ileum and caecum there is a junction called ileocaecal junction and from that junction a finger like projection protruded downward called as vermiform appendix.
- **Colon:** It is the longest part of the large intestine, Shaped like an inverted 'U'. The main function of colon is absorption of water. When the gastric content passes through various parts of colon water is absorbed and it becomes a hard fecal matter. Colon is divided into four sections as seen in Figure 1:
  - *Ascending colon*: It starts from the caecum at the bottom right hand side of the abdomen and ascends (i.e., goes upward) toward the liver.
  - *Transverse colon*: The transverse means 'across'. This part of the colon extends across the abdomen from right to left.
  - *Descending colon*: It descends (goes downwards) on the left hand side of the abdomen.
  - *Sigmoid colon* : It is the last part of the large intestine, and is located on the bottom left hand side of the abdomen. It is the S-shaped connection between the descending colon and the rectum.
  - *Rectum*: The rectum is the final part of the large intestine. It is where stool (feces) is stored before being passed as a bowel motion.

Functions of Large Intestine

- Absorption of water and electrolytes, as feces travels through the colon, the lining of the colon absorbs most of the water and some vitamins and minerals.
- The bacteria which is seen in the intestine called as normal flora helps in the production of vitamin K which helps in preventing bleeding disorders.

Regions of Abdomen

There are nine quadrants in the abdomen, they are as follows:

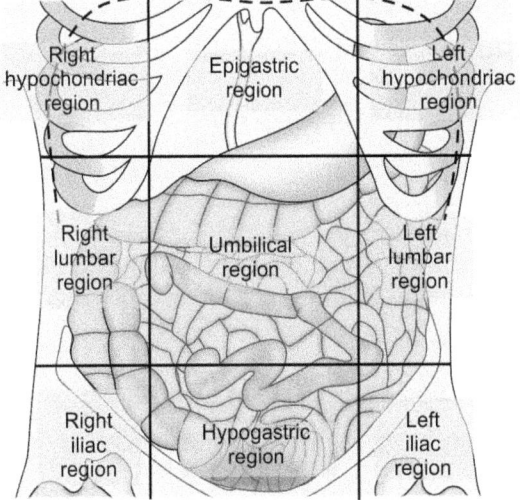

Specified pain sites in common conditions

Right hypochondriac	Epigastric	Left hypochondriac
Gallstones Stomach ulcer Pancreatitis	Stomach ulcer Heartburn Indigestion, hernia	Biliary colic Duodenal ulcer Hepatitis
Right lumbar	**Umbilical**	**Left lumbar**
Kidney stones, urinary infection, constipation hernia	Pancreatitis Early appendicitis Stomach ulcer Umbilical area	Kidney stones Constipation, IBS
Right iliac	**Hypogastrium**	**Left iliac**
Appendicitis Constipation Pelvic and groin pain	Urine infection Diverticulitis Inflammatory disease Fibroid and miscarriage Pelvic pain	IBS and crohn's disease Ovarian cyst Diverticular disease Pelvic pain

DIAGNOSTIC MEASURES

Blood Examination

- Complete blood count
- Serum electrolytes
- Serum bilirubin total 0.3-1.5 mg/dL
- Serum bilirubin direct normal value 0-0.3 mg/dL
- SGOT (Serum glutamic oxaloacetic transaminase) Normal level = 5-40 U/L
- SGPT (serum glutamic-pyruvic transaminase) normal level = 5-50 U/L
- CEA: The carcino embryonic antigen (CEA) test measures the amount of this protein that may appear in the blood of some people who have certain kinds of cancers, especially cancer of the large intestine (colon and rectal cancer). It may also be present in people with cancer of the pancreas, breast, ovary, or lung.

Upper GI Series

It is also called as barium meal or barium swallows. Client must allow to swallow the barium to rule out any abnormalities in the upper GI tract.

Nursing Care

- NPO from midnight
- Explain the patient the taste of barium is chalky
- Provide more fluids to wash out barium after the procedure

Lower GI Series or Barium Enema

Barium is instilled into the colon as enema.

Nursing Care

- Give soap and water enema in the morning of the test
- Provide more fluids after the procedure to wash out barium from the body because it is nephrotoxic.

Endoscopy

Direct visualization of the esophagus, stomach and duodenum by the insertion of a lighted endoscope to rule out any abnormalities or bleeding.

Nursing Care

- NPO for 6-8 hours
- Discourage speaking during the procedure.

Colonoscopy

Endoscopic visualization of large intestine.

Nursing Care

- Explain the patient that while inserting the endoscope a feeling of press might be experienced.
- Observe for any rectal bleeding.

Sigmoidoscopy

Sigmoidoscopy is an endoscopic procedure used to see inside the sigmoid colon and rectum.

Nursing Care

- Explain the procedure to the patient.
- Explain to the patient an urge to defecate or abdominal cramping may be experienced during the procedure.

Gastric Analysis

Gastric analysis is a method to measure secretion of hydrochloric acid under basal (Baseline) and augmented (stimulated) conditions. Insertion of a nasogastric tube to examine fasting gastric contents for acidity and volume.

Nursing Care

- NPO for 6-8 hours before the test.
- Avoid antacids and anticholinergics before the test.
- Avoid smoking before the test.
- While collecting the sample do not allow the gastric acid to touch with saliva to prevent buffering, so expectorate before sample collection (The pH of saliva is 7.4 and the pH of gastric acid is 1.5-3.5).

Liver Biopsy

A specially designed needle is inserted into the liver to remove a small piece of tissue for study purpose.

Nursing Care

- NPO 6-8 hours before the test.
- Instruct the client to hold breath during the procedure.
- Position the patient to right lateral side or spine with hand flexed behind the head or make the person lies face up on a table and rests the right hand above the head (percutaneous liver biopsy).

Oral Cholecystogram or Cholecystography

Oral cholecystography is a procedure used to visualize the gallbladder by administering radiopaque contrast agent that is excreted by the liver. It is used to assess the patency of biliary duct.

Nursing Care

- Check for any allergy to dye (iodine)
- Offer a low fat meal before the test
- Observe the side effect of dye (diarrhea).

GAVAGE AND LAVAGE

Gastric Gavage (Feeding)

Gastric gavage is the introduction of food or fluids into the stomach for the nourishment of the body by means of a tube passed through the nose or mouth or through a surgically created hole in the person's neck, chest, stomach or intestine.

Indications

- Gastrointestinal diseases and surgery.
- Hypermetabolic states such as burns, multiple trauma, sepsis or cancer.
- Certain neurological conditions such as stroke or coma.
- Any surgery to neck, head or esophagus.

Types

Nasogastric Tube (NG Tube)

A tube is placed in either nostril, passed down the pharynx through the esophagus and to the stomach.

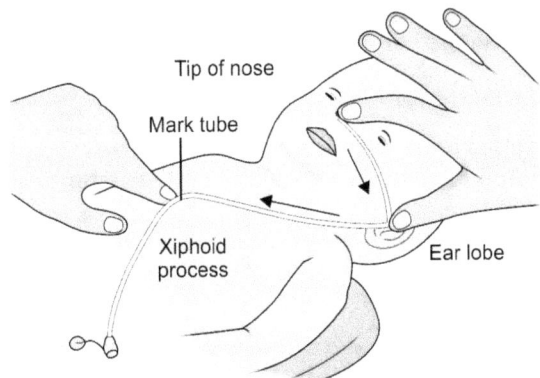

Fig. 3: Nasogastric tube

- To measure the lengths of the tube calculate the length from the tip of nose to the ear lobe and from the ear lobe to the xiphoid process as seen in Figure 3.
- The length of tube is 36-45 inch.
- Example of NG tube is Levin's single lumen catheter, salem-sump tube.

Nursing Care

- Check the length of the tube before insertion.
- Check the patency of the tube, either by aspirating the gastric contents or dip the tube in a glass of water or auscultate the sound after pushing the air.
- Aspirate the gastric contents before each feeding, do not discard the aspirated content to prevent metabolic alkalosis, so reinsert the content back.
- After gastrectomy place an NG tube to prevent gastric decompression and that should be left open. Expect bloody drainage for first 24 hours. If there is any clot in the tube, administer bicarbonate beverages in order to dislodge the clot (e.g. A drop of Cola or Sprite).
- While removing the NG tube instruct the patient to hold the breath or follow valsalva maneuver (to prevent the friction inserting on the tube by epiglottis).
- Check the amount of feeding in each time (Suppose doctor ordered to give 90 mL of feed every 4 hours, before the next feeding if you are getting 40 mL back then remaining 50 mL need to administer).

Nasojejunal Tube (NJ Tube)

A tube is inserted via the nostril through the stomach into the jejunum as seen in Figure 4.

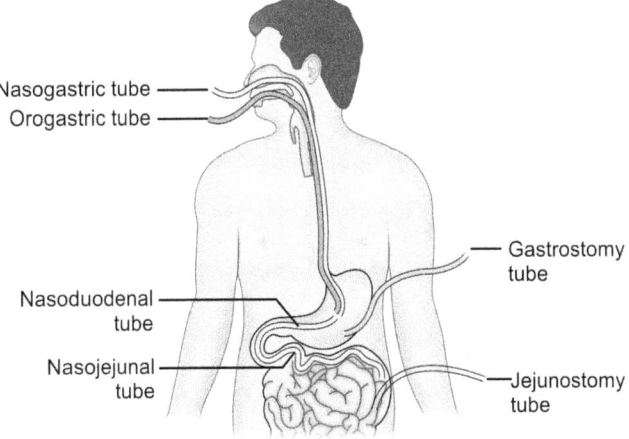

Fig. 4: Nasojejunal tube

- To facilitate proper placement of the tube, fowlers position up to the stomach, right side position through the stomach and supine position up to the jejunum.
- NJ tube is inserted under fluoroscopic guidance.
- Example of NJ tubes are miller Abbott or cantor tube.

Gastrostomy Tube

- The tube goes directly into the stomach through the skin, it is surgically inserted into the abdominal wall.
- It is used for the delivery of enteral nutrition.
- Monitor and maintain the skin integrity.
- Administer feeding in high Fowler's position and maintain head of bed elevation 30 minutes after meals.

Jejunostomy Tube

- The tube is surgically implanted in the upper section of the small intestine called the jejunum which is just below the stomach.
- It is used to be fed directly into the intestinal tract, the patient must always be fed with an enteral feeding pump.

Gastric Lavage (Washing)

A procedure used to empty the stomach of its contents performed using a flexible rubber tube that is passed through the mouth and advanced to the stomach. The procedure includes the instillation of a balanced salt solution into the stomach via the tube. It is an effective procedure used for the treatment of toxic ingestion. An alternative for gastric lavage is the oral administration of activated carbon or charcoal (50-100 gm).

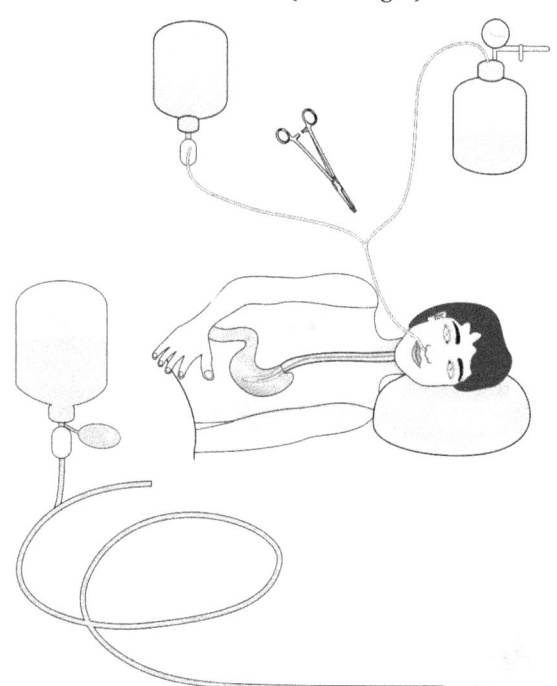

- Insert a large bore double lumen orogastric catheter.
- Aspirate gastric contents.
- Use a small cycle lavage of 50-100 mL and aspirate it.
- Monitor for complications such as aspiration pneumonia, hypoxia, bradycardia.

ENEMA

It is the process of cleansing the lower gastrointestinal tract by the injection of liquid into the lower bowel through the rectum (as seen in the below picture). It is otherwise known as a technique for the evacuation of stool.

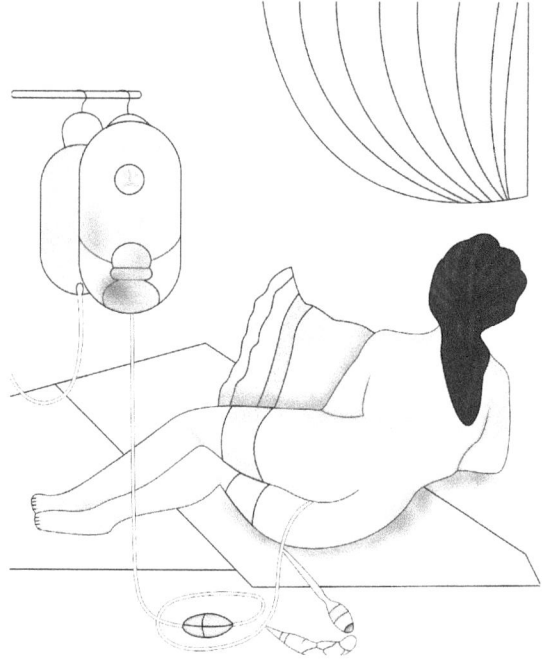

Types of Enema

Cleansing Enema

- It is also known as soap and water enema.
- The length of insertion of rectal tube is 4–5 inch.
- The height, if enema can is 18 inch (45 cm).
- Amount of solution is 500-1000 mL
- Temperature of solution is 105-110° F.

Retention Enema

- It is also known as proctoclysis enema.
- Amount of solution 150-200 mL (Oil used instead of water).
- Temperature of solution is normal body temperature.

Nursing Care

- Explain the procedure to the patient.
- Provide proper positioning (left lateral or sim's lateral position).

Nursing Care

- Maintain a proper airway.
- Make the patient to lie on left side.

- Teach the patient in case of self enema administration (use left lateral position).
- Drape the patient properly and use water proof pad under the buttocks.
- Instruct the client to hold the solution for at least 30 minutes in case of retention enema.
- Observe for any abdominal cramping, if any cramping develops in between enema administration do not stop the enema, reduce the height of enema can to decrease the force or speed of instillation.
- Monitor the color and amount of stool.
- Observe the electrolyte levels if the patient is undergoing repeated enema.

DISORDERS

Cancer Mouth

Cancer which occurs in lips and oral cavity, if any sore or mouth ulcer which is not healed for prolonged time should be further rule out for cancer or CEA.

Causes

- Smoking
- Alcoholism
- Substance abuse

Clinical Manifestation

- Red color patches or erythroplakia
- White color patches or leukoplakia
- Bleeding from the mouth
- Numbness in the mouth
- Difficulty in swallowing
- Hoarseness of voice

Nursing Care

- Provide side-lying position
- Avoid suctioning in lip surgery
- Provide mouth care with normal saline or sodium bicarbonate solution
- Avoid the use of commercial mouth preparations, lemon or glycerine swabs
- Prepare the patient for chemotherapy and radiation therapy

Cancer Esophagus

Cancer which is seen in the esophagus or food pipe.

Causes

- Cigarette smoking
- Alcoholism
- Repeated GERD (gastroesophageal reflux disease)
- Hypotonia of the sphincter

Clinical Manifestation

- Dysphagia
- Substernal burning sensation after drinking hot fluids
- Weight loss
- Barium swallow shows a mass.

Nursing Care

- Provide NG tube feeding.
- Expect bloody drainage for the first 12 hours and gradually changes to yellow or green.
- Provide semi fowler's position before and after 2 hours of feeding.

Gastritis

It is the acute inflammation of the gastric mucosa; it may be acute or chronic:
- Acute gastritis (due to food allergy or NSAID or steroid therapy).
- Chronic gastritis (due to any rotavirus infections or repeated *H. pylori* infections).

Clinical Manifestation

- Nausea and vomiting
- Diarrhea
- Abdominal pain
- Vitamin B_{12} deficiency in case of chronic gastritis.

Nursing Care

- Monitor for dehydration
- Provide oral rehydration therapy
- Administer IV fluids
- Administer vitamin B_{12} injections for life long to prevent pernicious anemia.

Peptic Ulcer

Ulcer or open sore that develop on the inside lining of esophagus, stomach and the upper portion of small intestine. The most common symptom of a peptic ulcer is abdominal pain.

Causes

- Repeated *H. pylori* infection
- Stress (peptic ulcer is also known as stress ulcer)
- Prolonged use of NSAID or steroids
- Smoking and alcoholism

Peptic ulcers include:
- *Gastric ulcers* that occur on the inside of the stomach.
- *Esophageal ulcers* that occur inside the hollow tube (esophagus) that carries food from your throat to your stomach.

- *Duodenal ulcers* that occur on upper portion of small intestine (duodenum).

Gastric Ulcer

Ulcer formation in the mucosal lining of stomach, common site is antrum of stomach.

Clinical Manifestations

- Pain in the epigastric region, radiating to back and usually occurs immediately after food.
- Weight loss
- Bleeding
- Decreased hemoglobin and hematocrit levels.
- Black tarry stool

Esophageal Ulcer

Ulcer formation on the mucosal lining of the esophagus or food pipe.

Clinical Manifestation

- Pain when swallowing or trouble swallowing
- Heartburn (pain behind the breastbone)
- Nausea and vomiting
- Chest pain

Duodenal Ulcer

Ulcer formation on the mucosal lining of the duodenum, first 2 cm of duodenum.

Clinical Manifestation

- Pain in the midepigastric region
- Burning or cramping pain occurs within 2-4 hours after meal and relieved by food intake.

Diagnosis

- Endoscopy
- Barium swallow
- Gastric analysis (in gastric ulcer pH is normal and in duodenal ulcer pH is low).
- Guaiac test (stool occult blood positive).

Nursing Care

- Administer antacids
- Teach the patient proper stress management strategies
- Administer medications 1 hour before food or 2 hour after food or empty stomach
- Avoid ulcerogenic foods such as caffeine, alcohol or highly seasoned food items
- Avoid stressful situations
- Avoid bedtime snacks
- Prepare the patient for surgical correction.

Medical Management of Gastric Ulcer

1. **Antacids:** There are two types:
   - *Aluminium containing antacids:* E.g. Amphogel, the side effect of aluminium containing antacid is constipation.
   - *Magnesium containing antacids:* E.g. Milk of magnesia, the side effect is diarrhea.

   MD in AC

M	Magnesium containing antacid
D	Diarrhea
A	Aluminium containing antacid
C	Constipation

2. **H_2 receptor antagonist:** E.g. Ranitidine, cimetidine, famotidine.
3. **Proton pump inhibitor:** E.g. pantoprazole, omeprazole, omez, esmoprazole.
4. **Sucralfate:** E.g. Sucralfate or sucrafil, it forms a paste on the ulcer area which does not allow the food to contact with ulcer area.

Surgical Management of Gastric Ulcer

- *Vagotomy*, removal of the vagus nerve, the sensory part to decrease the pain.
- *Bilroth I (gastroduodenostomy)*, removal of the diseased portion of the stomach and remaining part anastomosed to the duodenum.
- *Bilroth II (gastrojejunostomy)*, removal of diseased portion of the stomach and remaining part anastomosed to the jejunum.

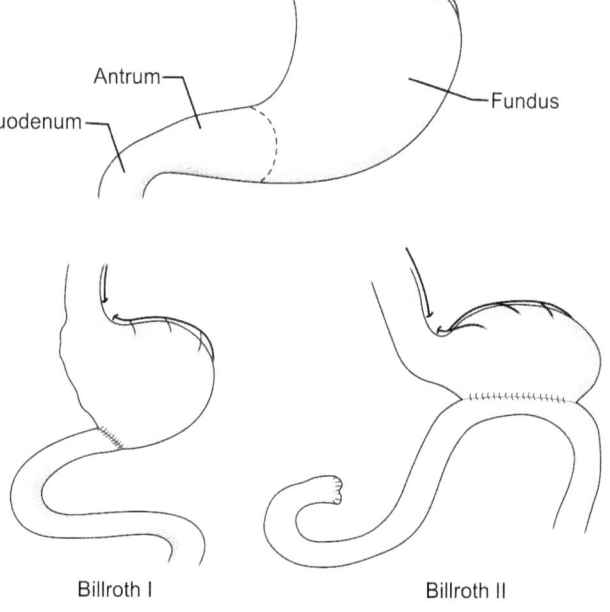

- **Gastrectomy:** Removal of 60–80% of stomach.

Cirrhosis of Liver

Liver

Liver is the largest excretory organ. The weight if liver is 1.5 kg, in cirrhosis of liver the weight is up to 10 kg.

Functions of Liver

- Production of bile
- Storage of iron
- Detoxification of toxins
- Conversion of waste products of metabolism

Portal Circulation

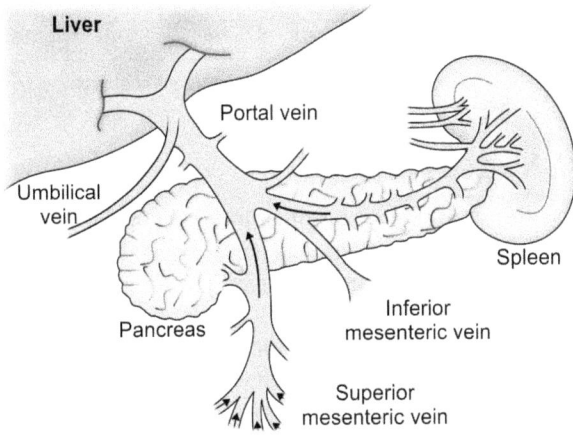

Fig. 5: Portal circulation

The deoxygenated blood enters into the liver from the gastrointestinal tract through the portal veins for detoxification. This circulation is called as portal circulation as seen in Figure 5.

Cirrhosis of Liver (COL) is the progressive damage to the liver cells due to any viral, bacterial or due to any toxic effects of drugs.

Types

1. *Laennec's cirrhosis:* It is also called as alcoholic cirrhosis, due to alcoholism
2. *Biliary cirrhosis:* Due any biliary infection
3. *Post necrotic cirrhosis:* Due to any viral infection
4. *Cardiac cirrhosis:* Due to any right ventricular failure.

Clinical Manifestation

- Nausea and vomiting
- Hepatomegaly and Jaundice
- Pain in the right upper quadrant
- Spider angiomas (swollen blood vessels)
- Palmar erythema (redness over the hands, trunk, etc)
- Asterixis (flapping tremor or liver flap)
- Fetor hepaticus (ammonia odor in breath)
- Changes in mood

Complications

1. **Ascites:** Accumulation of blood or fluid in the peritoneal cavity.

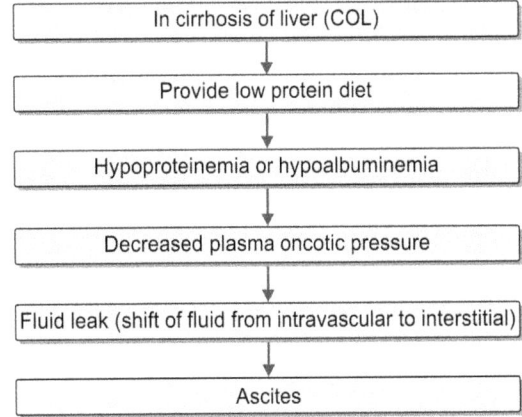

2. **Esophageal varices (vomiting of blood)**
   Why there will be vomiting of blood in the last stage of cirrhosis of liver or alcoholism?

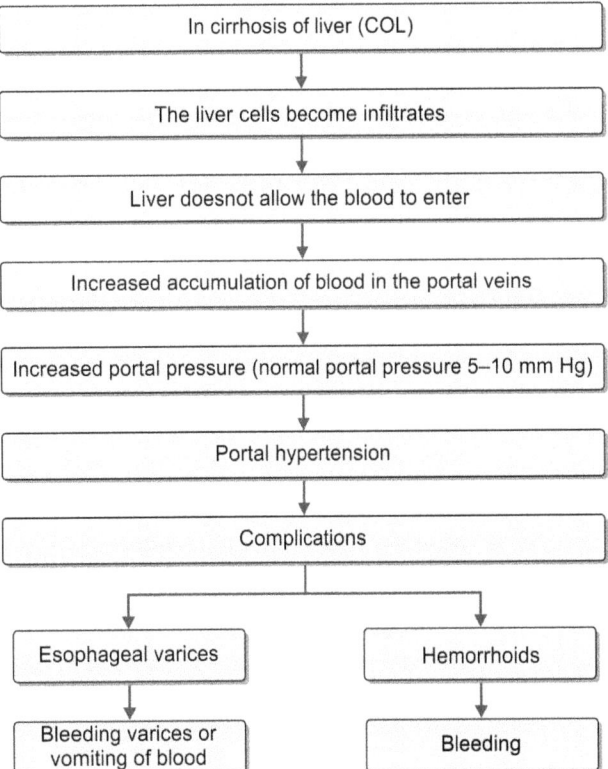

3. **Coagulation disorders**

   Why the doctors instruct the nurse to monitor for coagulation studies (PT with INR)?

   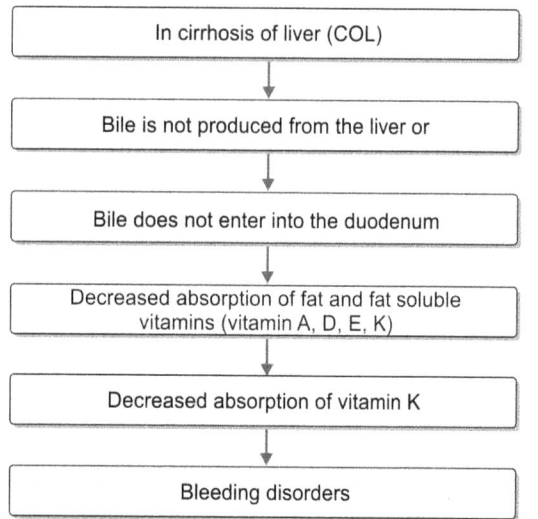

4. **Asterixis**

   It is also known as flapping tremor.
   Why the doctor instruct the nurse to give low protein diet in cirrhosis of liver?

   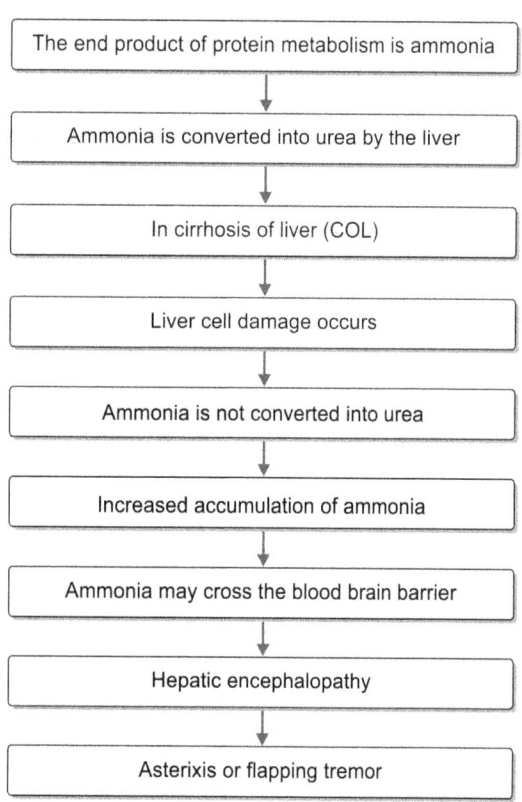

5. **Fetor hepaticus**

   Why the doctors instruct the nurse to administer lactulose syrup for COL?

   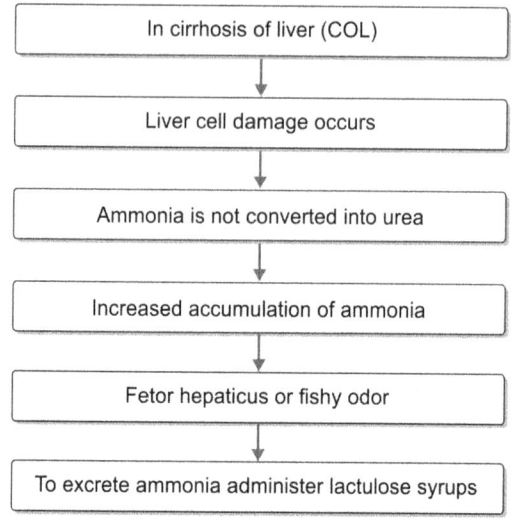

Nursing Care

- Monitor for any complications such as bleeding.
- Administer vitamin K as per order to prevent bleeding.
- Monitor coagulation profile.
- Provide low protein diet.
- Provide emotional support.
- Restrict sodium intake 200–500 mg per day.
- Measure the abdominal girth.
- Provide high fowler's position.
- Administer lactulose syrups to excrete ammonia from the body through the feces.
- Administer albumin injections to overcome hypoalbuminemia thereby increases the plasma oncotic pressure and prevent fluid leak.
- Prepare the patient for abdominal paracentesis (insertion of a needle into the peritoneal cavity through the abdomen and remove the excess fluids, position the patient supine with slight elevation of head).
- Prepare the patient for shunt creation (peritoneal venous shunt, permits the ascitic fluid back into the venous system through a silicon catheter.

Esophageal Varices

It is the dilated and tortuous veins on the either side of the esophagus, bleeding varices are an acute emergency.

Causes

- Portal hypertension
- Cirrhosis of liver

Clinical Manifestation

- Bleeding or vomiting of blood
- Melena
- Signs of shock in case of severe bleeding
- Black tarry color stool

Nursing Care

- Monitor for bleeding
- Blakemore- Sengstaken tube or Sengstaken-Blakemore tube is used for the treatment of oesophageal varices, if the patient feels respiratory distress while inflating the tube removes the tube immediately or cut the tube immediately, so keep scissors ready in the emergency tray while dilating.
- Administer cold saline to stop bleeding
- Administer IV fluids
- Provide head of bed elevation
- Administer vasoconstrictors to control bleeding
- Prepare the patient for sclerotherapy or endoscopic ligation.

Hemorrhoids

It is the swollen or dilated veins in the anal canal; it may be internal hemorrhoids (above the anal sphincter), external (below the anal sphincter) or prolapsed hemorrhoids.

Causes

- Increased intra-abdominal pressure
- Pregnancy
- Heavy manual labor
- Portal hypertension
- Cirrhosis of liver
- Excessive straining for stools

Clinical Manifestation

- Rectal bleeding
- Rectal pain
- Rectal itching

Nursing Care

- Treat the underline cause
- Apply cold packs in the anal area
- Encourage high fiber diet
- Administer stool softeners (lactulose or dulcolax)
- Administer medications such as sitcom (euphorbia prostrate) or pilex to reduce the size and swelling.
- Prepare the patient for hemorrhoidectomy (surgical removal of hemorrhoids).
- After hemorrhoidectomy provide ice packs to reduce swelling, sitz bath to reduce the discomfort, and medication to get relief from pain.
- Provide flat position for the first hour following surgery to reduce the risk of anesthesia induced headache.
- Provide flat position in case of any respiratory distress postoperatively.
- Avoid heavy lifting for 2-3 weeks.

Cholecystitis

Cholecystitis is inflammation of the gallbladder. Gallbladder is a small, pear-shaped organ on the right side of your abdomen, beneath your liver as seen in Figure 6. The gallbladder secretes bile to the duodenum which helps in the absorption of fats:

- Acute cholecystitis is due to gallbladder stones (cholelithiasis).
- Chronic cholecystitis is due to bile infection (inefficient bile emptying).

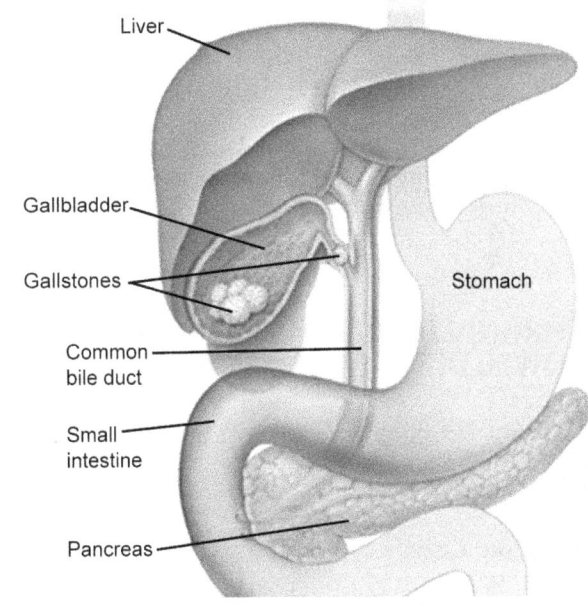

Fig. 6: Structure of gallbladder

Causes

- Gallbladder stones
- Any tumor
- Blockage in the bile duct

Clinical Manifestation

- Nausea and vomiting
- Indigestion
- Pain in the right upper quadrant
- Tenderness on the abdomen while palpation
- Fever
- Murphy's sign (when the examiner fingers are passed below the hepatic margin the patient cannot take a breath because of severe pain)
- Severe epigastric pain radiates to back and scapula 2-4 hours after eating a fatty meal
- Manifestations of jaundice.

Nursing Care

- Prepare the patient for cholecystectomy or choledocostomy.
- Cholecystectomy is the removal of gallbladder and insertion of a 'T' tube into the common bile duct, if common bile duct (CBD) exploration is performed.
- Choledocostomy is the removal of gallbladder stone and insertion of a 'T' tube into the common bile duct, if common bile duct (CBD) exploration is performed.
- Provide semi-fowler or sideline position.
- Monitor the function of 'T' tube.
- Monitor the amount of drainage, normal drain 300-500 mL for the first 24 hours (up to 750-900 mL) followed by 200 mL per day.
- Monitor the color of stool. (After the insertion of 'T' tube there will be manifestations of light colored stool, if there is any clay colored stool it indicates some obstruction in the 'T' tube).
- Educate the patient after the removal of 'T' tube the stool will appear as normal color.
- Ensure that the 'T' tube is connected to the closed gravity drainage system.
- Instruct the patient to resume their normal activities within 2 weeks in case of laparoscopic surgery.

CHRONIC INFLAMMATORY BOWEL DISORDERS

It is the chronic inflammation of all parts of the digestive tract. It primary includes ulcerative colitis and Crohn's disease.

Ulcerative Colitis

It affects mainly the colon and rectum. Inflammation primarily affects the rectosigmoid junction and spread upward.

Causes

- Stressful situation
- Autoimmune
- Hereditary

Clinical Manifestations

- Severe diarrhea, 15-20 liquid stools per day containing blood, mucus and pus.
- Weight loss
- Abdominal pain and cramping

Crohn's Disease

It is also called as regional enteritis; it affects both small intestine and large intestine (ileum, caecum and ascending colon).

Causes

- Unknown
- Food allergy
- Autoimmune

Clinical Manifestations

- Nausea and vomiting
- Pain in the right lower quadrant
- 3-4 semi-solid stools per day with cast, mucus and pus
- Steatorrhea (presence of fat in the feces)
- Abdominal pain and distension.

Nursing Care

- Monitor the fluid electrolyte levels
- Administer high calorie, high vitamin, low fiber diet.
- Administer antidiarrheals (Loparamide, Lomotil, Imodium).
- Perform stool examination.
- Administer antimicrobials such as metronidazole, sulfasalazine, etc.
- Administer corticosteroids.
- Administer immunosuppressants such as cyclosporine (Panimun-bioral), azathioprine (Azoran).
- Prepare the patient for bowel surgeries.

Intestinal Obstruction

Any obstruction in the passage of intestinal contents is called as intestinal obstruction.

Causes

- Due to any hernia or volvulus (mechanical obstruction)
- Due to any impairment in nerves supply (neurogenic obstruction)
- Due to any electrolyte imbalances such as hypokalemia
- Due to any impairment in blood supply (vascular obstruction).

Clinical Manifestation

- High pitched bowel sounds above the level of obstruction and low pitched bowel sound below the level of obstruction.
- In case of small intestinal obstruction non-fecal type of vomiting and in case of large intestinal obstruction fecal type of vomiting (presence of feces or waste products in vomitus).

Nursing Care

- Maintain fluid and electrolyte balance
- Provide high fowler's position
- Auscultate for bowel sound or peristaltic movements
- Prepare the patient for bowel surgeries.

Diverticulum and Diverticulosis

Diverticulum is an outpouching of the intestinal mucosa, occurs commonly in the sigmoid colon. Diverticulosis is the multiple outpouching of the intestinal mucosa. Diverticulitis is the inflammation of diverticulum.

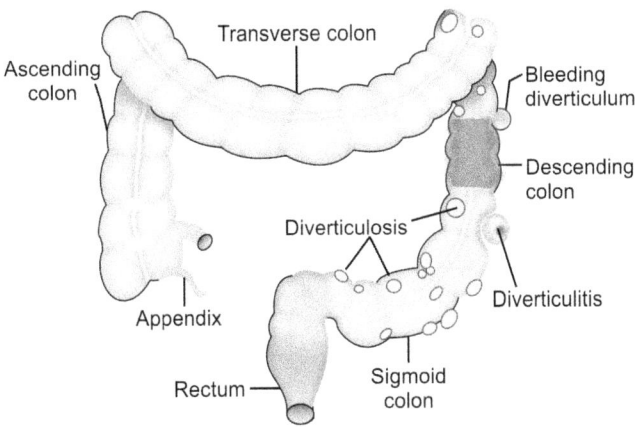

Causes

- Unknown
- Eating low fiber rich diets
- Straining due to prolonged constipation

Clinical Manifestation

- Alternate diarrhea and constipation
- Pain in the left lower quadrant
- Rectal bleeding
- Fever in diverticulitis

Nursing Care

- In case of diverticulosis provide high fiber diet with no seeds.
- In case of diverticulitis provide low fiber diet.
- Avoid use of laxatives and enema.
- Prepare the patient for bowel surgeries.

Colon Cancer

Colon cancer is cancer of the large intestine (colon), the lower part of the digestive tract. Adenocarcinoma is the most common type of colon cancer which metastasis to liver. It is the second most common cancer in men and women.

Causes

- Hereditary
- Familial tendency
- Diverticulitis
- Ulcerative colitis

Clinical Manifestation

- Alternate diarrhea and constipation
- Weight loss
- Anorexia
- Abdominal distension
- Rectal bleeding or blood in the stool

Nursing Care

- Monitor the laboratory reports (CEA).
- Monitor stool occult blood for positive.
- Perform barium enema test, it shows a mass.
- Prepare for sigmoidoscopy, it shows a mass.
- Prepare the patient for digital rectal examination, it shows a mass.
- Provide chemotherapy and radiation therapy.
- Prepare the patient for bowel surgeries.

BOWEL SURGERIES

AP Resection (Abdominoperineal Resection)

An abdominoperineal resection is a surgery in which the anus, rectum, and sigmoid colon are removed. This procedure is most often used to treat cancers located rectum or anus. Once the anus and rectum are removed, a permanent colostomy is created.

Ileostomy

An Ileostomy is the opening of the ileum through the abdominal wall usually on the right lower side of abdomen. It is most commonly performed in ulcerative colitis.

Kock Pouch

An intra-abdominal reservoir is created inside the abdomen with a nipple valve which acts as a reservoir for the fecal matter as seen in Figure 7. A catheter is inserted through the stoma to remove the fecal matter.

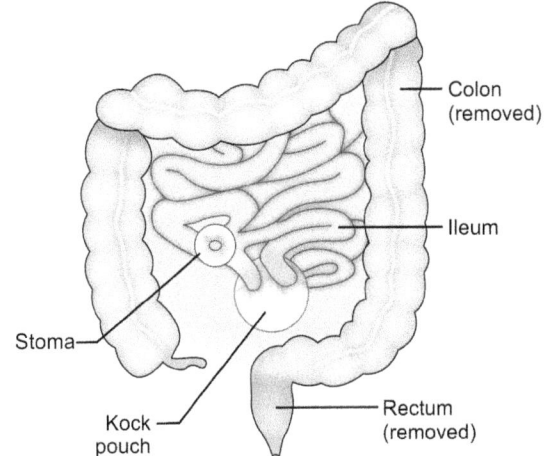

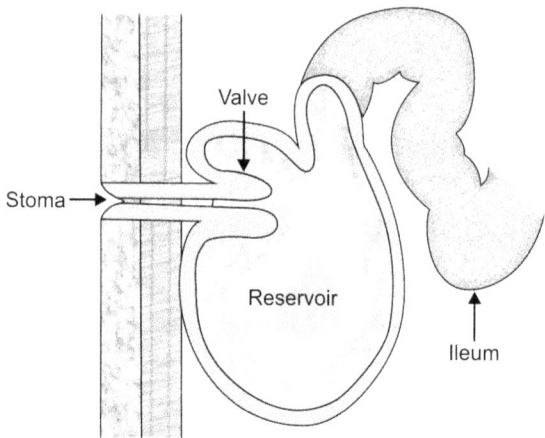

Fig. 7: Kock pouch

Colostomy

Colostomy is a surgical procedure which brings the end of the large intestine or colon into the abdominal wall through an opening or stoma. There are mainly two types of colostomy. Temporary colostomy is created in the ascending or transverse colon and permanent colostomy is created on the sigmoid colon or descending colon.

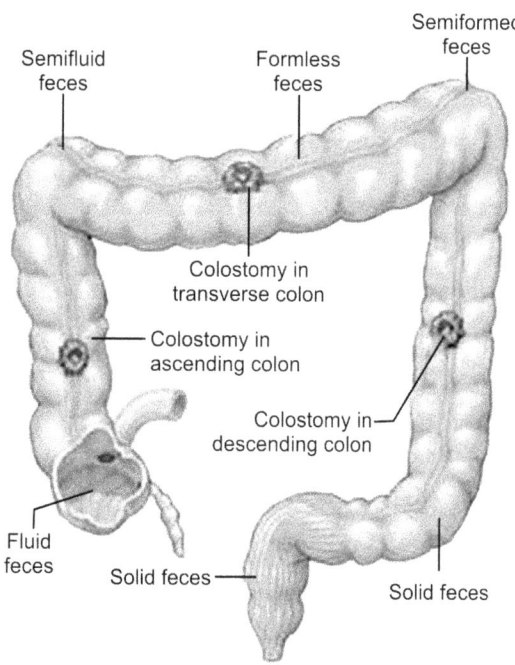

Nursing Care (Preoperative)

- Monitor the laboratory values
- Monitor the fluid and electrolyte balance
- Administer antibiotics 3-5 days prior to surgery
- Administer cleansing enema before surgery
- Administer vitamin C and vitamin K to prevent post-operative complications.

Nursing Care (Postoperative)

- Monitor the stoma site for any discharge or bleeding.
- Cleanse the skin around stoma with mild soap and water.
- Change the pouch or seal only when necessary, but empty the pouch frequently when it is half filled.
- Assess the stoma color for any infection, normally the stoma is moist and pink.
- Irrigate the colostomy as per order.
- Provide high fowler's position or toilet seat position while irrigating.
- Irrigate with normal saline (600-1000 mL).

Teaching Points

- Report any change in the odor and color of stoma
- Report any bleeding from stoma.
- Expect mucus or serosanguineous drainage for first 24 hours.
- Teach the patients that charcoal tablets or anti-flatulent preparations may help to reduce odor.
- Limit intake of foods that have strong odors, such as onions, fish, eggs, cheese and asparagus.
- Eat a low-residue diet for the first couple of months to reduce the strain on your bowels and stoma. It might be a good idea to avoid certain foods, such as popcorn or celery seeds.
- Once you have fully recovered (usually around three months after surgery), there are no restrictions on your diet.
- Teach colostomy irrigation.

Colostomy	Ileostomy
Created on the large intestine (colon)	Created on the small intestine (ileum)
Can irrigate colostomy	Cannot irrigate ileostomy
Stools are hard	Stools are liquid type

CA STOMACH (STOMACH CANCER)

Stomach cancer is also known as gastric cancer, is a condition in which malignant cells form in the lining of stomach. CA stomach is more common in people over 65 years of age(common in men between 50-70 years). There are mainly two types of stomach cancer.

- ***Adenocarcinoma***: Starts in the gland cells that line the stomach, is a most common type, more than 90% of stomach cancers are adenocarcinoma.

- **Squamous cell cancers:** These are the skin type cells that sit between the gland cells and the stomach lining.

Causes

- Diet low in quantity of vegetables
- Repeated *H. pylori* infections
- Eating high salted and smoked foods
- Smoking
- Absence of HCL in stomach (achlorhydria)
- Excessive tyramine rich diet

Clinical Manifestation

- Weight loss
- Fatigue, indigestion and feeling of fullness in the stomach
- Palpable epigastric mass
- Nausea and vomiting
- Hemetemesis
- Guaiac test positive

Nursing Care

- Monitor for the presence of CEA.
- Prepare for gastroscopy, barium meal and biopsy examinations.
- Prepare for radiation therapy, chemotherapy and surgical correction.
- Prepare the patient for gastric surgeries.
- In general, total removal of the stomach (gastrectomy) is performed in patients with cancer affecting the upper third of the stomach. Partial gastrectomy can be performed in cases where the cancer is located lower.

DUMPING SYNDROME

Dumping syndrome is a common complication seen after gastrectomy. It is due to the abrupt emptying of the stomach contents into the intestine. Earlier it occurs as a result of fat digestion and later due to carbohydrate indigestion. It appears within 15–30 minutes after meals and last for 20–60 minutes.

Causes

- Gastrectomy
- Esopahgectomy

Clinical Manifestation

- Feeling of fullness
- Abdominal discomfort
- Nausea and vomiting
- Rapid heart rate and palpitation

Nursing Care

- Avoid high concentrated sweats.
- Provide small meals in a day (6 small meals in a day).
- Avoid fluids during the meals or with the meals.
- Provide supine or recumbent position at least half hour after meals.

HEPATITIS

Hepatitis is a medical condition characterized by inflammation of the liver and results in jaundice. It can be caused by viral or non-viral causes. There are different types of hepatitis such as hepatitis A, B, C, D, E and G.

Causes

- Any viral infections
- Alcoholism
- Toxic effects of drugs
- Autoimmune

Clinical Manifestation

- Appearance of jaundice
- Fever, nausea, vomiting
- Dark urine
- Painful joints
- Edema

Stages of Hepatitis

Pre-icteric Stage

- It is the first stage of hepatitis
- Includes flue like symptoms such as cold, fever.

Icteric Stage

- It is the second stage of hepatitis
- Appearance of jaundice, elevated bilirubin level (more than 1.5 mg/dL)
- Increased SGOT and SGPT
- Increased alanine transaminase (ALT)
- Increased aspartate transaminase (AST)
- Increased alkaline phosphatase

Post-icteric Stage

- It is the final stage of hepatitis
- The serum levels returns
- Urine and stool color returns to normal.

	Hepatitis A	Hepatitis B	Hepatitis C
Mode of transmission	Communicable hepatitis. Transmission is fecal-oral route, contaminated food and water	Infectious hepatitis (dangerous). Blood and blood products, sexual contacts, mother to fetus	Post-transfusion hepatitis. Blood transfusion or dialysis common in CRF
Diagnosis	HAV (Hepatitis A virus)	HbSAg (Hepatitis B virus antigen)	HCV (Hepatitis C virus)
Incubation period	Incubation period 2–6 weeks (15–45 days)	6–24 weeks (50–180 days)	2–26 weeks (5–50 days)
Vaccine	Vaccine is Havrix A	Engerix B	No vaccine
Prevention	Disposal of waste. Proper handwashing	Blood precautions universal precautions	Proper donor screening, universal precaution

Nursing Care

- Provide proper nutrition
- Provide high calorie, high carbohydrate, high protein and high vitamin diet
- Provide proper isolation
- Administer immunoglobulins as per order
- Monitor the laboratory values
- Administer corticosteroids
- Administer vaccines as per order
- Perform proper donor screening while administering blood
- Administer liver supplements such as limarin (Silymarin) or udiliv (Ursodeoxycholic Acid) to maintain liver enzymes normal.

Teaching Point

- Teach the patient about the importance of avoiding alcohol
- Proper disposal of waste
- Maintain proper hand washing and sanitation techniques
- Avoid unwanted sexual activities to prevent the transmission
- If anyone is exposed to infection take immediate precautions or treatment (if any nurse gets needle prick injury from hepatitis B patient immediately take post-exposure prophylaxis of hepatitis B immunoglobulin)
- Educate the patient about proper dietary instructions.

HERNIA

Hernia is the protrusion of an organ through the weakened abdominal wall. The most common site is the groin accounted for nine out of 10 hernias.

Causes

- Weakened muscles of abdomen
- Increased abdominal pressure
- Heavy lifting
- Persistent coughing or sneezing

Clinical Manifestation

- A visible lump or a swollen area
- Abdominal pain and abdominal distension during exertion or bowel movements
- A heavy or uncomfortable feeling in the gut, particularly when bending over
- Digestive upsets, such as constipation
- The lump disappears when the person is lying down and it enlarges upon coughing, straining or standing up.

Types of Hernia (Fig. 8)

- *Inguinal hernia:* The intestine or bladder protrudes through the abdominal wall or to the inguinal canal in the groin, most common type, about 96 % or groin hernias are inguinal.
- *Femoral hernia:* The intestine enters the canal carrying the femoral artery into the upper thigh. Femoral hernias are most common in women, especially those who are pregnant or obese.
- *Umbilical hernia:* A part of the small intestine passes through the abdominal wall near the navel. Common in newborns.
- *Incisional hernia:* The intestine pushes through the abdominal wall at the site of previous abdominal surgery.
- *Hiatal hernia:* The upper stomach squeezes through the hiatus, an opening in the diaphragm through which the esophagus passes.
- *Reducible hernia:* It can be manually placed into the abdominal cavity.
- *Irreducible hernia:* It cannot be placed back into the abdominal cavity.

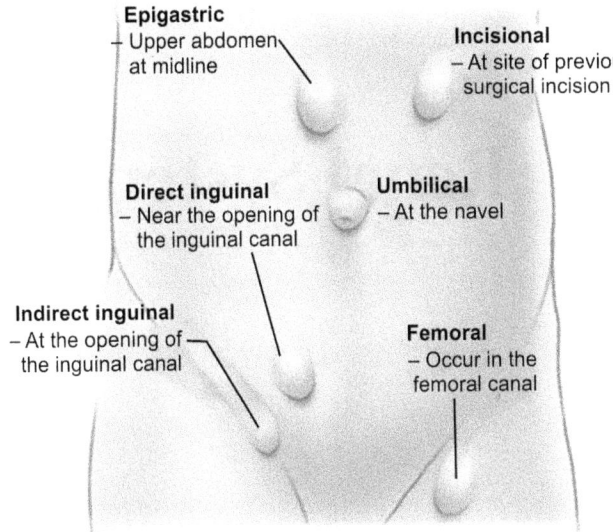

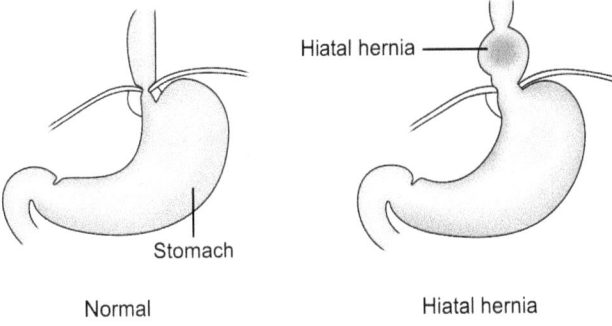

Fig. 8: Major sites of hernia

Nursing Care

- Avoid coughing
- Apply ice pack to scrotal area to decrease edema and swelling
- Provide scrotal support
- Avoid heavy lifting for 6 weeks
- Anticipate bleeding for the first 6 hours
- Assist to splint incision while coughing or sneezing.

HIATAL HERNIA

It is also called as esophageal hernia or diaphragmatic hernia. It is the protrusion of the stomach upward into the thorax through an abnormal opening in the diaphragm.

Causes

- Congenital weakness of muscles in the diaphragm
- Increased abdominal pressure.

Clinical Manifestation

- Regurgitation
- Heart burn after meals
- Dyspnea
- Dysphagia
- Feeling of fullness in stomach

Nursing Care

- Administer antacids as per order
- Avoid spicy foods
- Avoid anticholinergics because it may delay stomach emptying
- Prepare the patient for surgical correction (Fundoplication, wrapping a portion of stomach (fundus) along with esophageal sphincter).

CHAPTER 8

Renal System

Chapter Objectives

- Key notes in the renal system
- Anatomy of renal system
- Various diagnostic measures
- Disorders in the renal system
- Dialysis

KEY TERMS

VMA test   BPH
GFR   Prostatis
ARF   Cystitis
CRF   Dialysis

KEYNOTES

- The weight of the kidney is 290 gm (150 gm in male and 130 gm in female).
- Normal glomerular filtration rate = 125 mL/minute.
- Normal urine specific gravity = 1.010–1.020.
- The position used for renal biopsy = prone position.
- In chronic renal failure the GFR is less than 60 mL/minute.
- The priority nursing care of a patient with increased serum potassium (>6.5 mg/dL) is place the patient in cardiac monitor.
- The excellent method to rule out kidney function is Creatinine Clearance Rate.
- Withhold cardiac glycosides (Digoxin) for a patient on hemodialysis.
- Urinary tract infection is more common in females.
- The size of female urethra is 3–5 cm and male urethra is 18 cm.
- In case of urinary tract infection Norfloxacin and Nitofurantoin are the drug of choices.
- The classical manifestations of UTI are increased frequency and urgency, burning micturation, voiding in small amount and lower abdominal pain.
- The classical manifestation of urethritis in males is mucopurulent discharge from penis.
- The classical manifestation of urethritis in females is lower abdominal discomfort.
- The classical manifestation observed in pyelonephritis is costovertebral angle tenderness and flank pain.
- The main clinical manifestation observed in bladder injury is referred pain to shoulders (due to phrenic nerve irritation).
- The main clinical manifestation observed in glomerulonephritis is hematuria, dark cola-colored or red brown urine.
- The main clinical manifestation observed in hydronephrosis is flank pain radiating to groin.
- The main clinical manifestations observed in Renal Calculi are renal colic pain originates in lumbar region and radiating around the sides and down to testicles in male and uterus in females and ureteral colic pain radiating to genital and thigh (pain is sharp severe with sudden onset).

- Salbutamol nebulization is the earliest method to decrease serum potassium in patients with CRF associated hyperkalemia.
- Muchrcke's lines is the characteristic red bands that develop on nails of the patient with CRF.
- Mulberry stones refer to calcium oxalate stones.
- The bladder capacity of a normal adult is 1 liter.
- Normal urine output of an adult is 1500 mL.
- Normal pH of urine is 4.5–7 (Acidic).
- Normal pH of vaginal fluid is 3.8–4.5 (Acidic).
- Normal pH of seminal fluid is 7–8 (Alkaline).

ANATOMY OF URINARY SYSTEM

The urinary system consists of the kidneys, ureters, urinary bladder, and urethra as seen in Figure 1. The kidneys filter the blood to remove wastes and produce urine. The ureters, urinary bladder, and urethra together form the urinary tract, which acts as a pumping system to drain urine from the kidneys, store it, and then release it during urination.

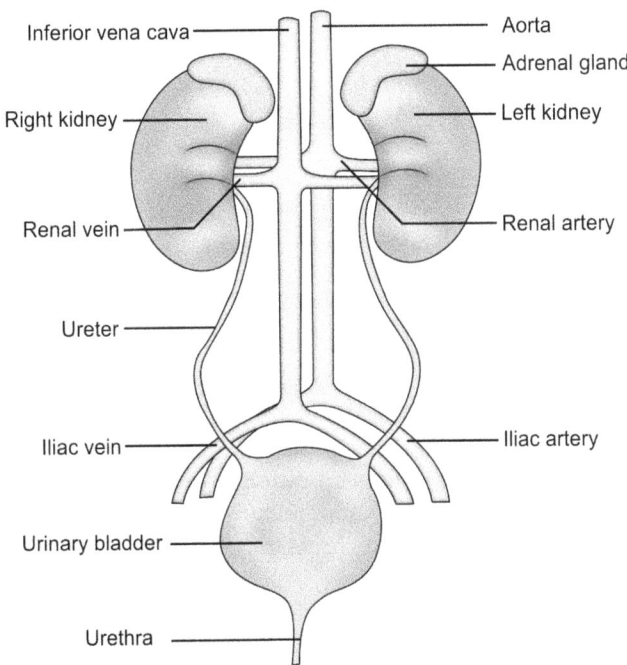

Fig. 1: Anatomy of urinary system

Kidney

The kidneys are a pair of bean-shaped organs found along the posterior wall of the abdominal cavity. It is located in between the last thoracic and first three lumbar regions. The left kidney is located slightly higher than the right kidney because the right side of the liver is much larger than the left side. The kidneys, unlike the other organs of the abdominal cavity, are located posterior to the peritoneum and touch the muscles of the back. The kidneys are surrounded by a layer of adipose that holds them in place and protects them from physical damage.

Functions of kidney are:
- **Maintain acid-base balance**
  In case of any acidosis the kidney will retain HCO_3 and thereby it will maintain acid-base balance.
- **Helps in erythropoiesis**
  Erythropoietin is a hormone produced by the kidney helps in the production of RBC.
- **Secrete Renin in order to control the BP.**
- **Synthesis of vitamin D for the calcium absorption and regulation of parathyroid gland.**
- **Excrete waste products and bacterial toxins.**

Ureters

The ureters are a pair of tubes that carry urine from the kidneys to the urinary bladder as seen in Figure 1. The ureters are about 10 to 12 inches long and run on the left and right sides of the body parallel to the vertebral column. Gravity and peristalsis of smooth muscle tissue in the walls of the ureters move urine toward the urinary bladder. The ends of the ureters extend slightly into the urinary bladder and are sealed at the point of entry to the bladder by the ureterovesical valves. These valves prevent urine from flowing back toward the kidneys.

Urinary Bladder

The urinary bladder is a sac-like hollow organ used for the storage of urine as seen in Figure 1. The urinary bladder is located along the body's midline at the inferior end of the pelvis. Urine entering the urinary bladder from the ureters slowly fills the hollow space of the bladder and stretches its elastic walls. The walls of the bladder allow it to stretch to hold anywhere from 600 to 800 milliliters of urine.

Urethra

The urethra is the tube through which urine passes from the bladder to the exterior of the body as seen in Figure 1. The female urethra is around 2 inches long and ends inferior to the clitoris and superior to the vaginal opening. In males, the urethra is around 8 to 10 inches long and ends at the tip of the penis. The urethra is also an organ of the male reproductive system as it carries sperm out of the body through the penis.

The flow of urine through the urethra is controlled by the internal and external urethral sphincter muscles. The internal urethral sphincter is made of smooth muscle and opens involuntarily when the bladder reaches a certain set level of distension. The opening of the internal sphincter results in the sensation of needing to urinate. The external urethral sphincter is made of skeletal muscle and may be opened to allow urine to pass through the urethra or may be held closed to delay urination (Fig. 2).

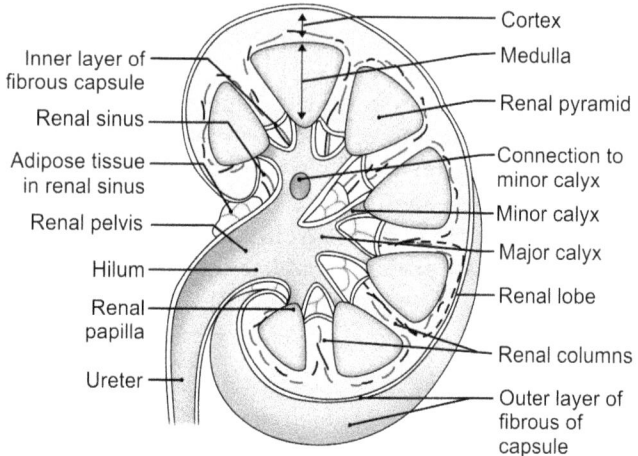

Fig. 2: Cross-section of kidney

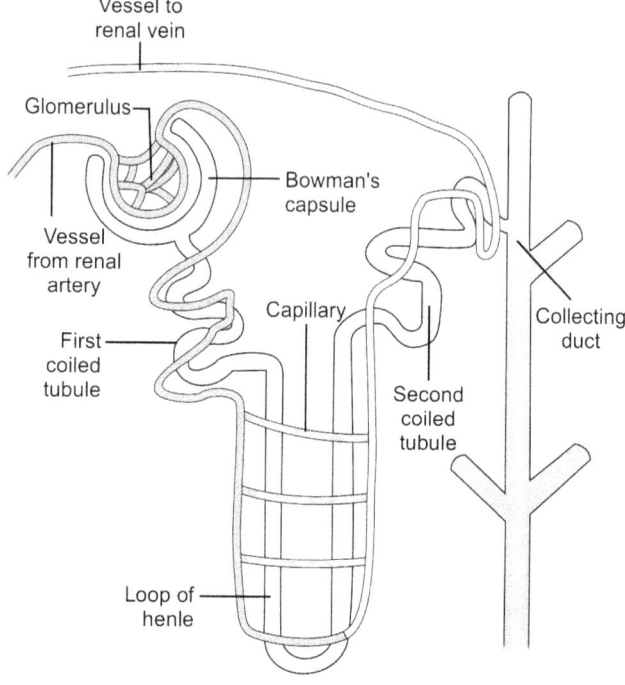

Fig. 3: Structure of nephron

Structure and Function of the Nephron

The nephron is a long tube that runs from the cortex into the medulla and back again to the cortex before joining another tube called the collecting duct. The nephron starts as a small cup-like structure known as the Bowman's capsule and leads into what is known as the first convoluted tubule (also known as the proximal convoluted tubule as seen in Figure 3). It descends into the medulla as the loop of Henle then back into the cortex to become the distal convoluted tubule. These tubules drain into the collecting duct. Several convoluted tubules drain into each collecting duct, these collecting ducts empty into the renal pelvis. From the renal pelvis the excretory product, urine, drains into the ureter. The ureter from each kidney empties into the bladder, and urine leaves the body via the urethra.

There is a branch of the renal artery, the afferent arteriole, entering the small cup-like space of the Bowman's capsule as a network of blood capillaries. This network is known as the glomerulus. Emerging from this network, the capillaries re-unite to form a small arteriole, known as the efferent arteriole. As the efferent arteriole continues it twines around the proximal and distal convoluted tubule. The efferent arteriole divides into capillaries at several points along the length of the tubules, absorbing various substances. These capillaries eventually reunite to drain into the renal vein. The efferent arteriole is smaller than the afferent arteriole. This difference in diameter helps to raise the glomerular pressure and aids in ultra-filtration.

DIAGNOSTIC MEASURES

- **Blood Examination**
  - Serum Potassium (Normal value = 3.5–5.1 mEq/L)
  - Serum Sodium (Normal value = 135–145 mEq/L)
  - Serum Bicarbonate (Normal value = 22–29 mEq/L)
  - Serum Blood Urea Nitrogen (Normal value = 8–25 mg/dL)
  - Serum creatine (Normal value = 0.6–1.3 mg/dL)
  - PSA test (Normal value = <4 ng/mL)
  - pH determination (Normal value = 4.6–7.5)
- **Specific Gravity Determination**
  - Normal urine specific gravity 1.010–1.020
  - In case of increased urine output the specific gravity is decreased.
  - In case of decreased urine output the specific gravity is increased.
- **Creatinine Clearance Rate**
  - It is an excellent method to rule out kidney function. It reflects the GFR.
  - In a normal individual the creatinine clearance rate is increased.
- **Urine Analysis**
  - Appearance of urine
  - Odor of urine
  - Color of urine

- pH of urine
- Osmolarity
- **VMA Test (Vanillyl Mandelic Acid)**
  - 24 hours urine is collected
  - Used to diagnose pheochromocytoma
  - Determines catecholamine level in urine
  - Avoid caffeine, cocoa, vanilla, cheese and fruits 2 days before the test.
- **X-ray KUB**
- **Renal Angiography**
  - Check for any allergy to dye
  - Encourage fluid intake after the procedure, because the dye is nephrotoxic.
  - After the procedure instruct the patient to maintain supine position with leg straight.
- **Renal scanning**
  - Intravenous injection of radioisotope for visual imaging.
  - Assess for any allergy to dye.
  - It helps to rule out the renal blood flow, glomerular filtration rate and tubular function.
- **Cystoscopy**
  - It helps to rule out the inflammation, calculi and tumor.
  - Increase the fluid intake
  - Encourage deep breathing exercise to relieve bladder spasm.

DISORDERS

Acute Renal Failure

- It is also called as acute kidney injury.
- It is the rapid lose of kidney function from the renal cell damage which results in hypoperfusion of the calls.
- It is reversible.
- If is characterized by oliguria. (Urine output less than 400 mL/day).

Causes

Pre-renal Cause

- Dehydration
- Decreased cardiac out put
- Shock
- Diuretic therapy

Intra-renal Cause

- Intra renal infection
- Nephrotoxicity
- Renal parenchyma damage
- Vascular disorders

Post-renal Cause

- Bladder neck obstruction
- Bladder cancer
- Bladder calculi

Nephrotoxic drugs are
- Amphotericin B
- Tetracycline
- Gentamycin
- Cyclophosphamide
- Methotrexate
- Cyclosporine
- Acetaminophen

Clinical Manifestation

Oliguric Phase

- Increased blood urea nitrogen
- Increased creatinine
- Decreased urine specific gravity
- Decreased GFR
- Hyperkalemia
- Hypervolemia
- Hypocalcemia
- Hyperphosphatemia

Diuretic Phase

- Gradual decrease in blood urea nitrogen and creatinine
- Hypokalemia
- Hyponatremia
- Hypovolemia

Recovery Phase

- Increased GFR
- Complete recovery may take 1–2 year

Nursing Care

- Monitor vitals
- Monitor urine output (Oliguria)
- Monitor the signs and symptoms of fluid overload (Hypertension, pulmonary edema, pleural effusion).
- Monitor the signs of uremia (The signs and symptoms of ARF are primarily caused by the retention of nitrogenous waste products like urea, uric acid, etc, in the blood, it may cross the brain barrier and causes changes in the level of consciousness).
- Monitor the signs of metabolic acidosis (Kussmauls respiration).
- Administer prescribed diet (low–moderate protein to reduce the work load of kidney).

- Alert on the nephrotoxic drugs.
- Prepare the patient for dialysis.

CHRONIC RENAL FAILURE (CRF)

It is slow progressing irreversible kidney disease characterized by GFR ≤ 60 mL/mt for 3 months or longer (Normal GFR is 125 mL/mt, if the GFR is less than 20 it is called as End Stage kidney disease).

It affects all the major body systems and result in accumulation of nitrogenous waste in the body. CRF requires dialysis or kidney transplantation to maintain the life.

Causes

- Recurrent infection
- May follow ARF
- Hypertension
- Diabetes mellitus
- Renal artery occlusion

Clinical Manifestation

1. Activity intolerance (due to fatigue)
2. Anemia (erythropoietin is a type of hormone produced by the kidney. it helps in the production of RBC. In case of CRF erythropoietin is not produced, so anemia occurs).
3. Gastrointestinal bleeding
   (In CRF the urea is broken down to Ammonia and this ammonia is an irritant and it will cause GI bleeding)
4. Hyperkalemia and hypertension
5. Hyperphosphatemia
6. Hypocalcemia
   (Phosphorus and calcium are reciprocally related, due to hyperphosphatemia there will be hypocalcemia)
7. Pruritus (itching)
   As a result of CRF the urate crystals will deposit in the body and excrete through the skin and it results in uremic frost and causes itching)
8. Increase in the creatinine level
9. Metabolic acidosis
10. Neurological manifestations.

Nursing Care

- Provide proper nutrition (moderate protein diet).
- Administer epoetin alfa or neo recormon (erythropoietin).
- Check for any bleeding and provide skin care.
- Provide high calorie low potassium diet.
- Administer phosphate binders (calcium carbonate).
- Provide calcium supplements.
- Monitor serum creatinine level.
- Monitor for metabolic acidosis (kussmauls respiration or fruity breath)
- Assist the patient for renal replacement therapies.

UREMIC SYNDROME

Accumulation of nitrogenous waste in the blood caused by kidneys inability to filter out the waste products, it occurs as a complication of ARF and CRF.

Clinical Manifestation

- Oliguria
- Presence of protein, RBC, cast in urine
- Alteration in the level of consciousness
- Increase in the urea, uric acid, phosphorus, etc.

Nursing Care

- Monitor the vitals
- Monitor the serum electrolytes
- Provide low quantity but high quality protein diet.
- Assist the patient for renal replacement therapies.

RENAL REPLACEMENT THERAPIES

It consist of:
1. Hemodialysis
2. Peritoneal dialysis
3. Continuous renal replacement therapy
4. Kidney transplantation

HEMODIALYSIS

It the process of cleansing the clients blood for removing the accumulated waste products.

Principles

1. Osmosis (movement of fluid across a semi permeable membrane from the area of lower concentration of particles to the higher concentration of particles).
2. Diffusion (movement of particles from an area of higher concentration to lower concentration).
3. Ultrafiltration (it is an artificially created pressure gradient system.

Nursing Care

- Monitor vitals (mild elevation of temperature is common because the blood is passing through a machine. If there is excessive rise in temperature it indicates sepsis).
- Assess for any fluid overload.

- Monitor for any bleeding (because heparin is added to the solution).
- Withhold antihypertensive, cardiac glycosides (Digoxin) and antibiotics during dialysis.

Common Sites used for Hemodialysis

1. **Subclavian and femoral catheter**
   - It is used for a short period of time, when the fistula becomes ready. It will keep for 6 weeks.
   - Instruct the patient do not sit more than 45 degree.
2. **External arterio-venous shunt**
   - Two silastic cannulas are surgically inserted into an artery and vein in the forearm or leg to form an external blood path.
3. **Internal arterio-venous fistula**
   - A permanent method for a client with CRF. It will take 4-6 week for maturity. Check for the maturity of the fistula for the presence of thrill or auscultate for bruit.
4. **Internal arterio-venous graft**
   - An artificial graft is made of bovine carotid artery of Gore Tex. After creating the graft monitor for any arterial steal syndrome (blood will flow to the vein from the artery and thereby causes decrease in the blood flow to the extremities).

COMPLICATIONS OF HAEMODIALYSIS

1. **Air embolism**
   During dialysis, asses for any shortness of breath, if there is any shortness of breath it is due to air embolism (pulmonary embolism).
   Nursing care
   - Stop the dialysis
   - Administer oxygen
   - Keep the patient in sideline position (left side position and head down in order to trap the emboli in right atrium).
2. **Disequilibrium syndrome**
   Due to rapid change in the composition of blood or shift of fluid there will be confusion and seizures.
   Nursing care
   - Slow or stop dialysis
   - Prepare to administer intravenous hypertonic solution
3. **Dialysis encephalopathy**
   Aluminum toxicity occurs from dialysate solution and also from the aluminium containing antacid which may lead to mental changes, seizures, speech disturbances, etc.

PERITONEAL DIALYSIS

Peritoneum will act as a dialysate membrane (semi permeable membrane).

Principles

- Osmosis
- Diffusion
- Ultra filtration

Peritoneal membrane is large and porus allowing the solution and fluids to move via osmosis.

Contraindication

- Peritonitis
- Recent abdominal surgery
- Any diverticulum or bowel surgery

Procedure

- A siliconized rubber catheter, Tenckhoff catheter is inserted 3-5 cm below umbilicus.
- 1-2 liter of dialysate is infused by gravity for 20-30 minutes.
- Monitor for complication:
  - Peritonitis (cloudy dialysate shows infection)
  - Abdominal pain
  - Insufficient out flow
  - Leakage around catheter site.

Continuous Renal Replacement Therapy (CRRT)

- CRRT provides continuous ultra-filtration for 8-24 hours.
- This is indicated for a patient who cannot tolerate dialysis or chronically ill patients.
- It does not require a dialysis machine.

KIDNEY TRANSPLANTATION

- A human kidney from compactable donor is implanted into a recipient.
- Kidney transplantation is done for irreversible kidney damage.
- The recipient should receive immunosuppressant for life long.

Donor

- The donor should be screen for ABO incompatibility, human leukocytic antigen, mixed lymphocytic culture.
- In case of living donor he must have excellent health and two functioning kidney.
- In case of cadaver he should meet the criteria of a brain death and should be younger than 70 years.

Preoperative Nursing Care

- Check the blood investigation
- Administer immunosuppressant two days before transplantation.

- Maintain strict aseptic technique.
- Verify that the hemodialysis should complete 24 hour before transplantation.

Postoperative Nursing Care

- Check for urine output (urine output usually begins immediately if donor was living donor, it may be delayed for few days or longer in case of cadaver)
- Hemodialysis may perform until the kidney function established.
- Monitor the lab reports
- Check for graft rejection (occurs at the time of anastomosis).
  Acute rejection (occurs within 6 weeks).
  Chronic rejection (occurs within months to years).

Signs and Symptoms of Graft Rejection

- Temperature higher than 100F
- Edema
- Hypertension
- 2-3 lbs weight gain in 24 hours
- Increased WBC
- Increased blood urea nitrogen(BUN) and creatinine.

CYSTITIS

- It is an inflammation of the bladder result from infection, obstruction of urethra.

  The most common causative organisms are:
- E. coli
- Enterobacter
- Pseudomonas
- Serratia specious

  Cystitis is more common in women because women have shorter urethra than the men and it is located close to rectum. Sexually active and pregnant women are more vulnerable to cystitis.

Signs and Symptoms

- Frequency and urgency
- Burning on urination
- Incomplete emptying of bladder
- Cloudy dark and foul smelling urine
- WBC count more than 1 lakh cells/cubic meter
- Increased specific gravity and pH of urine.

Causes

- Bladder distension
- Calculus
- Micro-organisms
- Poor fitting vaginal diaphragms
- Use of spermicidal
- Allergens or irritants

Nursing Care

- Increase fluid intake (3000 mL/day)
- Administer prescribed medication
- Maintain an acidic pH
- Discourage caffeine products such as coffee, tea, cola
- Avoid alcohol.

Client Education

- Void every 2-3 hours, if pregnant void every 2 hours
- Continue antibiotics for 7-14 days.

RENAL CALCULI

- Calculi are stones that can form anywhere in the urinary tract.
- Urolithiasis refers to formation of urinary calculi in the ureters.
- Nephrolithiasis refers to formation of calculi in the nephrons or kidney.
- When calculi occluded the ureters and blocks the flow of urine the ureters dilates producing hydroureter.

Causes

- Family history of stone formation
- Diet high in calcium, vitamin D, protein, oxalate, purine, etc
- Obstruction and urinary stasis
- Use of diuretics
- Dehydration
- Immobilization
- Hypercalcemia
- Hyper parathyroidism
- Increased serum uric acid

Clinical Manifestation

- Renal colic which originate in the lumbar region and radiates around side of testicle in men and bladder in women.
- Ureteral colic which radiates toward the genitalia and thigh
- Sharp severe pain
- Nausea and vomiting

- Low grade fever
- Hematuria

Management

- Monitor intake and output
- Encourage fluid 3 L/day
- Administer IV fluids
- Strain urine for the presence of stone, send the stone for analysis.
- A special diet is prescribed for the patient:
  - In case of calcium phosphate stone acid ash diet because calcium stones are alkaline.
  - In case of cystine stone alkaline ash diet.
  - In case of calcium oxalate stone and struvite stone acid ash diet.
  - In case of uric acid stone alkaline ash diet.
- E.g. **Alkaline ash diet**:- diet increases the pH of urine or diet reduces acidity of urine most vegetables, rhubarb
- E.g. **Acid ash diet**: Diet reduces the pH of urine, diet make the urine more acidic meat, fish, cranberry, etc.

Surgical Management

- **Cystoscopy**
  - It is done for the stones in the bladder or lower ureter.
- **Extracorporeal shortwave lithotripsy (ESWN)**
  - A non-invasive technique in which the stones are breaking down into small piece.
- **Percutaneous lithotripsy**
  - Invasive procedures in which the stones are break down under fluoroscopic guidance.
- **Ureterolithotomy**
  - A surgical procedure perform if lithotripsy is not effective.
- **Partial or total nephrectomy**

PROSTITIS

Inflammation of the prostate gland, it may be acute or chronic.

Signs and Symptoms

- Frequency and urgency of urination
- Urethral discharge
- Lower back pain
- Dysuria
- Hematuria

Nursing Care

- Encourage the fluid intake
- Administer antibiotics

Benign Prostatic Hyperplasia (BPH)

It is the enlargement of prostate gland. It will compress urethra resulting in partial or complete obstruction. It is commonly seen after 50 years.

Signs and Symptoms

- Inability to start or continue urination
- Inability to start to pass urine in straight stream
- Post voidal dribbling

Management

- Encourage the fluid 2–3 L/day
- Administer medication (Dutasteride, tamsulosin, finasteride).
- Encourage the patient to perform Digital Rectal Examination (DRE).
- Encourage the patient to do PSA test (prostate specific antigen)
- If the medical management is unsuccessful instruct the patient to undergo TURP.

PROSTATE CANCER

- Second most common cancer death in male above 55 years of age.
- Exact cause is unknown.
- Management is estrogen therapy, radiation therapy and surgery.
- The surgical management are:
  - Transurethral resection of prostate (TURP)
  - Supra pubic prostatectomy
  - Retropubic prostatectomy
  - Perineal prostatectomy

Nursing Care

- Expect hematuria for 2–3 days
- Irrigate catheter with normal saline
- Administer anticholinergic (Propantheline bromide)
- Report bright red and thick blood in catheter.

Sample Questions

1. **During digital rectal examination, a key sign of prostate cancer is:**
   a. A hard prostate, localized or diffuse
   b. Abdominal pain
   c. A boggy, tender prostate
   d. A non-indurated prostate

2. **The nurse is caring for a patient who is admitted with Acute Renal Failure. The appearance of U-wave in the ECG should alert the:**
   a. Hyperkalemia
   b. Hypokalemia
   c. Hypernatremia
   d. Hyponatremia

Answers

1. **Ans. is a, A hard prostate, localized or diffuse**
   On digital rectal examination; a key sign of prostate cancer are a hard prostate.

2. **Ans. is b, Hypokalemia**
   U-wave can be seen in patient with hypokalemia and in hyperkalemia prolonged PR interval can been seen.

CHAPTER 9

Musculoskeletal System

Chapter Objectives

- Keynotes in the musculoskeletal system
- Anatomy of musculoskeletal system
- Various diagnostic measures
- Tractions
- Disorders in the musculoskeletal system

KEY TERMS

CRP   ROM
MRI   Cast
RA   Tendon
THR   Gout

KEYNOTES

- The musculoskeletal system is also known as locomotor system.
- There are about 206 bones in human body.
- There are 33 vertebral bones in our body (24 + sacrum + coccyx).
- Largest bone is femur and smallest bone is stapes.
- The fossa seen behind knee joint is popliteal fossa.
- Antecubital fossa is seen above the elbow joint.
- Calcium and phosphorus are two important minerals required for bone growth.
- The common type of fracture seen in old age is pelvic fracture.
- The common type of fracture seen in children is green stick fracture.
- Cartilage is a form of connective tissue.
- Tendon is a structure which connect muscle to bone.
- Ligament is a structure which connect bone to bone.
- The priority nursing care of a patient with open fracture is control bleeding to prevent hypovolemic shock.
- The priority nursing care of a patient with cast application is frequent neurovascular assessment.
- To assess the blood circulation under the cast monitor the capillary refill by pressing and releasing the fingers.
- Administer more fluids for a patient with fracture.
- Knee joint is an example for synovial joint.
- The drug of choice for gout is colchicines.
- The diet for osteoporosis is high calcium diet.
- The health teaching for osteoporosis patient is take safety measures.
- Musician's nerve is ulnar nerve.
- Largest tarsal bone is calcaneum.
- Soleus is known as peripheral heart.
- First cervical vertebrae are otherwise called Atlas.
- Kyphosis of dorsal spine is known as Dowager's hump.
- Pott's fracture related to fibula.
- The first bone to ossify in our body is clavicle.
- The second bone ossify in our body is mandible.
- The cause of winging of scapula is paralysis of serratus anterior.
- Largest carpal bone with a rounded end is capitates.
- Erb's palsy (is the paralysis of the arm caused by injury to the upper group of arms main nerves) is also called Potter's tip hand or police man tip hand.
- Achilles reflex is downward jerk of the foot.
- Lordosis is the inward curvature of the portion of the lumbar and cervical vertebral column.
- Kyphosis is also called as round back or Kelso's hunchback.

- Most common site for bone marrow aspiration—iliac crust.
- Which vitamin that helps in the absorption of calcium? Vitamin D.

ANATOMY

Human musculoskeletal system consists of bones, muscles, tendons and ligaments.

Skeletal System

The skeletal system consists of 206 bones that make up the frame of our body called as skeleton as seen in Figure 1. Skeletal system consists of bony structures and joints.

Functions

- Skeleton supports our body
- It protects our internal organs
- Attach the muscles to our body
- Storage of minerals (calcium and phosphorus)
- Produce blood cells.

Bones

Bones are also known as osseous tissues. These are the hardest structure or material of our body. The process of bone formation is called as ossification. It begins from the third month of fetal life and is completed by late adolescence.

Types of Bone

- **Long bones:** Made of compact bones, composed of cancellous bones (femur, humerus).
- **Short bones:** Cancellous bones covered by thin layers of compact bone (carpals, tarsals).
- **Flat bones:** Two layers of compact bones (skull, ribs).
- **Irregular bones:** Sizes and shapes vary (vertebrae, mandible).

Formation of a New Bone (Ossification)

There are three types of cell present in bone that are of particular interest—osteoblasts, osteocytes and osteoclasts, which are respectively responsible for the production, maintenance and resorption of bone.
- **Osteoblasts:** Mononucleated "bone-forming" cells found near the surface of bones. They are responsible for making *osteoid*, which consists mainly of collagen. The osteoblasts then secrete alkaline phosphatase to create sites for calcium and phosphate deposition, which allows crystals of bone mineral to grow at these sites. The osteoid becomes mineralized, thus, forming bone.

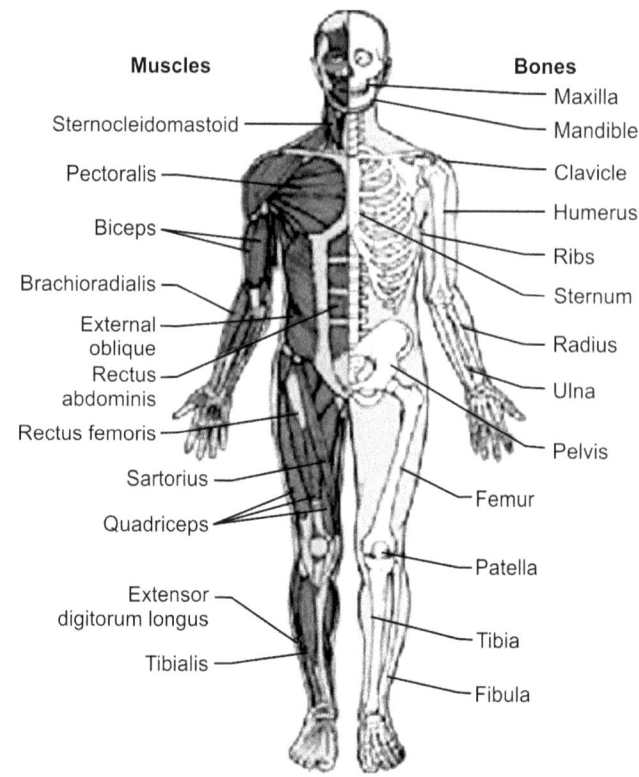

Fig. 1: Anatomy of musculoskeletal system

- **Osteocytes:** These are osteoblasts that are no longer on the surface of the bone, but are instead found in lacunae between the lamellae in bone. Their main role is homeostasis—maintaining the correct oxygen and mineral levels in the bone.
- **Osteoclasts:** Multinucleated cells responsible for bone resorption. They travel to specific sites on the surface of bone and secrete acid phosphatase, which unfixes the calcium in mineralized bone to break it down. The replacement of cartilage by bone is known as endochondral ossification.

Stages of Bone Healing

Four Stages of Bone Healing

- **A hematoma is formed:** Blood vessels are ruptured when the bone breaks; as a result of this, a blood filled swelling called a hematoma forms. Bone cells deprived of nutrition dies out.
- **The break is splinted by a fibrocartilage callus:** An early event of tissue repair is growth of new capillaries into the clotted bloods at the site of damage and disposal of death tissues occurs, the fibrocartilage callus that contains several elements, such as cartilage matrix, bony matrix and collagen fibers and acts to splints the broken bone, closing the bone.

- ***The bony callus is formed:*** More osteoblasts and osteoclasts migrate into the area and multiply, the fibrocartilage callus is gradually replaced by one mode of spongy bone called bony callus (Fig. 2)
- ***Bone remodeling occurs:*** Over the next few weeks to month depending on the bone's size and site of the break, the bony callus is remodelled in response to the mechanical stresses placed on it, so that it forms a strong permanent patch at the fractured site.

Joints

Joints are formed when two or more bones meet. This is also referred to as an articulation.

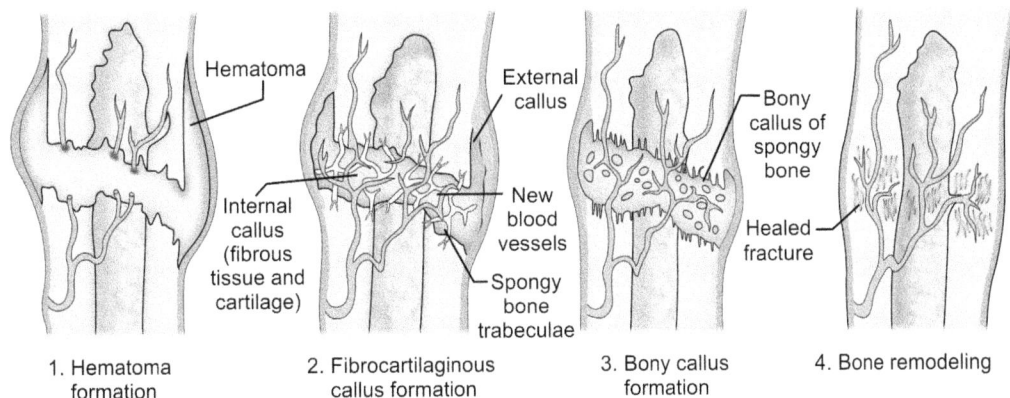

Fig. 2: Stages of bone healing

Types of Joints

There are three primary types of joint articulation:
- **Synovial joints:** Freely movable, the joints do not touch each other, e.g. knee joint, shoulder joint.
- **Cartilaginous joints:** Slightly movable, e.g. vertebral bodies of the spine.
- **Fibrous joints:** Immovable, e.g. skull sutures.

Muscles

Muscles are bundles of parallel muscle tissue fibers. As these fibers contract (shorten in length), they produce movement of or within the body. The movement may take the form of bringing two bones closer together, pushing food through the digestive system, or pumping blood through blood vessels. In addition to producing movement, muscles also hold the body erect and generate heat. There are about 700 named muscles in our body.

Types of Muscles

There are three types of muscles:
1. **Visceral Muscle:** Visceral muscle is found inside of organs such as stomach, intestines, and blood vessels. The weakest of all muscle tissues, visceral muscle makes organs contract to move substances through the organ. The visceral muscle is controlled by the unconscious part of the brain, it is known as involuntary muscle. It cannot be directly controlled by the conscious mind. The term "smooth muscle" is often used to describe visceral muscle because it has a very smooth, uniform appearance when viewed under a microscope. This smooth appearance starkly contrasts with the banded appearance of cardiac and skeletal muscles.
2. **Cardiac Muscle:** Found only in the heart, cardiac muscle is responsible for pumping blood throughout the body. Cardiac muscle tissue cannot be controlled consciously, so it is an involuntary muscle.
3. **Skeletal Muscle:** Skeletal muscle is the only voluntary muscle tissue in the human body—it is controlled consciously. Every physical action that a person consciously performs (e.g. speaking, walking, or writing) requires skeletal muscle. The function of skeletal muscle is to contract to move parts of the body closer to the bone that the muscle is attached to. Most skeletal muscles are attached to two bones across a joint, so the muscle serves to move parts of those bones closer to each other.

Movement of Muscles (seen in following pictures)

- *Abduction* (ab = away from)—movement away from midline of the body.
- *Adduction* (ad = toward)—movement toward midline of the body.
- *Flexion* (flex = to bend)—act of bending or being bent.
- *Extension* (extens = to stretch out)—movement that brings limb into or toward a straight condition.
- *Dorsiflexion* (dors = back of body)—backward bending, as of hand or foot.
- *Plantar flexion* (plant = sole of foot)—bending sole of foot; pointing toes downward.
- *Eversion* (e = outward)—turning outward.
- *Inversion* (in = inward)—turning inward.

- *Pronation*—to turn downward or backward as with the hand or foot.
- *Supination*—turning the palm or foot upward.
- *Elevation*—to raise a body part, as in shrugging the shoulders.
- *Depression*—a downward movement, as in dropping the shoulders.
- *Circumduction* (circum = around)—movement in a circular direction from a central point as if drawing a large, imaginary circle in the air.
- *Opposition*—moving thumb away from palm; the ability to move the thumb into contact with the other fingers
- *Rotation*—moving around a central axis.

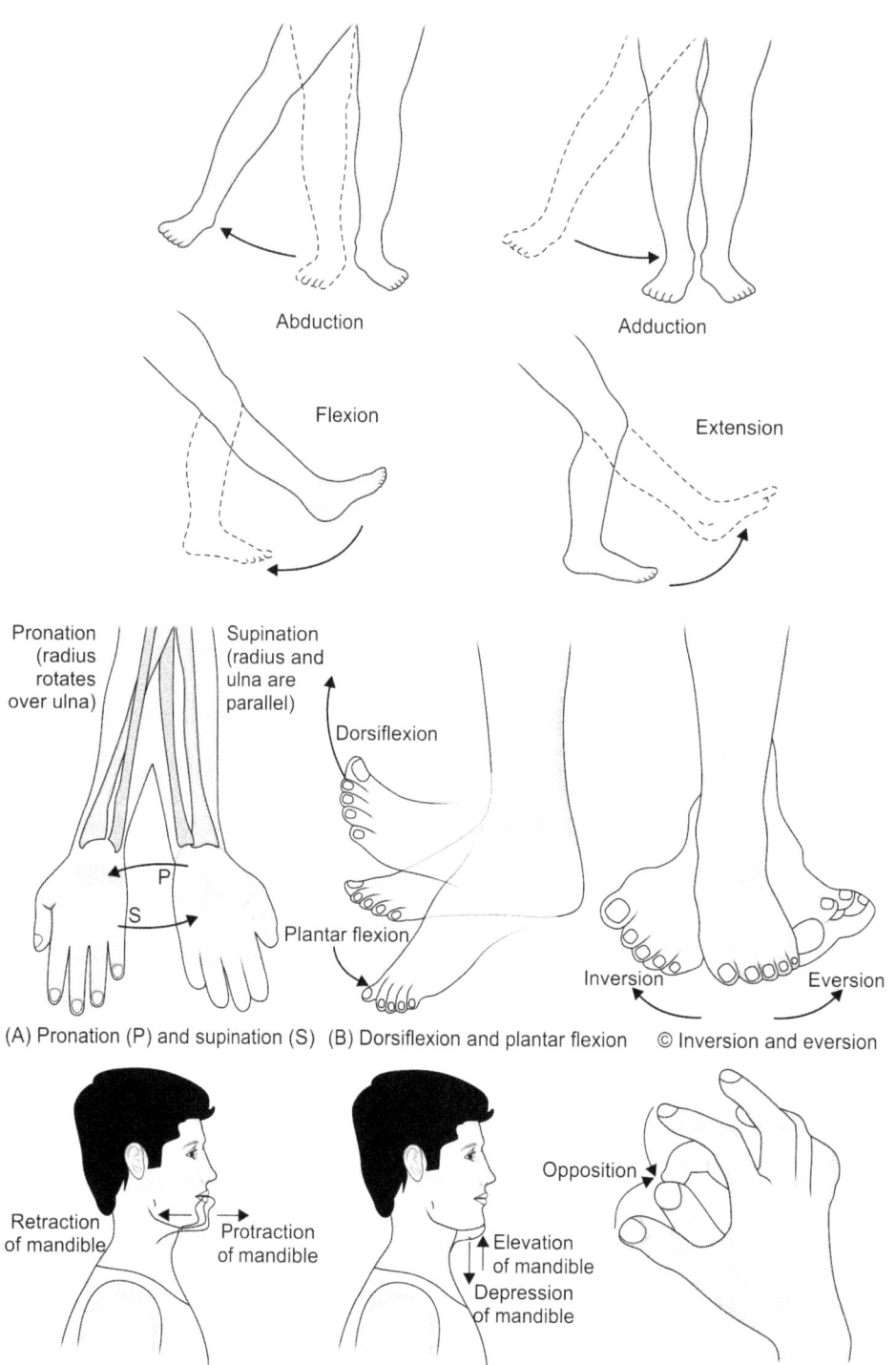

Type of Exercise or Nursing Interventions

- *Active exercise:* The individual moves the part by his own.
- *Passive exercise:* The physiotherapist moves the part.
- *Isometric exercise:* It is an active exercise in which the relaxation and contraction of muscle without any joint movement helps to maintain muscle strength.
- *ROM (range of motion exercise):* The movement of joints through its full range of motion to prevent contractures and to maintain good muscle strength. The instrument used to measure ROM is Goniometer.
- *Aerobic exercises,* such as cycling, walking, running, hiking, and playing tennis, focus on increasing cardiovascular endurance.
- *Anaerobic exercises,* such as weight training, increase short-term muscle strength.
- *Flexibility exercises,* such as stretching, improve the range of motion of muscles and joints.

DIAGNOSTIC MEASURES

- *X-rays:* Radiographic examination of the bones to detect any injury or tumor
- *CRP (C-reactive protein)*—it is a type of protein produced by the liver, increased CRP indicates infection. Normal CRP is 0–3 mg/dL, if it is less than 1 indicates low risk for cardiovascular disorders and if it is 3 or more indicates high risk for cardiovascular disorders.
- *RA factor (rheumatoid factor)*—normal RA factor is 0–39 IU/ml. If it is between 40 and 79 indicates weakly reactive and, if it is greater than 80 indicates highly reactive.
- *Serum uric acid:* Increased serum uric acid is seen in gout. Normal serum uric acid is 3.5–8 mg/dL.
- *Arthrography:* X-ray record of a joint usually taken after the joint has been injected by a contrast medium.
- *Bone scan:* Nuclear medicine procedure in which the patient is given a radioactive dye and then scanning equipment is used to visualize bones. It is especially useful in identifying stress fractures, observing progress of treatment for osteomyelitis and locating cancer metastasis to the bones. Instruct the client to void immediately before the test.
- *Arthroscopy:* Examination of the interior of a joint by entering the joint with an arthroscope. The arthroscope contains a small television camera that allows the physician to view the interior of the joints on a monitor during the procedure. Some joint conditions can be repaired during arthroscope. Maintain pressure dressing over the site for 24 hours after the test and advice the patient to limit activities for several days.
- *Arthrocentesis:* Insertion of a needle into the joints to aspirate synovial fluid for diagnostic as well as therapeutic purposes.
- *Myelography:* Study of the spinal column after injecting opaque contrast material particularly useful in identifying herniated nucleus prolapsed or IVDP. LP is used to remove a small amount of CSF (Cerebrospinal fluid) and dye is mixed and reinserted. The dye may be oil-based, air-based or water-based. If an oil-based dye or water-based dye is used provide flat with head of bed elevation 30–45 degree to prevent the upward displacement of dye. If an air-based dye is used provide head lower than trunk position.
- *Electromyography:* Study and record the strength and quality of the muscle contraction as a result of electrical stimulation.
- *Muscle biopsy:* Removal of muscle tissue for pathological examination.

Complications of Immobility or Fracture

- Renal calculi (calcium calculi)
- Pulmonary embolism (fat embolism)
- Constipation
- Deep vein thrombosis
- Skin breakdown.

How fracture leads to pulmonary embolism?

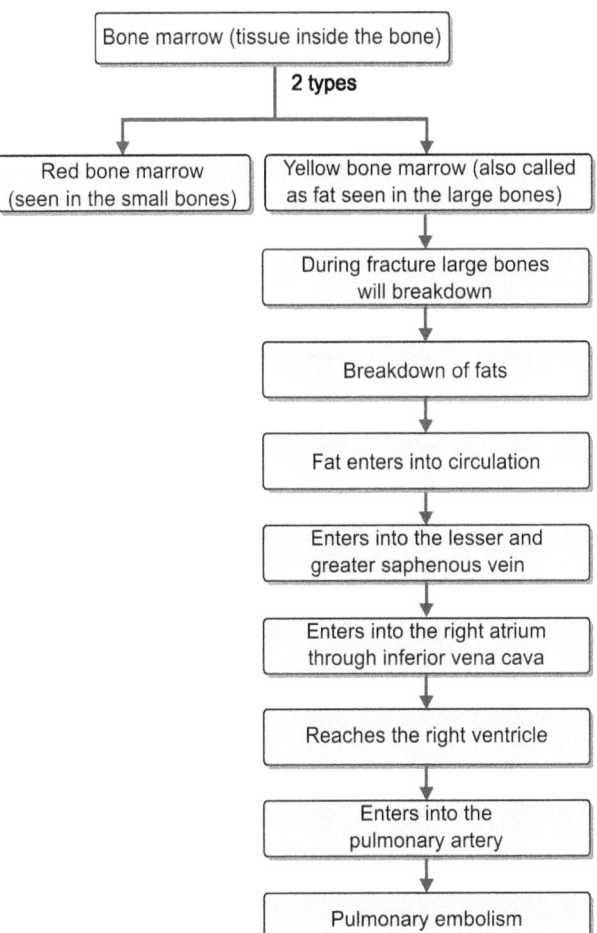

Assistive Devices for Walking

Canes

A cane is a walking stick used as a mobility aid as seen in Figure 3. Cane can help to redistribute the weight of a weak leg or lower leg to improve walking or stability.

Nursing Care

- Teach the client to hold the hands opposite to the affected extremity and advance the cane at the same time, the affected leg move forward.

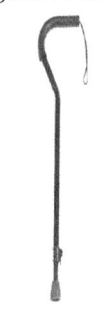

Fig. 3: Canes

Crutches

Crutches are a type of mobility aid with a long stick with a crosspiece at the top used as a support under the armpit by a lame person as seen in Figure 4.

Nursing Care

- Top of the crutch is 2 inch below the axilla and tip of the crutch is 6 inch in front and sideways.
- Weight should not be worn by the axilla to prevent damage to the brachial plexus and to prevent paralysis of arm.

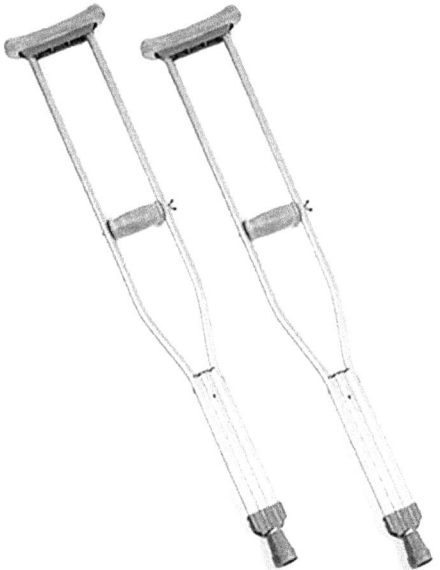

Fig. 4: Crutches

Type of Crutch Gaits (www.walkeasy.com)

- **4-point alternate crutch gait:** Right crutch, left foot and left crutch, right foot.
- **2-point alternate crutch gait:** Right crutch and left foot, left crutch and right foot (most closely resembles normal walking).
- **3-point alternate crutch gait:** Both crutches and the weaker leg move forward simultaneously, then the stronger extremity is moved forward while placing most of the body weight on the arms.
- **Swing to crutch gait:** Bear weight on good leg (legs), advance both crutches forward simultaneously, lean forward while swinging the body to a position even with crutches.
- **Swing-through crutch gait:** Advance both crutches forward; lift legs off the ground and swing forward landing in advance of the crutches (fastest of all gaits).

Representation of Crutch Gaits

2-point gait	3-point gait	4-point gait	Swing through/tripod
Partial weightbearing boot feet	Non-weightbearing (left foot)	Partial weight bearing both feet	Weightbearing both feet (or one foot)
Provides less support	Requires good balance	Maximal support provided	Requires arm strength
Faster than a 4-point gait	Required arm strength Faster gait	Requires constant shift of weight	Requires coordination/balance
	Can use with walker		Most advanced gait
4. Advance right foot and left crutch	4. Advance right foot	4. Advance right foot	4. Lift both feet/swing forward/land feet in front of crutches
3. Advance left foot and right crutch	3. Advance left foot and both crutches	3. Advance left crutch	3. Advance both crutches (partial wt. or more on right foot)
2. Advance left foot and right crutch	2. Advance right foot	2. Advance left foot	2. Lift both feet/swing forward/land feet in front of crutches
1. Advance left foot and right crutch	1. Advance left foot and both crutch	1. Advance right crutch	1. Advance both crutches (partial wt. or more on right both)
Beginning stance	Beginning stance	Beginning stance	Beginning stance

While climbing the stairs (upstairs) good leg first, downstairs bad leg first……..

(Good goes to heaven……………Bad goes to hell……..)

Walker

It is a mechanical device with four legs (Fig. 5). A walker or walking frame is a tool for disabled or elderly people who need additional support to maintain balance or stability while walking.

Nursing Care

- Teach the client to hold the upper bar of the walker at each side, then move the walker forward and step into it.

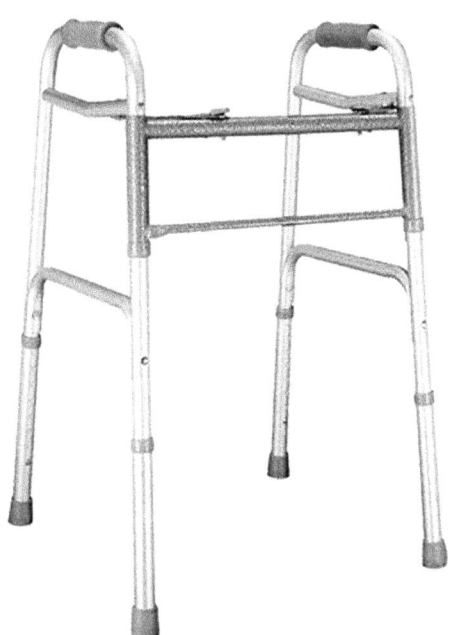

Fig. 5: Walker

TRACTION

Traction is a pulling force used to immobilize the fractured area. It is also used to decrease the muscle spasm and correct immobility.

Types of Traction

1. Skin traction
2. Skeletal traction

Skin Traction

Weight attached to the skin and secured by an elastic bandage. A maximum of 5 kg weight is applied by this method. It is an intermittent traction.

Types of Skin Traction

1. **Buck's traction:** It is used in the fracture of hip for immobilizing the leg.

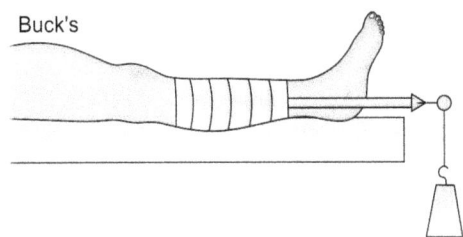

2. **Russell traction:** Creating an upward pull from the knee.

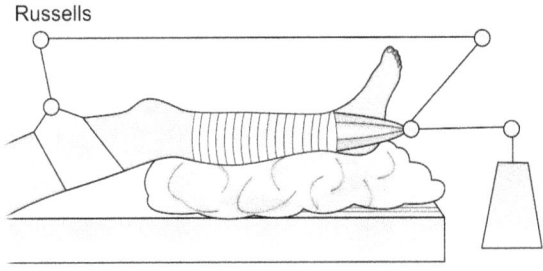

3. **Pelvic traction:** Pelvic gridle with extension straps attached to ropes and weight, used in back pain and pelvic fracture.

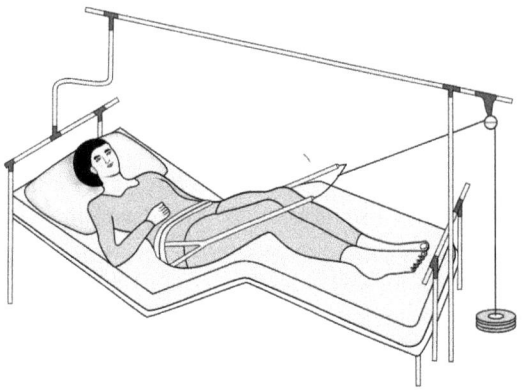

Pelvic traction

4. **Cervical traction:** Weight is attached to the head to reduce the muscle spasm and alignment, elevate the head of bed to provide countertraction.

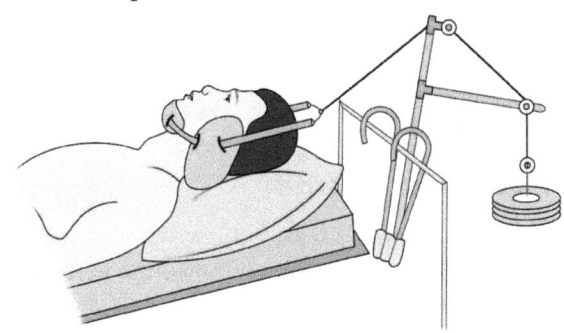

Cervical traction

Skeletal Traction

Traction applied to the bone by using pins, wires or screws. The weight, if skeletal traction is 35–40 lbs (11–18 kg). It is a continuous traction. Skeletal traction requires an invasive procedure in which pins, screws, or wires are surgically installed for use in longer term traction requiring heavier weights.

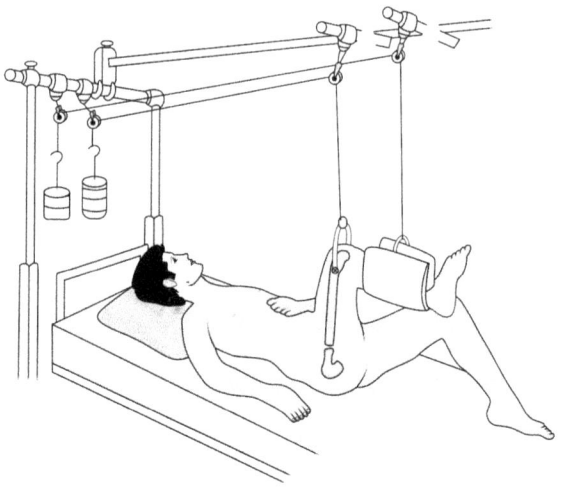

Skeletal traction

Nursing Care

- Monitor the neurovascular assessment, assess the extremity for any impairment in blood supply and nerve supply.
- Monitor the skin for any breakdown or infection.
- Monitor the pin site for any infection or redness.
- The standard solution used to clean the pin site is chlorhexidine.
- Encourage to perform plantar flexion and dorsiflexion exercises.
- Monitor for any sign and symptoms of DVT.
- Assist with the activities of daily living.
- Administer pain medications.
- Provide emotional support to overcome fear and anxiety.

DISORDERS

Rheumatoid Arthritis

Rheumatoid arthritis is a chronic systemic disease characterized by pain and inflammation of the joints. Rheumatoid arthritis commonly affects the hands, knees and feet. Generally, both sides of the body are affected. It is commonly seen in women between 30 and 45 years of age.

Causes

- Idiopathic
- Autoimmune disorder
- Excessive stress

Clinical Manifestation

- Join distribution is symmetrical, bilateral, commonly affecting the smaller and peripheral joints of the hands, wrist, elbows, shoulder, hip, etc.
- Stiffness in the joints, especially in the morning
- Painful and swollen joints
- Fatigue
- Sleep disturbances
- Muscles weakness.

Nursing Care

- Monitor the laboratory values (increased ESR, increased CRP and RA factor positive).
- Administer medications (NSAIDs, such as ibuprofen or indomethacin).
- Administer disease-modifying antirheumatic drugs (DMARDs), such as azathioprine or methotrexate.
- Administer gold compounds or chrysotherapy, such as sodium thiomalate or aurothioglucose IM weekly once
- Administer corticosteroids, such as prednisolone
- Encourage to perform range of motion exercise several times in a day
- Encourage to stop the exercise at the point of pain
- Provide prone position several times in a day to prevent hip or knee contractures
- Avoid physical or emotional support
- Encourage the patient to take a well-balanced nutrition
- Assist the client to perform activities of daily living (ADL).
- In case of acute rheumatoid arthritis, provide cold treatment and, in case of chronic rheumatoid arthritis, provide hot treatment.

OSTEOARTHRITIS

Osteoarthritis is a chronic non-systemic disorder characterized by inflammation of weight-bearing joints. It is common seen after the age group of 45 years (increase with aging). In osteoarthritis, the cartilage becomes brittle and breaks down and the deterioration of cartilage can lead to degeneration of joints.

Causes

- Unknown
- Previous injury or trauma

- Advanced age
- Family history of osteoarthritis

Clinical Manifestation

- Stiffness and joint pain
- Pain aggravated by movement and relieved by rest
- Heberden's node (small bony overgrowth at the interphalangeal joints)
- Crepitus (a grating or crackling sound while moving the joints)

Nursing Care

- Encourage the client to move the extremities (it is important to maximize the health of cartilage and to maintain joint movement and strength)
- Administer medications (analgesics and corticosteroids)
- Provide heat treatment

OSTEOPOROSIS

Osteoporosis is a progressive bone disorder characterized by demineralization of the bones. Osteoporosis literally means holes in the bones.

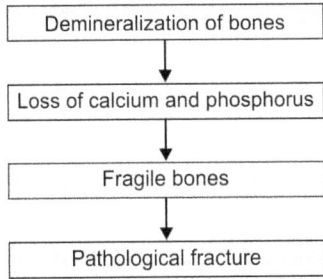

The priority nursing care of a patient with osteoporosis is prevention of risk for pathological fracture. Osteoporosis is more commonly affecting the wrist, hip and vertebral column.

Types

- ***Primary osteoporosis:*** Due to primary cause, in males, it is due to low testosterone levels and in females at the postmenopausal period.
- ***Secondary osteoporosis:*** Due to secondary cause, e.g. use of thyroid reducing hormones, prolonged use of steroids and the use of aluminum-containing antacids (decreases Ph).

Clinical Manifestation

- Back pain
- Pelvic pain
- Kyphosis of the dorsal spine (Dowager's hump)
- Low calcium and phosphorus
- Pathological fracture

Nursing Care

- Prevention of risk for pathological fracture
- Use side rails to prevent fall
- Provide assistive devices for walking
- Instruct the client to take diet rich in protein, calcium, vitamin C and D
- Provide more fluids to prevent renal calculi

OSTEOMYELITIS

Osteomyelitis is the inflammation of the bone and surrounding tissues. The most common causative organism is *Staphylococcus aureus*.

Causes

- Bacterial infection
- Infection of the fractured site

Clinical Manifestation

- Localized pain and swelling
- Fever
- Drainage from the wound
- Increased ESR and WBC count

Nursing Care

- Administer analgesics as ordered
- Provide antibiotic therapy
- Prepare the patient for sequestrectomy (removal of the dead tissue)
- Immobilize the affected part
- Provide sterile dressing

OSTEOMALACIA

Osteomalacia is a disorder characterised by softening of the bones due to the deficiency of vitamin D.

Causes

- Deficiency of vitamin D or cholecalciferol
- Certain gastric surgeries
- Due to celiac disease
- Certain drugs, such as dilantin or phenobarbital

Clinical Manifestation

- Bone pain and muscle weakness
- Changes in the gait

Nursing Care

- Administer vitamin D supplements
- Instruct the patient take the calcirol or vitamin D3 along with milk, because the milk is a rich source of calcium and it enhance the easy absorption.
- Provide foods rich in vitamin D, such as oily fish (salmon, mackerel, and sardines) and egg yolks. Also, look for foods that are fortified with vitamin D, such as cereal, bread, milk and yogurt.

GOUT

Gout is a metabolic disorder characterized by increased in the uric acid level which results in inflammation of joints. It is a disorder of purine metabolism.

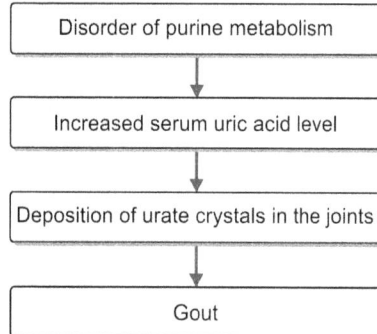

Causes

- Increased uric acid level
- Consume too much alcohol or beer
- Consume a diet high in 'purines', such as meat, sweetbreads, offal, shellfish, and fructose (found in fruit juices and soft drinks sweetened with corn syrup)
- Prolonged use of diuretics

Clinical Manifestation

- Joint pain, joints of the foot, especially great toe and angle
- Redness and swelling
- Limited movement
- Tachycardia

Nursing Care

- Monitor serum uric acid level
- Administer colchicines (Goutnil), a standard drug for gout, discontinue in case of diarrhea
- Administer allopurinol or zyloric or febuget (febuxostat)
- Provide diet in low in quantity of purine
- Avoid organ meats, sardines, sweatbread, etc.
- Limit alcohol use
- Increase fluid intake 2-3 liter per day
- Teach regular exercise pattern

FRACTURE

A fracture is a break or crack in the continuity of the bone. A fracture occurs when force exerted against a bone is stronger than the bone can structurally withstand.

Causes

- Trauma
- RTA
- Osteoporosis

Types

- **Open fracture:** The bone is exposed into the air through a break in the skin.
- **Closed fracture:** The skin over the fracture area remain intact, the bone has not pierced into the skin.
- **Green stick fracture:** It is a common type of fracture seen in children, one side of bone is broken down and other side bends.
- **Comminuted fracture:** The bone is shattered into small pieces. This type fracture tends to heal very slowly.
- **Complicated fracture:** The structures surrounding the fracture are injured. There may be damage to the veins, arteries or nerves, and there may also be injury to the lining of the bone (the periosteum).
- **Compression fracture:** This occurs when two bones are forced against each other. The bones of the spine, called vertebrae, can have this type of fracture. Older people, particularly those with osteoporosis, are at higher risk.
- **Hairline fracture:** The most common form is a stress fracture, often occurring in the foot or lower leg as a result of repeated stress from activities, such as jogging or running.
- **Avulsion fracture:** The muscles are anchored to bone with tendons, a type of connective tissue. Powerful muscle contractions can wrench the tendon free and pull out pieces of bone. This type of fracture is more common in the knee and shoulder joints.

Clinical Manifestation

- Pain aggravated with movement
- Redness and swelling
- Deformity
- Loss of function.

Nursing Care

- Keep the person still, do not move them
- Control bleeding in case of an open fracture
- Never try to straighten the broken bone
- Apply splint to support the limb

- Raise the fractured area, if possible and apply some ice packs to reduce selling
- Monitor for any complications, such as fat embolism, compartment syndrome, avascular necrosis and osteomyelitis (Compartment syndrome occurs when pressure increases in one or more compartment leads to reduced blood flow and tissue damage).
- Monitor the neurovascular assessment
- Provide proper care of traction
- Provide high protein diet to promote wound healing
- Encourage more fluids to prevent constipation and renal calcium calculi.

HIP FRACTURE

A hip fracture is a break in the upper end of femur (thigh bone), the head neck and tronchanteric area of the femur. It is associated with advanced age and osteoporosis.

Causes

- Osteoporosis
- Cancer
- Stress
- Old age

Clinical Manifestation

- Severe pain in the hip and groin
- Affected limb appears shorter and externally rotated
- Stiffness, bruising and swelling the affected area
- Inability to bear weight

Nursing Care

- Apply traction to immobilize the area
- Prepare the patient for ORIF (open reduction and internal fixation)
- Prepare the patient for THR
- Perform neurovascular assessment
- Monitor the complications of immobility

Nursing Care of Total Hip Replacement (THR)

The upper femur and the socket of pelvic bone are replaced with prostheses (AMP or Austin Moore prosthesis). Total hip replacement may be a good option if arthritis or a prior injury has damaged the joint, affecting its function even before the fracture.

- Maintain abduction of the affected limb at all times with two pillows between the legs.
- Prevent external rotation by placing trochanter rolls along the feet.
- Prevent hip flexion by keeping the head of bed flat or raise the bed to 45 degree for meals if allowed.
- Turn only to the non-operated side.
- Use log rolling technique while moving the patient.
- Do not use low chairs.
- Early ambulation on the second postoperative day.
- Avoid weightbearing until allowed.
- Do not cross the legs.
- Use raised toilet seats.
- Do not bend down to put on shoes.

INTERVERTEBRAL DISC PROLAPSE (IVDP)

The human vertebral column consists of 24 articulating vertebrae and 9 fused vertebrae, so a total of 33 vertebral bones. They are:

Cervical	7
Thoracic	12
Lumbar	5
Sacrum	5
Coccyx	4

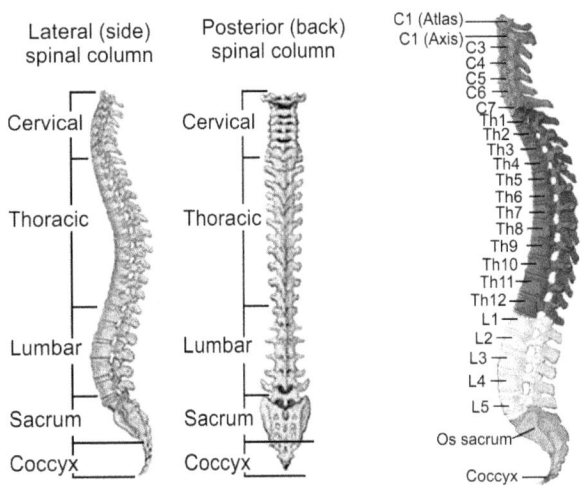

Intervertebral disc prolapse is also known as herniated nucleus prolapses (HNP). It is the protrusion of nucleus into the spinal canal causing compression of the spinal nerve root. It is commonly seen in males. The common site is between L_4 and L_5.

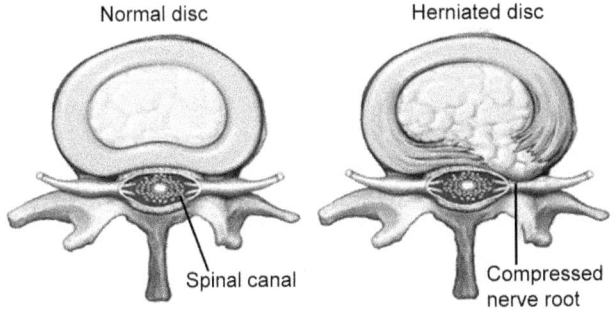

Top views of vertebrae

Causes

- Heavy lift pulling
- Trauma or RTA

Clinical Manifestation

Lumbar Region: Occurs in 80% of Cases

- Back pain radiating across the buttocks and down the legs
- Spasm of the back muscle
- Weakness of the leg and foot of the affected side
- Numbness and decreased reflexes
- Changes in bowel and bladder function
- Positive straight leg raise test (pain on raising the leg)

Cervical Region: 20% of Cases

- Shoulder pain radiating down the arm and hand
- Respiratory failure
- Paralysis of four extremities

Nursing Care

- Provide proper bed rest
- Provide cervical or pelvic traction
- Administer anti-inflammatory drugs
- Administer muscle relaxants
- Apply cervical collar
- Administer corticosteroids
- Prepare the patient for surgical corrections.

Surgical Correction

Chemonucleolysis

Chemonucleolysis is a non-surgical treatment for a bulging disc that involves the injection of an enzyme into the vertebral disc with the goal of dissolving the inner part of the disc, the nucleus pulposus.

The procedure uses chymopapain, an enzyme from the papaya fruit, to dissolve the displaced disc material that is putting pressure on the spinal nerve. The theory is that if chemonucleolysis can successfully alleviate back pain from a bulging disc, it could prevent the need for invasive surgery, such as a spinal fusion.

Nursing Care

- Administer premedications
- Administer diphenhydramine or benadryl
- Administer corticosteroids as per order
- Observe for any reactions or anaphylactic shock.

Laminectomy

A Laminectomy is a surgical incision (cut) into the vertebra (backbone) to get access to the structures associated with the spinal cord. It is usually performed in the cervical and lumbar regions, and less often in the thoracic region. If the surgery is at the lumbar region provide flat position and if the surgery is at the cervical region provide slight elevation of head end of bed and apply cervical collar.

Spinal Fusion

- Spinal fusion is surgery to permanently join together two or more bones in the spine so there is no movement between them.
- If the surgery is at the lumbar region keep the bed flat for first 12 hours and prone position.
- If the surgery is at the cervical region slight elevation of head of bed and apply cervical collar.
- Assist with ambulation on the third or fourth post-operative day
- A lumbo-sacral brace will be needed for the first four months and after that a lighter corset for one year, it may take one year for the graft to become stable.
- No bending, lifting, stooping or sitting for prolonged time.

CHAPTER 10

Hematological System

Chapter Objectives

- Keynotes in the hematological system
- Composition of blood
- Various diagnostic measures
- Disorders in the hematological system

KEY TERMS

RBC   Cells
WBC   Platelet
HOP   Plasma
RACE Anemia

KEYNOTES

- Schilling's test is used to rule out pernicious anemia.
- Pernicious anemia occurs as a deficiency of vitamin B_{12}.
- Red beefy tongue is seen in pernicious anemia.
- Other name of vitamin B_{12} is cyanocobalamin.
- Coombs test is used to rule out Rh-incompatibility.
- Sickledex test is used to rule out sickle cell anemia.
- Antidote of iron is deferoxamine mesylate (Desferal).
- Action of deferoxamine in thalassemia is excretion of iron.
- Confirmatory test for thalassemia is Hb electrophoresis.
- Usual cause of microcytic hypochromic anemia is decreased iron intake.
- The priority nursing care of a patient with sickle cell anemia is hydration.
- Universal blood donor is O negative (O^-).
- Universal blood recipient is AB positive (AB^+).
- Largest plasma protein is albumin.
- Average life span of red blood cells (RBCs) is 120 days.
- Average life span of sickled RBC is 5–20 days.
- Average life span of platelet is 9–10 days.
- Average life span of white blood cells (WBCs) is 10–20 days.
- Largest lymphatic organ is spleen.
- Spleen is called as the slaughter house of RBC.
- About 200 mL of blood is stored in the spleen in every minute during the circulation.
- Shape of RBCs is biconcave disc-shaped.
- The classical manifestation of anemia is palpitation.

INTRODUCTION

Hematology is a branch of science which deals with the study, diagnosis, treatment and prevention of blood-related disorders. Hematological system consists of blood and blood forming organs, such as liver, spleen, bone marrow, etc.

BLOOD

Normal blood volume in an individual is 70–80 mL/kg (5–6 liter). Blood is a circulating fluid in our body which carries oxygen and removes the waste products of metabolism.

Composition of Blood

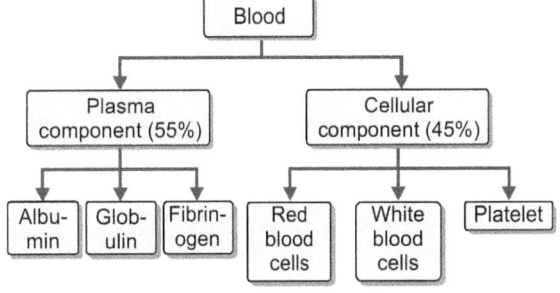

Plasma

About 55% of the blood component is plasma. It is a pale yellow colored liquid component of blood in which the blood cells are suspended. It consists of albumin, globulin and fibrinogen.

- **Albumin:**
  - It is the largest plasma protein. It maintains plasma oncotic pressure.
  - Normal serum albumin is 3.5–5 g/dL.
  - If it is less than 3.5, it is malnutrition.
  - If it is less than 2.5, it shows severe catabolism and muscle wasting.
  - Hypoalbuminemia is condition characterized by decreased albumin in blood.
  - The classical manifestation of hypoalbuminemia is edema resulting from fluid leak, secondary to decreased plasma oncotic pressure.
- **Globulin**
  - It is also a group of plasma protein which is produced by the liver and immune system.
  - It has higher molecular weight than albumin.
  - Globulin helps in the transportation of nutrients and steroids in our body.
  - Globulins are insoluble in plain water and soluble in salt water.
  - Normal serum globulin level is 2.5–4.5 g/dL.
  - Increased albumin level leads to decreased globulin levels (e.g. dehydration).
- **Fibrinogen**
  - It is a plasma protein which is produced by the liver cells.
  - It is also called as Factor I.
  - Fibrinogen helps to control bleeding, it is a clotting factor.
  - Normal fibrinogen level is 150–400 mg/dL.
  - Increased fibrinogen level is associated with cardiovascular disorders.

Cells

About 45% of the blood consists of cellular component. It consists of RBCs, WBCs and platelet.

- **RBCs (red blood cells)**
  - It is also called as erythrocytes.
  - It carries oxygen to different parts of our body.
  - Hemoglobin is a protein inside the RBC responsible for the carrying of oxygen.
  - RBC is produced by the bone marrow.
  - Normal RBC level is 4.7–6.1 million cells in males and 4.2–5.4 million in females.
  - Normal hemoglobin level 14–18 g/dL in males and 12–14 g/dL in females.
  - The life span of normal RBC is 120 days.
  - Increased RBC level leads to polycythemia.
  - Decreased RBC level leads to anemia.
- **WBCs (white blood cells)**
  - It is also called as leukocytes.
  - WBC maintains our immunity, protecting body against infection.
  - It is produced by the bone marrow.
  - Normal WBC count is 4000–11000 cells.
  - Increased WBC count seen in bacterial infection.
  - Decreased WBC count seen in viral infection.

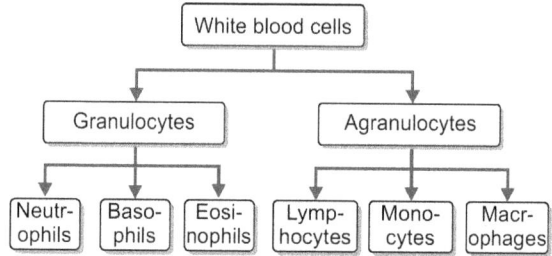

Granulocytes (polymorphonuclear leukocytes):
- **Neutrophils:** Defend against bacterial or fungal infection; Normal count is 45–70%.
- **Basophils:** Responsible for allergic and antigen response by releasing the chemical histamine which causes dilation of blood vessels; Normal count is 0–2%.
- **Eosinophils:** Primarily deals with parasitic infection; Normal count is 1–4%.

Agranulocytes (mononuclear leukocytes):
- **Lymphocytes:** Maintains immunity of body, consist of three types. **B-lymphocytes** produce antibodies in humoral immune response, **T-lymphocytes** responsible for cell-mediated immune response and **cytotoxic cells** that participate in innate immune response.
- **Monocytes:** Involved in long-term phagocytosis, constitute 4–8% of the WBC.
- **Macrophages:** They are monocytes that have migrated out of the blood stream and into the body tissues. They take up and destroy necrotic cell debris and foreign material, including virus, bacteria, etc.
- **Platelets**
  - They are also called as thrombocytes.
  - Platelets are colorless blood cells that help in blood clotting.
  - Normal platelet count is 150000–450000 cells.
  - Decreased platelet leads to severe bleeding.
  - Increased platelet leads to severe coagulation.
  - The life span of platelet is 9–10 days.

BONE MARROW

- Bone marrow is a spongy tissue inside the bone.
- Bone marrow produce blood cells, it is the blood cell factory.

- There are two types of bone marrow—**red bone marrow** is seen in small bones helps in hematopoiesis and **yellow bone marrow** also known as fat seen in long bones.
- Any breakdown in large bones results in fat embolism or pulmonary embolism.

COAGULATION FACTORS

Factor I	Fibrinogen
Factor II	Prothrombin
Factor III	Tissue factor or thromboplastin
Factor IV	Calcium
Factor V	Proaccelerin (Labile factor)
Factor VII	Proconvertin (Stable factor)
Factor VIII	Antihemophilic factor A Antihemophilic globulin
Factor IX	Antihemophilic factor B Plasma thromboplastin component, Christmas factor
Factor X	Stuart-Prower factor
Factor XI	Plasma thromboplastin antecedent Hemophilia C Rosenthal syndrome
Factor XII	Hageman factor
Factor XIII	Fibrin stabilizing factor Laki-Lorand factor

BLOOD GROUPS

Groups	Antigen	Antibody
A	A antigen on red cells	B antibody in the plasma
B	B antigen on red cells	A antibody in the plasma
AB	Both A and B antigen	No A and B antibody in plasma
O	No A and B antigen	Both A and B antibody in plasma

In addition to the A and B antigens, there is a third antigen called the Rh factor, which can be either present (+) or absent (–). In general, Rh-negative blood is given to Rh-negative patients and Rh-positive blood or Rh-negative blood may be given to Rh-positive patients.
- The universal red cell donor is O negative.
- The universal plasma donor is AB positive.

Groups	Donate to	Receive blood from
A$^+$ (positive)	A$^+$, B$^+$	A$^+$, A$^-$, O$^+$, O$^-$
O$^+$ (positive)	O$^+$, A$^+$, B$^+$, AB$^+$	O$^+$, O$^-$
B$^+$ (positive)	B$^+$, AB$^+$	B$^+$, B$^-$, O$^+$, O$^-$

Contd.

Groups	Donate to	Receive blood from
AB$^+$ (positive)	AB$^+$	Everyone
A$^-$ (negative)	A$^+$, A$^-$, AB$^+$, AB$^-$	A$^-$, O$^-$
O$^-$ (negative)	Everyone	O$^-$
B$^-$ (negative)	B$^+$, B$^-$, AB$^+$, AB$^-$	B$^-$, O$^-$
AB$^-$ (negative)	AB$^+$, AB$^-$	AB$^-$, A$^-$, B$^-$, O$^-$

- The universal blood donor is O negative.
- The universal blood recipient is AB positive.

HEMOLYSIS OR HEMOLYTIC REACTION

Hemolysis is the destruction or breakdown of the red blood cells. Hemolysis is usually evident as a pink or red tinge in the serum or plasma. The classical manifestation of hemolytic reaction is jaundice. There are mainly two causes of hemolysis:
1. *In-vivo hemolysis* may be due to pathological conditions, such as autoimmune hemolytic anemia or transfusion reactions.
2. *In-vitro hemolysis* may be due to improper specimen collection, specimen processing or specimen transport.

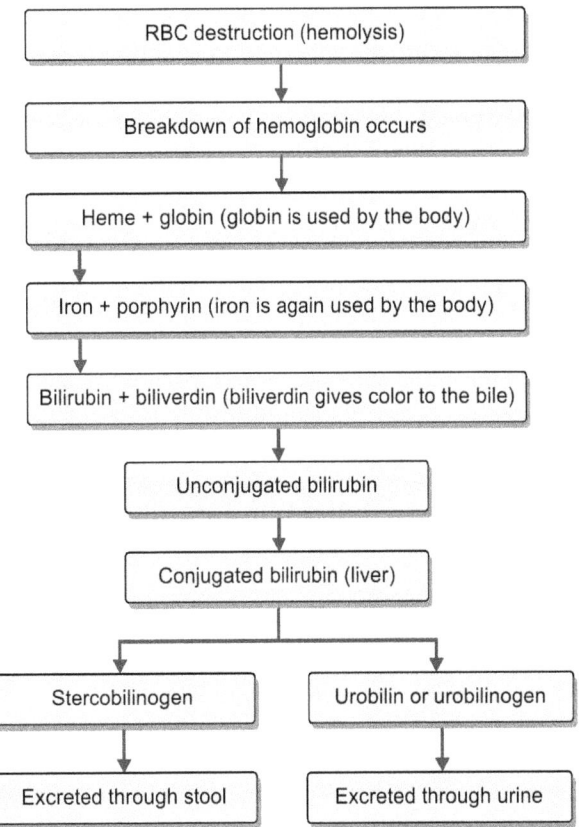

BLOOD TRANSFUSION

The process of transferring blood from one person to another is called as blood transfusion.

Nursing Care (Important Points to Consider)

- The blood is administered through a micron mesh filter called as blood set.
- During blood transfusion, monitor for any allergic reactions.
- Urticaria is a type of skin rash or reaction, is an allergic reaction occurs during blood transfusion.
- Administer premedications, such as Avil (chlorpheniramine maleate) of betnesol (betamethasone) as ordered.
- During blood transfusion, be with the patient for the first 15 minutes, because the reactions is most commonly seen in first 15 minutes.
- The maximum time of blood transfusion is 2-4 hours (platelet 20 minutes).
- The patient who is receiving more banked blood (blood from blood bank), have more chances of hyperkalemia because in the blood bank the preservative which is used to store blood is potassium citrate or sodium citrate.
- During blood transfusion, monitor for any shortness of breath, due to pulmonary embolism.
- During blood transfusion, do not add or touch with dextrose solution because dextrose causes hemolysis.
- Monitor for any fluid or circulatory overload during or after blood transfusion, in case of any fluid overload administer loop diuretics.
- During blood transfusion, monitor for any back pain, in case of any hemolytic reaction the broken down RBC will enter into the kidney cells and results in back pain.
- Monitor BP before during and after blood transfusion.
- Monitor for any TRALI (transfusion-related acute lung injury); where the transfused blood reacts with the person leading to blockages in the blood vessels in the lungs. Symptoms include difficulty in breathing and low blood oxygen levels. This can be life-threatening.

Nursing Care of Patient undergoing Iron Therapy

- Iron is best absorbed on an empty stomach. Yet, iron supplements can cause stomach cramps, nausea and diarrhea in some people. It may take with a small amount of food to avoid this problem.
- Milk, calcium and antacids should NOT be taken at the same time as iron supplements. One should wait for at least 2 hours after having these foods before taking the iron supplements.
- Food should NOT take with iron therapy are:
  - High fiber foods, such as whole grains, raw vegetables and bran.
  - Food or drinks with caffeine.
- Taking vitamin C supplement or drinking orange juice with iron pill. This can help the fast iron absorption of iron into the body.
- Side effect of iron therapy are constipation and diarrhea (very common).
- The stools are tarry-looking as well as black.
- Liquid forms of iron may stain your teeth.
- Try mixing the iron with water or other liquids (such as fruit juice or tomato juice) and drink the medicine with a straw.
- Iron stains can be removed by brushing your teeth with baking soda or peroxide.
- While administering iron injections, follow Z track method, fully stretch the skin to one side for easy absorption and to prevent irritation.
- Do not massage the site after iron injections.
- In case of IV infusion of iron, follow 1 mL per minute.

DISORDERS

Anemia

It is a condition in which there is a deficiency of red cells or hemoglobin in the blood, resulting in pallor and weariness.

Causes
- Blood loss
- Decreased or faulty RBCs production.
- Destruction of RBCs

Types
- Iron deficiency anemia
- Pernicious anemia
- Aplastic anemia
- Sickle cell anemia (hemolytic anemia)
- Thalassemia (hemolytic anema)

Iron Deficiency Anemia

It is caused by inadequate absorption of iron or excessive loss of iron.

Clinical Manifestations
- Pallor and chubby appearance
- Brittle hair
- Spoon-shaped nails
- Palpitation
- Dyspnea.

Diagnosis
- Decreased Hb and Hct (Hematocrit)
- Decreased serum iron level

Nursing Care
- Administer iron preparations.
- Oral iron preparation (Ferrum 200-325 mg).
- Educate the patient to clean the teeth after taking iron preparations because it may stain the teeth.
- Educate the patient that a black tarry color stool is common during iron therapy.
- Administer parenteral iron preparation, iron dextran injections or C-pink injections.
- Provide iron rich diets, such as green leafy vegetables, dried fruits, bread, cereals, liver, meat, etc.

Pernicious Anemia

It is a chronic progressive macrocytic anemia caused by absence or deficiency of intrinsic factor. Intrinsic factor is a glycoprotein which is seen in the intestinal mucosa. It helps in the absorption of vitamin B_{12}. So, pernicious anemia is due to the deficiency of vitamin B_{12}.

Clinical Manifestation
- Beefy red tongue
- Pallor
- Palpitation
- CNS symptoms like paralysis and paresthesia.

Diagnosis
Schilling test, 24 hours urine specimen is collected to monitor for vitamin B_{12}.

Nursing Care
- Administer vitamin B_{12} injections or intranasal sprays monthly for life long.
- Provide vitamin B_{12} rich food, such as citrus foods, dried fruits, green leafy vegetables, liver and organ meat.

Aplastic Anemia

It is also called as pancytopenia or bone marrow depression. Fatty replacement of the normal bone marrow may cause decreased RBCs, WBCs and platelets.

Classical Manifestation
- Anemia (due to decreased RBCs).
- Bleeding (due to decreased platelet).
- Infection (due to decreased WBCs).

Nursing Care
- Administer corticosteroids.
- Prepare the patient for bone marrow transplantation.

Hemolytic Anemia

It is a dangerous form of anemia in which there is increased destruction of RBC occurs. The classical manifestations of hemolytic anemia are jaundice and hypoxia.

Types

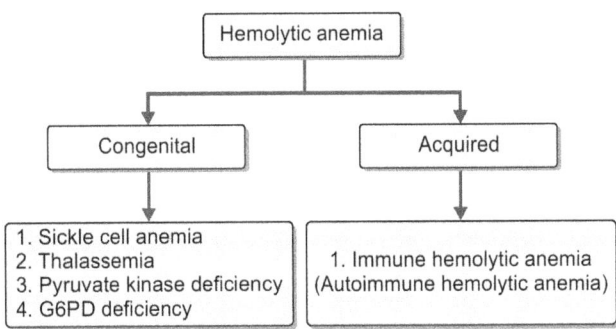

Sickle Cell Anemia

It is an autosomal recessive disorder in which the structure of hemoglobin becomes abnormal. The complication of sickle cell anemia is severe hypoxia and dehydration. The life span of RBCs is 120 days and the shape of normal RBC is round and pliable. The life span of sickled RBCs is 6-20 days and the shape of sickled RBC is rigid and inflexible. It may clog together and result is blockage of blood vessel.

Clinical Manifestation
- Colic abdominal pain
- Splenomegaly
- Frequent infections
- Dactylitis (hand foot syndrome, inflammation of entire digit)
- Delayed growth and development
- Renal failure

Diagnosis
- Decreased Hb level.
- Sickledex test (a drop of blood mixed with solution, the mixture turns to cloudy indicates presence of sickled RBC).

Nursing Care
- The priority nursing care of a patient with sickle cell anemia is hydration oral or IV.
- Avoid tight clothing.
- Avoid activities that interfere with oxygenation, such as mountain climbing, flying in unpressurized aeroplane, etc.
- Administer urea to prevent sickling (hydroxyurea or myelostat).
- Administer Desferal or Deferoxamine mesylate.
- Provide HOP management
  - H: Hydration
  - O: Oxygenation
  - P: Pain management.

Thalassemia

It is an autosomal recessive disorder characterized by destruction of globin chain of hemoglobin. It is also known as Cooley's anemia. It is commonly seen in Mediterranean people, Greek, Italian, etc.

Clinical Manifestation
- Severe anemia
- Frontal bossing
- Maxillary prominence
- Greenish-yellow skin tone.

Nursing Care
- Monitor for iron overload.
- Provide chelation therapy.
- Administer Deferoxamine mesylate or Desferal for iron overload.

(G6PD) or glucose-6-phosphate-dehydrogenase deficiency: An X-linked recessive disorder characterized by hemolysis. In G6PD deficiency, the RBCs are missing an important enzyme called G6PD. G6PD is part of the normal chemistry inside RBCs. In G6PD deficiency, if RBCs come into contact with certain substances in the bloodstream, the missing enzyme causes the cells to rupture (burst) and die.

Clinical Manifestation
- Jaundice
- Activity intolerance

Nursing Care
Prepare the patient for blood transfusion.

Pyruvate kinase deficiency: In this condition, the body missing an enzyme called **pyruvate kinase**. Lack of this enzyme causes RBCs to breakdown easily.

Clinical Manifestation
- Hemolytic anemia
- Gall bladder stones
- Infections
- Splenomegaly
- Leg ulcers

Nursing Care
- Prepare the patient for blood transfusion.
- Prepare the patient for splenectomy.

Immune hemolytic anemia: Immune hemolytic anemia occurs when antibodies form against the body's own RBCs and destroy them. This happens because the immune system mistakenly recognizes these blood cells as foreign. It occurs as a result of blood transfusion reaction, drug induced or due to any cancer.

Clinical Manifestation
- Pallor
- Brittle nail
- Headache
- Shortness of breath

Nursing Care
- Administer corticosteroids
- Administer immunoglobulin IV as per order
- Prepare the patient for splenectomy

Polycythemia

It is a disorder characterized by increased RBC level.

Clinical Manifestation
- Ruddy complexion of the skin and mucous membrane
- Hypertension
- Headache
- Gout due to increased serum uric acid

Diagnosis
- Increased Hb and Hct
- Increased bilirubin.

Nursing Care
- Monitor for bleeding
- Administer more fluids 3-4 liter/day.
- Administer busulfan to depress the bone marrow
- Avoid iron preparations.
- Avoid person with infection.
- Prepare the patient for phlebotomy, removal of 350-500 mL of blood.

Hemophilia

It is considered as a Royal disorder. It is a bleeding disorder characterized by deficiency of clotting factor.

Types
- Hemophilia A: Deficiency of factor VIII, antihemophilic factor.
- Hemophilia B: Deficiency of factor IX, Christmas factor.
- Hemophilia C: Deficiency of factor XI.

Clinical Manifestation
- Prolonged bleeding after a minor injury.
- Prolonged bleeding after cutting the cord, circumcision and dental extraction.
- Hemarthrosis (bleeding into the joints).

Nursing Care
- Administer cryoprecipitate
- Avoid ASA or aspirin preparations.
- Administer deficient factor.
- Provide RICE therapy
  - R: Rest
  - I: Ice application
  - C: Compression
  - E: Elevation.

Idiopathic Thrombocytopenic Purpura

It is a disorder of platelet in which the platelet count is less than 1 lakh. It is characterized by petechiae and ecchymosis (without any reason there is thrombocytopenia and manifested as purpura).

Clinical Manifestation
- Blood in body secretions
- Melena
- Hematuria
- Epistaxis
- Spider-like appearance.

Nursing Care
- Administer steroids
- Prepare the patient for platelet transfusion
- Take prompt measures to control bleeding
- Avoid ASA, acetylsalicylic acid
- Administer immunoglobulin.

Disseminated Intravascular Coagulation

Disseminated intravascular coagulation (DIC) is a rare, life-threatening condition that prevents blood from clotting normally. The blood clots reduce blood flow and can block blood from reaching to other body organs. It is the diffused fibrin deposition in the arteries or capillaries which results in bleeding from the internal organs, such as kidney, brain, heart, adrenal, etc.

Causes
- Commonly seen in PIH (pregnancy-induced hypertension) and cancer
- Hypothermia
- Burns

Clinical Manifestation
- Petechiae
- Ecchymosis
- Prolonged bleeding after child birth
- Coma, convulsions
- Decreased BP

Nursing Care
- Monitor the platelet count
- Monitor PT and APTT
- Prepare the patient for blood transfusion
- Avoid IM injections.

Infectious Mononucleosis

It is a viral infection caused by Epstein-barr virus. It is seen in the saliva of the infected person, so it is also known as kissing disease. It is commonly seen in adolescents and young adults.

Clinical Manifestation
- Enlargement of the lymph nodes
- Lethargy
- Sore throat
- Tonsillitis
- Increased WBC count.

Nursing Care
- Administer antibiotic therapy, a short course of penicillin in case of beta hemolytic streptococci.
- Monitor for complications, such as splenic rupture or Vincent's angina (also known as *streptococcal pharyngitis* or *bacterial gingivitis*).

CHAPTER 11

Integumentary System

Chapter Objectives

- Keynotes in the integumentary system
- Anatomy and structure
- Disorders in the integumentary system
- Burns
- Shock

KEY TERMS

Skin, MSH, Melanin, Acne, Burns, Shock, Epidermis, Clubbing

KEYNOTES

- The weight of skin is 5-10 lbs.
- Curling ulcer is seen in burns patient.
- Rule of nine is applicable in burns.
- The characteristic feature of the shock phase in burns is shift of plasma volume from intravascular to interstitial space.
- Clubbing is the enlargement of fingers and toes, nails become convex appearance is seen in pulmonary and cardiovascular conditions.
- Melanocyte which produces a pigment called melanin is responsible for the skin color.
- Beau's line is a transverse groove in nails seen in systemic disorders.
- Alopecia is loss of hair.
- A benign, often itchy growth that appears like a 'stuckon' wart is seborrheic keratosis.
- A raised red and itchy patch on the skin that arises suddenly called as hives.
- Shingles infection is also called as herpes zoster, caused by chickenpox virus.
- Ringworm also called as tinea, a fungal infection of skin.
- Shigellosis is a bacterial infection of the digestive tract manifested as diarrhea.
- Removal of a small piece of tissue for examination is called skin biopsy.
- Replacement of damaged skin with a healthy skin to provide protection is called skin graft.
- Redness on skin is the classical manifestation of stage I bed sore.
- Human amniotic membrane is also used for grafting.
- Koebner phenomenon is associated with psoriasis.

INTRODUCTION

The integumentary system is an organ consists of the skin, nails, hair and exocrine glands.

SKIN

It is the largest organ of the body consists of 20 square feet, 10 lbs. It forms the body's outer covering which protect us from microbes, chemicals and various physical damages.

Functions of Skin

- Helps in touch sensation
- Regulate body temperature
- Protection from microbes and harm.

Layers of Skin (Fig. 1)

There are three layers:
1. ***The epidermis,*** the outermost layer of skin, provides a waterproof barrier and creates our skin tone.
2. ***The dermis,*** beneath the epidermis, contains tough connective tissue, hair follicles and sweat glands.
3. ***The hypodermis*** (deeper subcutaneous tissue) is made of fat and connective tissue.

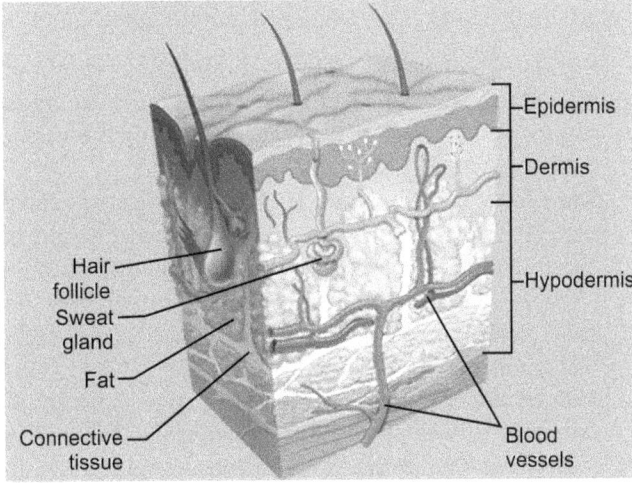

Fig. 1: Structure of skin

HAIR

Hair is an accessory organ of the skin made of columns of tightly packed dead keratinocytes found in most regions of the body. Hair helps to protect the body from UV radiation by preventing sunlight from striking the skin.

SWEAT GLANDS

They are also called as sudoriferous glands. There are two types of sweat glands—eccrine and apocrine sweat glands.
1. **Eccrine sweat glands:** They are found in almost every region of the skin and produce a secretion of water and sodium chloride. It is delivered via a duct to the surface of the skin and is used to lower the body's temperature through evaporative cooling.
2. **Apocrine sweat glands:** They are found mainly in the axillary and pubic regions of the body. The ducts of apocrine sweat glands extend into the follicles of hairs so that the sweat produced by these glands exits the body along the surface of the hair shaft. They are inactive until puberty, at which point they produce a thick, oily liquid that is consumed by bacteria living on the skin. The digestion of apocrine sweat by bacteria produces body odor.

SEBACEOUS GLANDS

They are exocrine glands found in the dermis of the skin that produce an oily secretion known as sebum. Sebum is produced in the sebaceous glands and carried through ducts to the surface of the skin or to hair follicles. Sebum acts to waterproof and increase the elasticity of the skin.

DISORDERS

Dermatitis

It is the irritation of the skin due to any specific substances.

Causes

- Allergens, such as chemicals
- Presence of fungus or yeast in the oily secretion.

Clinical Manifestation

- Pruritus
- Redness and itching
- Erythema
- Localized edema and vesicles

Nursing Care

- Apply wet dressing with Burow's solution, aluminum acetate in water to prevent irritation or rashes
- Apply corticosteroid creams, such as Betnesol or Candid creams
- Administer antihistamines, such as cetirizine or levo-cetirizine groups

Acne

Acne also called as acne vulgaris is the inflammation of the hair follicle. It is also called as pimple occurs at the time of puberty.

Causes

- Excessive oil production
- Due to any bacterial infection
- Pores plugged with dead tissues and oils.

Clinical Manifestation

- Small tender pimples
- Blackheads or whiteheads
- Painful lesions.

Nursing Care

- Administer medications as ordered (minocycline, isotretinoin, retinoids)
- Administer benzyl peroxide creams or clindamycin creams
- Instruct the patient to clean face
- Provide psychological support.

Psoriasis

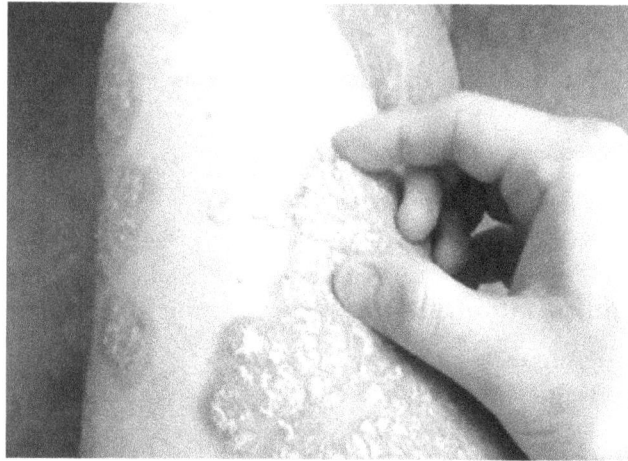

It is a chronic inflammation of the skin (chronic dermatitis).

Causes

- Familial tendency
- Stress
- Infection, such as tonsillitis
- Medications, such as lithium and beta blockers.

Clinical Manifestation

- Most commonly affecting the head, scalp and knees.
- Red scaly patches on scalp, elbows, knees and other parts of the body.
- Sharply circumscribed lesions.
- Shedding of scales of skin.
- Onycholysis or lifting of the free edge of the nail away from the skin below.
- Subungual hyperkeratosis or thickening of the skin below the nail.
- Itching.

Nursing Care

- Apply corticosteroid creams.
- Apply coal tar preparations, cortisone calcipotriol and other prescription creams.
- Administer medications, such as methotrexate (folitrax), neotigason, cyclosporine and calcipotriol.
- Prepare the patient for ultraviolet light therapy.
- Avoid sun exposure after coal tar application.

Skin Cancer

Skin cancer is the cancer that arises from the epidermis. It is commonly seen due to excessive sunlight exposure.

Types

- **Basal cell carcinoma:** This is the most common but least dangerous form of skin cancer. It most often occurs on the head and neck, followed by the upper body.
- **Squamous cell carcinoma:** This cancer grows over a period of weeks or months and may spread to other parts of the body if not treated quickly. It occurs most often on areas exposed to the sun. This can include the head, neck, hands and forearms. This cancer looks like thickened, red, scaly spots.
- **Melanoma:** Melanoma is the most dangerous form of skin cancer. Melanoma can grow quickly, developing over weeks to months. Nodular melanoma is a highly dangerous form of melanoma that looks different from common melanomas—they are raised from the start and are even in color (often red or pink and some are brown or black). This type of melanoma grows quickly and can be life-threatening if not detected and removed quickly.

Causes

- Excessive sunlight exposure.

Clinical Manifestation

- Lesions
- Large brownish spot in case of melanoma
- Red nodule
- Changes in wart or mole.

Nursing Care

- Provide protection against UV radiation.
- Use sunscreen lotions with SPF more than 30 and PABA (para aminobenzoic acid).
- Use ABCDE system to check the unusual wart or mole:
  - **Asymmetry:** Unevenness of the spot.
  - **Border:** Any change in the edge of the spot.
  - **Color:** The changes in the color of spot, shades of brown or black, red, white or blue.

- **Diameter**: The spot is larger than 6 mm across (about 1/4 inch) or is growing larger.
- **Evolution or elevation**: The spot may change in shape or size (enlarge) and a flat spot may become raised in a matter of a few weeks.

Herpes Zoster

Viral infection caused by herpes virus varicella zoster. It may cause inflammation of the dorsal root ganglia.

Clinical Manifestation

- Fever
- Pruritus
- CSF study shows increased protein level.

Nursing Care

- Administer cortisone
- Primary goal is to relieve itching and pain.

Burns

Burns are any injury to the skin occurs as a result of heat, electricity or chemicals.

Causes

- Chemicals: Ingestion or inhalation of acids or alkalies
- Thermal: Contact with flame or hot objects
- Electrical: Due to electricity
- Smoke or corrosive inhalation.

Types of Burns

- **First degree burns: Superficial burns**—In this type, if burns there is damage to the top layer, epidermis. Sensation is very painful.
- **Second degree burns: Partial thickness burns**—In this type of burns, there is damage to the first and second layer of skin. The burn site will be red, blistered and swelling. Sensation is also painful.
- **Third degree burns: Full thickness burns**—In this type of burns, there is damage to first, second and underlying tissues. The burn site is black colored. In some case, there will be damage to entire muscles and bones. Sensation is painless or has mild pain.

Rule of Nine (Fig. 2)

- Head and neck = 9%
- Each arm = 9%
- Trunk = 36% (anterior trunk 18 + posterior trunk 18)
- Each leg = 18%
- Genitalia = 1%

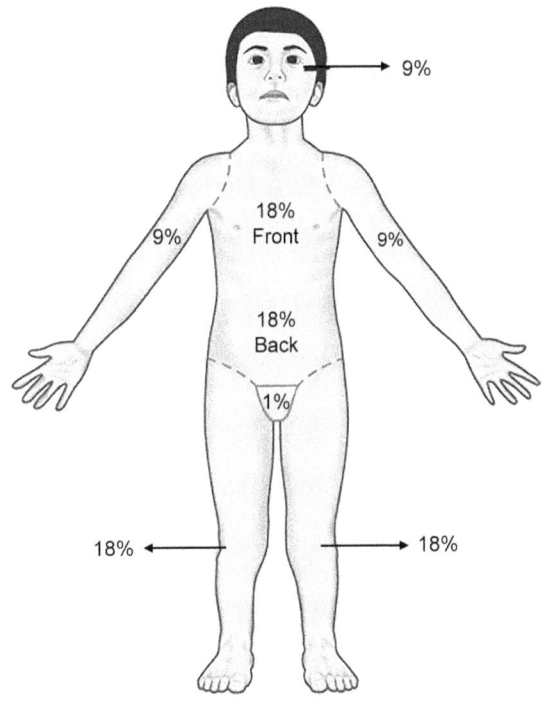

Fig. 2: Rule of nine

Stages of Burns

- **Emergent phase:** It is the first stage of burns; remove the person from the source of burns. In case of smoke inhalation maintain a patent airway; in case of chemical ingestion give gastric lavage.

RACE PASS

R: Rescue the patient
A: Alarm
C: Confinement
E: Extinguish
P: Pull the pin
A: Aim to the base of fire
S: Squeeze it
S: Swipe it

- **Shock phase:** It occurs first 24–48 hours after burns. In this phase, plasma volume shift to interstitial space causing hypovolemia, dehydration, hypotension, hyperkalemia, elevated Hct and metabolic acidosis.
- **Diuretic phase:** It occurs after 2–3 days of burns. Plasma return to the intravascular compartment characterized by increased BP, hypokalemia and increased urine output.
- **Recovery phase:** It occurs after diuretic phase, wound healing starts in this phase.

Nursing Care

- Administer IV fluids: Ringer lactate is administered as fluid replacement in order to replace the electrolytes.
- Administer antibiotics as ordered, topical antibiotics, such as silverex (silver sulfadiazine).
- Administer analgesic and tetanus toxoid injections, in case of severe pain administer morphine sulfate.
- Maintain strict intake output chart.
- Position the patient as comfort (in case of head, neck and face burns provide upright position).
- Provide proper nutritious diet to promote healing (high protein).
- In case of any skin graft, provide bed cradles and elevate the site when possible.
- Administer hypertonic solution in case of plasma volume depletion or vascular volume depletion.
- Use Parkland formula for fluid calculation (4 × percentage of body surface area burned × weight), administer half of the fluid in first 8 hours remaining half in next 16 hours.
- *Example: A patient having 20% burned is admitted in the hospital whose weight is 50 kg, calculate the amount of fluid administered in first 8 hours?*
- *Parkland formula = (4 × 20 × 50) = 4000 mL, so 2000 mL is administered in first 8 hours.*
- Monitor for any complications, curling ulcer is a type of stress ulcer seen in burns patient.
- Provide proper wound care with antiseptic solution (betadine).

Type of Solutions

Isotonic solution	Hypotonic solution	Hypertonic solution
0.9% Normal saline	0.25% Normal saline	Mixture solution
D5 (Dextrose 5%)	0.45% Normal saline	DNS (Dextrose normal saline)
RL (Ringer lactate)	0.225% Normal saline	Protein solution

Body Compartments

There are two compartments, intracellular and extracellular. The major cation in the extracellular compartment is sodium and major cation in the intracellular compartment is potassium.

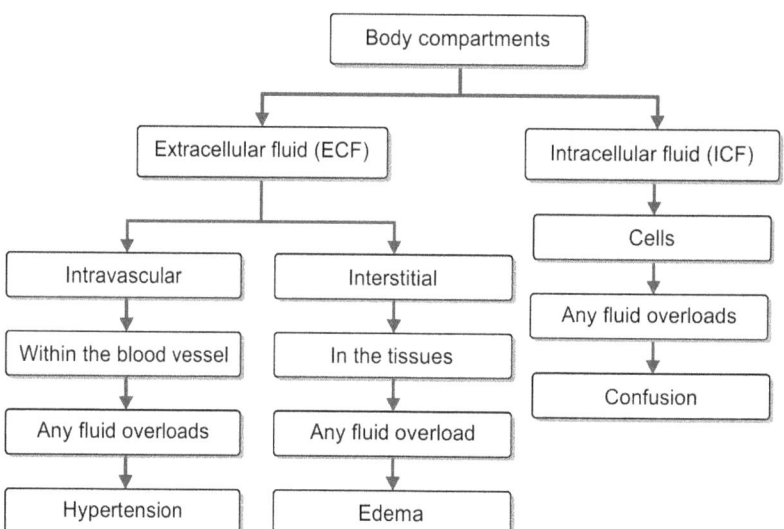

Bed Sore

Bed sores are also called pressure sores or pressure ulcers. These are injuries to skin and underlying tissue resulting from prolonged pressure on the skin. Bed sores most often develop on skin that covers bony areas of the body, such as the heels, ankles, hips and tailbone.

Stages of Bed Sore

- *Stage 1: Redness.*
- *Stage 2 (blister):* The epidermis or topmost layer of the skin is broken, creating a shallow open sore. Drainage may or may not be present.
- *Stage 3 (fascia):* The break in the skin extends through the dermis (second skin layer) into the subcutaneous and fat tissue. The wound is deeper than in stage two.
- *Stage 4:* The breakdown extends into the muscle and can extend as far down as the bone. Usually, lots of dead tissue and drainage are present.

Shock

Shock is a condition characterized by imbalance in the circulatory volume and demand. It is also known as a clinical state of cardiovascular collapse. Shock is a condition that results from severe illness or trauma which results in lack of oxygenation and circulatory volume depletion.

Causes

- Decreased intravascular hemorrhage (hypovolemia)
- Inappropriate peripheral vasodilation
- Trauma or severe illness.

Types of Shock

- *Cardiogenic shock:* Results from decreased myocardial contractility or cardiomyopathy or fluid volume excess.

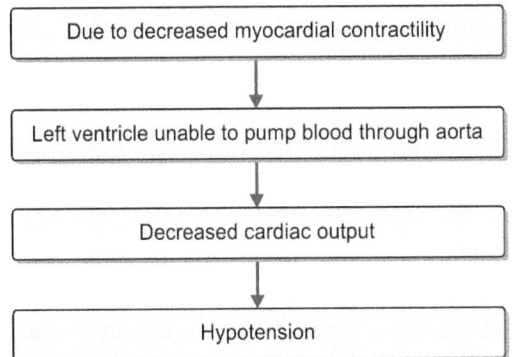

The **classical manifestation of cardiogenic shock** is JVD (jugular vein distension), edema and pulsus paradoxus (abnormal fall in systolic BP for more than 10 mm Hg).

- *Hypovolemic shock:* It means not enough blood volume. The main causes include bleeding, which could be internal (such as a ruptured artery or organ) or external (such as a deep wound) or dehydration. Chronic vomiting, diarrhea, dehydration or severe burns can also reduce blood volume and cause a dangerous drop in blood pressure.
- *Neurogenic shock:* Any injury to a person's spine may damage the nerves that control the diameter (width) of blood vessels. The blood vessels below the spinal injury relax and expand (dilate) and cause a drop in blood pressure.
- *Septic shock:* Any infection makes the blood vessels dilate, which drops blood pressure. For example, an *E. coli* infection may trigger septic shock.
- *Anaphylactic shock:* Any severe allergic reaction causes blood vessels to dilate, which results in low BP. The drug of choice in anaphylactic shock is adrenaline or epinephrine.

Clinical Manifestation

- Unconsciousness
- Low BP
- Weak and rapid pulse
- Weakness
- Pale, cold, clammy skin in hypovolemic shock and warm and dry in septic shock
- Rapid breathing or respiration due to hypoxia
- Decreased temperature in severe shock except in septic shock.

Nursing Care

- Maintain a patent airway
- Administer medications
- The drug of choice for shock is adrenaline or epinephrine to increase the force of myocardial contractility.
- Administer corticosteroids
- Administer positive inotropic drugs, such as dopamine
- Provide proper position (head down and legs up in order to shunt blood to heart and brains).

Chapter 12

Oncology

Chapter Objectives

- Keynotes in the oncology
- Staging and grading of cancer
- Chemotherapy and radiation therapy
- Type of cancers

KEY TERMS

CEA   Wilms tumor
BSE   Busulfan
TSE   Cisplatin
Teletherapy Brachytherapy

KEYNOTES

- Benign tumor of connective tissue is osteochondroma.
- Malignant tumor of connective tissue is chondrosarcoma.
- Sarcoma is the tumor of connective tissue.
- Tumor circumscribed in one area is known as benign tumor.
- The common type of cancer in males is prostate cancer.
- The common type of cancer seen in females is breast cancer and cervical cancer.
- Cardiotoxicity is associated with doxorubicin.
- Tinnitus is seen in patients taking cisplatin.
- Pulmonary function test is prescribed for a patient taking bleomycin.
- Lasix is an ototoxic drug.
- Reed-Sternberg cell is a classical feature of Hodgkin's lymphoma.
- Cisplatin is an alkylating agent.
- Folinic acid agents are synergistic agents administered along with methotrexate to prevent toxicity.
- Neurotoxicity is seen in patient taking vinca alkaloids.
- Monitor serum uric acid for a patient undergoing chemotherapy.
- One of the iatrogenic causes of cancer is the X-rays used for the treatment of cancer.

ONCOLOGY

Oncology is the study of cancer and its treatment. Cancer is a neoplastic disorder in which any cell which is growing outer than the predetermined boundary. Benign tumor is the tumor circumscribed in one area and malignant tumor is the tumor which metastasis to different parts of the body.

Route of Metastasis

- Blood-borne metastasis (blood route)
- Lymphatic spread

Warning Signs of Cancer

It is denoted by a word CAUTION.
- C: Changes in the bowel and bladder function
- A: A sore that does not heal
- U: Unusual urethral bleeding or discharge
- T: Thickening or lump in the breast
- I: Indigestion or dysphagia
- O: Obvious changes in the wart or mole
- N: Nagging cough

Grading of Cancer

- Grade I: Mild differentiation, mild dysplasia
- Grade II: Moderate differentiation, moderate dysplasia
- Grade III: Severe differentiation, severe dysplasia
- Grade IV: Undifferentiated, cells are not matured and destroyed.

Staging of Cancer

- Stage 0: Carcinoma in situ
- Stage I: localized tumor
- Stage II: Limited local spread
- Stage III: Extensive spread
- Stage IV: Distant metastasis.

Treatment of Cancer

- Chemotherapy
- Radiation therapy
- Surgery

Chemotherapy

The use of drugs for the treatment of cancer is called as chemotherapy.

Side Effects of Chemotherapy

- Alopecia—loss of hair
- Nausea
- Vomiting
- Excessive salivation

Complications of Chemotherapy

- Increases serum uric acid (due to cell damage)
- Decreases platelet count
- Bleeding
- Infection

Radiation Therapy

Radiation therapy is the use of X-rays or radiations for the treatment of cancer. Wash the irradiated area with mild soap and water.

Types

- Teletherapy: External beam radiation is used
- Brachytherapy: Radiations from implanted devices

CLASSIFICATION OF MEDICATIONS

1. **Antimetabolites**
    - It prevent metabolism of cells
    - For example, methotrexate (Folitrax, Oncotrex)
    - Administer along with folic acid to prevent toxicity
2. **Alkylating agents**
    - It breaks the DNA helix
    - For example, busulfan, cyclophosphamide, and cisplatin
    - Check serum uric acid level
    - Administer more fluids
3. **Antitumor antibiotics**
    - For example, doxorubicin, bleomycin
    - Monitor ECG changes for patient with doxorubicin therapy
    - Perform PFT for patient with bleomycin therapy
4. **Mitotic inhibitors**
    - Also called as plant alkaloids
    - For example, vincristine
5. **Hormonal therapy**
    - Tamoxifen citrate

TYPE OF CANCERS

Skin Cancer

Malignant lesion of the skin.

Clinical Manifestation

- Changes in the color and size of the lesion
- Pruritus
- Local soreness

Nursing Care

- Instruct to avoid sun exposure between 10 am and 4 pm
- Assess the grading and staging of cancer
- Instruct the patient to apply sunscreen lotion with SPF >15 (Sun Protecting Factor)

Multiple Myeloma

A malignant proliferation of the plasma cells within the bone.

Clinical Manifestation

- Bone pain
- Pathological fracture
- Elevated calcium and uric acid level
- Presence of bence jones protein in urine

Nursing Care

- Administer chemotherapy
- Check serum calcium level
- Monitor for BUN and creatinine level (renal failure)
- Administer more fluids (forcing fluid)

Lung Cancer

Malignant tumor of the bronchial and peripheral tissues, it is also called as bronchogenic carcinoma.

Clinical Manifestation

- Chest pain
- Blood tinged sputum
- Dyspnea

Nursing Care

- Maintain patent airway
- Provide Fowler's position
- Prepare the patient for surgical correction

Laryngeal Cancer

Most common upper respiratory malignancy, it is the malignant tumor of larynx.

Clinical Manifestation

- Progressive hoarseness of voice for more than 6 weeks
- Burning sensation while drinking hot fluids and orange juice
- Change in the voice quality.

Nursing Care

- Place the patient on Fowler's position
- High calorie high protein diet
- Prepare the patient for laryngectomy
- After laryngectomy, make the patient to accept the body image disturbance, because after surgery the sound of the patient will be monotonous.

Prostate Cancer

Slow growing malignancy of the prostate gland. Commonly seen in men after the age group of 50 years.

Clinical Manifestation

- Asymptomatic in early stage
- Hard and pea-shaped nodule is palpated through Digital Rectal Examination
- PSA (prostate specific antigen) will be elevated (normal PSA is < 4 ng/mL)

Nursing Care

- Prepare the patient to undergo Digital Rectal Examination (DRE)
- Prepare to administer medication
- Prepare the patient for TURP (Transurethral resection of the prostate)

Gastric Cancer

This is the malignant tumor of the mucosal ling of the stomach. It is due to the repeated *H. pylori* infection and high smoked and salted diet.

Clinical Manifestation

- Indigestion
- Feeling of fullness
- Epigastric pain and weight loss

Nursing Care

- Monitor hemoglobin and hematocrit levels
- Place the patient in Fowler's position after surgical correction.

Pancreatic Cancer

Malignant and rapidly growing adenocarcinoma of the pancreas, it is associated with increased age and a history of diabetes mellitus.

Clinical Manifestation

- Jaundice
- Clay-colored stools
- Glucose intolerance

Nursing Care

- Monitor the blood glucose level
- Prepare the patient for surgical correction.

Breast Cancer

Cancer which is seen in the breast and tissues surrounding the mammary gland.

Clinical Manifestation

- Mass felt during BSE (Breast Self-Examination)
- Nipple retractions
- Presence of lump on the breast
- Presence of lesions on mammography

Nursing Care

- Instruct the patient to perform BSE (perform under a shower or flow of water, ideal time is 7–10 days after menstrual period, monitor for any lump in the breast)
- Administer medication; the standard drug used for breast cancer is tamoxifen citrate.
- Estrogen receptor positive (ERP) seen in breast cancer
- Prepare the patient for mastectomy.
- After mastectomy, no IV injection, no blood pressure measurement and no venipunctures on the side of mastectomy and elevate the arm above heart level.
- The state seen in postmastectomy women is denial.

Testicular Cancer

Testicular cancer arises from the germinal epithelium from the sperm producing cells. Testicular cancer most often 15–40 years.

Clinical Manifestation

- Painless testicular swelling
- Dragging or pulling sensation is experienced in the scrotum.

Nursing Care

- Instruct the patient to perform testicular self-examination (TSE), usually performed after a warm shower when the scrotums are relaxed.
- Prepare the patient for orchiectomy

Cervical Cancer

Cancer which is seen in the cervix and pelvic structure.

Clinical Manifestation

- Painless vaginal postmenstrual and postcoital bleeding
- Foul smelling vaginal discharge
- Low back pain
- Leakage of urine and feces from the vagina.

Nursing Care

- Prepare the patient for laser therapy
- Monitor for vaginal discharge.

Ovarian Cancer

Ovarian cancer grows rapidly, spreads fast and is often bilateral.

Classical Manifestation

- Abdominal discomfort
- Vaginal bleeding
- Abdominal mass

Nursing Care

- Prepare the patient for radiation therapy
- Monitor for vaginal bleeding

Leukemia

They are a group of disorder involves the over production of leukocytes, usually at an immature stage in the bone marrow.

Clinical Manifestation

- Prolonged bleeding
- Anemia
- Increased temperature, palpitation and tachycardia
- Decreased hemoglobin, hematocrit and platelet count
- Enlarged lymph node, spleen and liver

Nursing Care

- Monitor for bleeding
- Administer antibiotics
- Administer blood
- Provide psychological support

Hodgkin's Lymphoma

Malignant neoplasm of the lymphatic tissue, it is common in adolescents.

Clinical Manifestation

- Enlarged cervical lymph nodes (nontender, firm and movable)
- Intermittent fever
- Night sweat

Nursing Care

- Prepare the patient for chemotherapy and radiation therapy.

Non-Hodgkin's Lymphoma

Tumor originating from the lymph tissue but control of the primary tumor is difficult. Primary site is GIT (gastrointestinal tract), ovaries, testis, CNS, liver, breast, etc.

Wilms' Tumor

Large encapsulated tumor in the renal parenchyma. Affect the left kidney first, peak age is 1-3 years.

Clinical Manifestation

- Hypertension
- Hematuria

Nursing Care

- Do not palpate the abdomen to avoid dissemination of cancer cells and metastasis.
- Handle the child carefully when bathing and giving care.

CHAPTER 13

Eye and Ear

Chapter Objectives

- Keynotes in eye and ear
- Anatomy and structure
- Disorders in eye
- Disorders in ear

KEY TERMS

POAG AH
PACG VH
Cochlea Stapes
IOP Snellen

KEYNOTES

- Lasix is an ototoxic drug (damages C8 cranial nerves).
- Streptomycin causes ototoxicity.
- The ideal way to remove the eye lenses is apply pressure to the eyelids.
- Diet for patient with Ménière's disease is low sodium and decrease fluid intake.
- Instruct the patient to suck a hard candy while hearing loud voice or flying from one altitude to another.
- One of the most common causes of adult hearing loss is otosclerosis.
- The other name of otosclerosis is stapes fixation.
- Visual acuity is tested with the help of eye chart, Snellen chart.
- Normal intraocular pressure (IOP) is 10–21 mm Hg.
- IOP varies throughout the day, it is slightly high in the morning.
- Glaucoma is a condition occurs due to increased IOP.
- To open the external auditory canal straight, hold the ear pinna upward and backward (adults) and downward and backward in children (less than 3 years) and after administering keep it for 2 minutes.
- How to speak with a patient having conductive hearing loss, speak in a normal tone.
- How to speak to a patient with impaired hearing, face to face and do not shout.
- The priority nursing care of a patient with glaucoma is instructing the patient to continue medication lifelong.
- Normal visual acuity is 6/6 (Snellen chart) or 20/20.
- Tears normally drain through small openings in the corners of the upper and lower eyelids called puncta and enter the nose through the nasolacrimal duct.
- Lack of tears in eyes will leads to dryness and infection.
- The commonly used artificial tears are refresh tears, tear drops, etc.
- Administer tropicacyl or tropicamide eye drops before ophthalmic examination in order to relax the muscles.
- After tropicamide application, there will be dilation of pupil, so assist the patient to bed or chair. Do not allow the patient to go alone or drive alone for at least 2–3 hours.
- Do not insert an otoscope blindly into the ear of the patient because it causes perforation.
- The proper place to instill eye drops is center of the eye, because blinking helps to spread the medicines to different parts of eye.
- The proper site to instill eye drop is lower conjunctival sac.
- PERRLA is related to eye (Pupils, Equal, Round, React to, Light and Accommodation).
- Accommodation is the ability of eye to change from distant to near objects and vice versa (ability to focus objects).

- The classical manifestation of retinal detachment is a sense of curtain falling over the eyes.
- Squint (also known as strabismus) is a condition that arises because of an incorrect balance of the muscles that move the eye, faulty nerve signals to the eye muscles and focusing faults (usually long sight).
- Accumulation of blood in the anterior chamber of eye is hyphema.
- Wash the eyes with water for 15–20 minutes if any chemical splash occurs.
- Acoustic neuroma is also known as vestibular schwannoma is a tumor of that develops from the balance and hearing nerve supplying the inner ear (vestibulocochlear nerve or C_8 cranial nerve).
- For what we have to do caloric test, what is its outcome? (for vestibular function and nystagmus seen on affected side of eye).

EYE

The eye is the most complex and important organ in our body. It is a 1 inch (2.5 cm) diameter structure which is seen in the anterior portion of the skull bone (orbit of the skull).

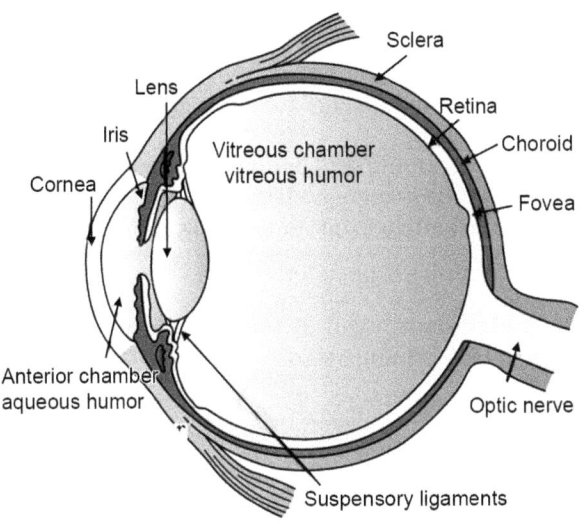

Fig. 1: Structure of eye

Layers of Eye

- External layer consists of cornea, sclera
- Middle layer consists of ciliary bodies and choroid
- Inner layer consists of retina

Cornea

It is a transparent part seen in front of the eye.

Sclera

It is the outer tough protective layer that covers the eye ball. It is normally white on color. Yellow color sclera is seen in jaundice, G6PD deficiency (Glucose-6-phosphate dehydrogenase deficiency), sickle cell anemia, etc.

Ciliary Bodies

Ciliary body is a group of circular muscles helps in maintaining the movement of eyeball and it produces aqueous humor, which maintains IOP (intraocular pressure).

Choroid

It is the vascular layer of the eye located between retina and sclera.

Retina

It is the light sensitive part of the eye located near to the optic nerve. It consists of rods and cons. Rods are responsible for peripheral vision or dim vision and cons help in color vision. Rhodopsin is a pigment produced by the rods helps in vision. Fovea is a place in the retina consist of most numerous number of con cells. Blind spot is a place in the retina in which there is no rods and cons.

Aqueous Humor

It is a clear watery fluid which is seen in the anterior and posterior chamber of the eye (anterior part of eye). as seen in the Figure 1. Anterior chamber is the place between iris and cornea and posterior chamber is the place between iris and lens. It maintains IOP (intraocular pressure). Normal IOP is 10–21 mm Hg. The instrument used to measure IOP is tonometry.

How Aqueous Humor Maintain IOP and How Glaucoma Occurs?

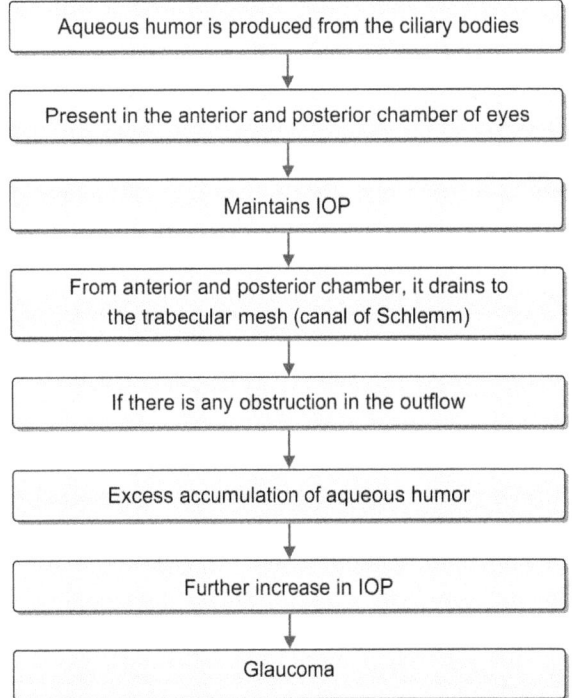

Vitreous Humor

It is a clear gel-like substance seen in the posterior part of eye which maintains shape to the eye (between the lens and retina).

Lens

It is a transparent structure behind the iris and in front of the vitreous body as seen in Figure 1. Any opacity in the lens is called as cataract. The cranial nerves responsible for eye movement are CN I (oculomotor), CN IV (trochlear) and CN VI (abducens). The cranial nerve responsible for vision is optic nerve (CN II).

Refraction

The bending of light rays towards the retina is called as refraction. Any error in refraction called as refractive errors. The common refractive errors are:
- *Myopia:* Short sight, *treatment is concave lens*
- *Hyperopia:* Long sight, *treatment is convex lens*
- *Presbyopia:* Loss of elasticity of lens due to aging, *treatment is bifocal or multifocal contact lenses*
- *Astigmatism:* Due to the irregular curvature of the cornea, so image fall on two different points on retina, *treatment is biconcave lens.*

DISORDERS

Cataract

Any opacity in the lens is called cataract.

Causes

- Increased exposure to UV light
- Smoking
- Family history of cataract
- Diabetes

Types

- Primary cataract: Congenital or senile cataract (due to aging)
- Secondary cataract: Maternal rubella infection or diabetes.

Clinical Manifestation

- Blurred vision
- Diplopia
- Permanent loss of vision in later stage.

Nursing Care

- Prepare the patient for cataract surgery
- Instruct the client to use sun glasses after surgery
- Avoid rubbing the eyes
- Do not lift weight more than 5 lbs, because it may increase IOP
- Report if there is any nausea or vomiting
- Avoid bending coughing or sneezing, because it may cause increase IOP.

GLAUCOMA

A group of ocular disorder characterized by increase in IOP (intraocular pressure).

Types

- Primary open angle glaucoma (POAG): It results from the gradual obstruction in the outflow of aqueous humor. It is painless and vision loss present (chronic and progressive damage).
- Primary angle closure glaucoma (PACG): It is the sudden obstruction in the outflow of aqueous humor. It is painful and vision loss present. It is acute emergency because of sudden pain.

Clinical Manifestation

- Diminished accommodation.
- In PACG, painful and blurred vision.
- In POAG, painless and vision loss present.
- Glaucoma is unnoticed in early stage because the central vision is unaffected.

Nursing Care

- Monitor IOP
- Administer beta blockers (timolol, glucomol, latanoprost eye drops).
- Avoid administering anticholinergics, such as atropine, because it further increase IOP.
- Instruct the patient to continue medication lifelong.

EAR

Ear is an important organ in our body which helps in hearing and maintaining balance.

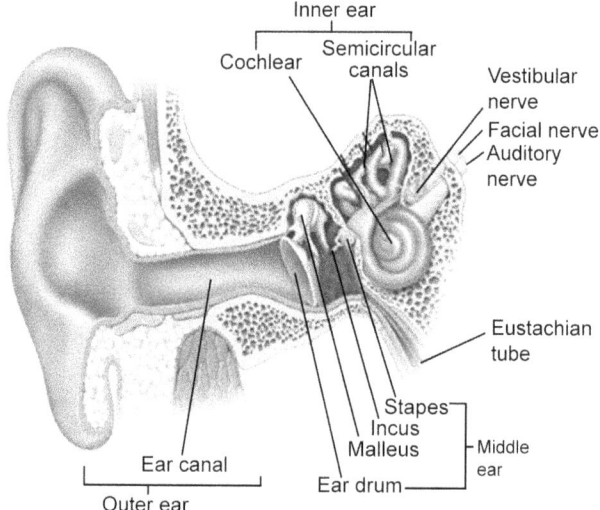

Fig. 2: Structure of ear

Layers of Ear (see Fig. 2)

- *External ear:* It consists of ear pinna, external auditory canal and tragus.
- *Middle ear:* It consists of ear ossicles, malleus, incus and stapes.
- *Inner ear:* It consists of semicircular canal, organ of corti and C8 cranial nerve.

Ear Pinna

It is also called as auricle which is the outer part of ear collects the sound waves. It is the visible part of ear.

Tragus

It is a small pointed eminence of the external ear or pinna. It is a fold of cartilage.

External Auditory Canal

It is a tube running from the external ear to the middle ear.

Ear Ossicles

Ear ossicles are the three bone layer in the middle ear (see Fig. 2). The malleus, incus and stapes transmit the sound waves to the inner ear from the tympanic membrane.

Organ of Corti

A spiral structure in the cochlea of the inner ear which produces nerve impulses in response to sound vibrations.

Eustachian Tube

A narrow tube connects the middle ear to the pharynx (nasopharynx), permitting the equalization of pressure on each side of the ear drum. If we open the mouth while hearing loud voice, it helps in equalization of pressure. So, we instruct the client to suck a hard candy or open the mouth while flying from one altitude to another.

Hearing Loss

There are two types of hearing loss:
- *Conductive hearing loss:* Due to any obstruction in the conduction of sound waves, e.g. foreign body or otosclerosis.
- *Sensorineural hearing loss:* Due to damage to C_8 (vestibulocochlear nerve).

Tuning Fork Test

Rinne's test and Weber's test are done to differentiate between conductive (middle and outer ear causes) and sensorineural hearing loss (damage to C_8 cranial nerve). These tests are always done together.

Rinne's Test

The vibrating tuning fork is presented first with the tines at the external auditory canal (front of the external auditory canal) for few seconds and then the base is pressed firmly on the mastoid process behind the ear. The patient is asked which is heard louder. In normal case, the sound is heard more when the tuning fork placed in front of the auditory canal because the air conduction is twice greater than bone conduction. If the client cannot hear when the tuning fork place in front of the external auditory canal, patient has conductive hearing loss.

Weber's Test

Place the base of vibrating tuning fork in the middle of the client's head, at the middle of forehead. Ask the patient whether the sound is heard equally in both ears. In normal case, the sound will be heard equally on both ears. If the client hears sound louder in one ear, it is called lateralization, which means client has conductive hearing loss in the lateralized ear and sensorineural hearing loss in the opposite ear.

DISORDERS

Otitis Media

It is an inflammation of the middle ear. It is also called as swimmer's ear.

Causes

- Any bacterial infection, streptococcal
- Repeated upper respiratory tract infections.

Clinical Manifestation

- Fever
- Redness
- Discharge from the ear

Nursing Care

- Administer antibiotics
- Provide heat treatment
- Instruct the patient to use ear plugs while swimming.

Otosclerosis

It is a disorder of the middle ear. It is one of the most common causes for adult hearing loss. It is also called as stapes fixation (bony overgrowth on the stapes). Incidence is more common in women.

Causes

- Hereditary (osteogenesis imperfecta)
- Virus infection especially measles

Clinical Manifestation

- Slow or progressive hearing loss, conductive hearing loss
- Pinkish discoloration of the tympanic membrane (Schwartz sign)
- Tinnitus (ringing sensation in ear)
- Negative Rinne's test and Weber's test show lateralization.

Nursing Care

- Administer antibiotics
- Prepare the patient for partial or complete stapedectomy

Ménière's Disease

It is also known as endolymphatic hydrops or abnormal fluctuations of endolymphatic fluids. Meniere's disease refers to the abnormal dilation of the endolymphatic system due to over production or decreased reabsorption of endolymphatic fluid.

Causes

- Bacterial or viral infection
- Any allergies
- Biochemical disturbances
- Vascular disturbances

Clinical Manifestation (Triad Symptom)

- Tinnitus
- Vertigo
- Fluctuating hearing loss

Nursing Care

- Administer antivertigo tablets
- Administer diuretics
- Provide low sodium diet
- The priority nursing care is provide safety measures [there will be damage to the C_8 cranial nerve (vestibulocochlear nerve), vestibule means balance and cochlear means hearing, so there is disturbance in balance].
- Provide assistive device for walking.

Foreign Body in Ear

Any ear wax or cerumen, vegetable, insect, objects like pencil eraser, etc. in the ear.

Clinical Manifestation

- Sensation of fullness in the ear
- Pain and redness
- Itching
- Bleeding

Nursing Care

- Do not use any ear candles
- Removal of ear wax by irrigation is a slow process, do not use water in case of vegetable matter.

Benign Paroxysmal Positional Vertigo (BPPV)

BPPV is a condition characterized by episodes of vertigo occurs when the head is moved. It is distressing condition commonly seen when doing any activity, getting up from bed.

Causes

- Due to any RTA or head injury
- Inner ear infections

Clinical Manifestation

- Loss of balance
- Vertigo and dizziness
- Nausea and vomiting

Nursing Care

- Administer antivertigo tablets (Betahistine or vertin, cinnarizine or Cinz)
- Provide assistive devices
- Instruct the patient to sit in the bed for some time when you get up.

CHAPTER 14

Immune System

Chapter Objectives

- Keynotes in the immune system
- Immunity
- Immune disorders
- AIDS

KEY TERMS

SLE
ANA
CRP
Kaposi's sarcoma
Allergen
Antigen
Antibody
Autoimmune

KEYNOTES

- Father of immunity or immunology is Paul Ehrlich.
- Immunity is maintained by antibodies and lymphocytes.
- The priority nursing care of a patient with immune deficiency is prevention of infection.
- Hypersensitivity reaction is a reaction which occurs in our body after the invasion of any allergen.
- Severe hypersensitivity reaction may results in anaphylactic shock.
- The drug of choice for anaphylactic shock is diphenhydramine or benadryl or epinephrine.
- Antibodies are produced in our body by immune systems.
- Antigen is otherwise known as allergen which enters in our body in the form of microorganisms or toxins.
- Night sweat is seen in acquired immune deficiency syndrome (AIDS).
- Kaposi's sarcoma is a type of cancer which is seen in AIDS patient.
- Zidovudine and lamivudine are examples of anti-retroviral medications given for AIDS patient.
- ANA titer is positive in AIDS patient.
- The confirmatory test for AIDS is western blot.
- The priority nursing care of a patient with neutropenia is limiting the number of visitors.
- In any allergic reactions or hypersensitivity reactions, there will be elevated ESR levels.
- Discoid lupus erythematosus is a chronic skin condition in which reddened scaly patches develop in sun exposed areas of the body, such as the face and hands.

INTRODUCTION

The study of immunity and immune disorders is known as immunology. Immunity is the ability of the body to fight against microorganisms. If any antigen enters our body, the antibody fails to resist against that it may results in allergic reactions. It may vary from mild to severe anaphylactic shock.

Immunity is otherwise known as a balanced state of having adequate biological defense to fight against infections and diseases.

Classification of Immunity

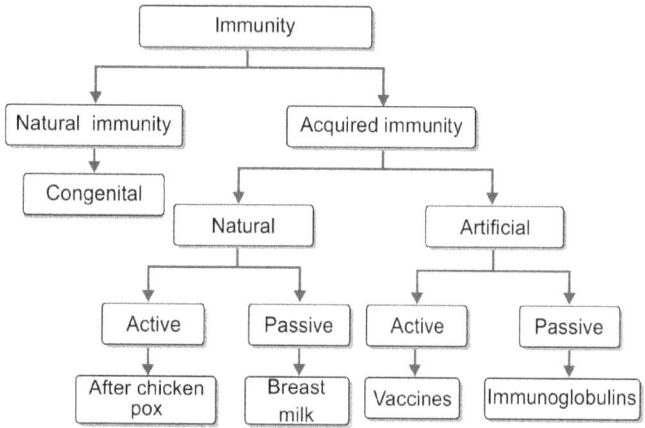

Immune Response

The immune response is how your body recognizes and defends itself against bacteria, viruses, and substances that appear foreign and harmful. There are two types of immune responses. They are:
- Cellular immunity
- Humoral immunity

Cellular Immunity

- It presents for prolonged period of time.
- It is an antigen-mediated response.
- Mediated by T lymphocytes
- For example, AIDS

Humoral Immunity

- It present for short period of time.
- It is mediated by B lymphocytes
- It is an antibody-mediated response
- For example, itching

Immunodeficiency

Absence of immunity (a state in which the immune system is weak or absent to fight against infection).

DIAGNOSTIC MEASURES

Skin Testing

- Administration of allergen intradermally in to the client's forearm to check for any allergic reactions.
- Keep ready the resuscitation tray while performing skin testing, if there is any anaphylactic reactions occur.

CRP (C-reactive Protein)

- It is a type of protein secreted in the liver.
- Increased CRP indicates infection.
- If it is less than 1 mg/dL, low risk for cardiovascular disorders.
- If it is greater than 3 mg/dL, high risk for cardiovascular disorders.

ANA (Antinuclear Antibody Titer)

- A test used to rule out any autoimmune disorders.
- Normal ANA titer is 1:20 or 1:40 depend on the titer.

Anti-dsDNA Blood Test (Antidouble-stranded DNA)

- A test used to rule out SLE (Systemic lupus erythematosus).
- Normal 70–200 units
- If it is less than 70, negative
- If it is greater than 200, positive

DISORDERS

Systemic Lupus Erythematosus (SLE)

It is a chronic progressive systemic inflammatory disease characterized by multisystem failure. It is a life-threatening autoimmune disorder.

Causes

- Unknown
- Autoimmune disease
- Stress, medications, etc.

Types

1. Systemic lupus erythematosus (SLE), affecting all major organs
2. Discoid lupus erythematosus (DLE), affecting mainly skin
3. Drug-induced lupus erythematosus (due to the chronic use of certain drugs, such as hydralazine, procainamide, quinidine, isoniazid, diltiazem, and minocycline)
4. Neonatal lupus erythematosus (seen in children)

Clinical Manifestation

- Butterfly-like rash on the face (malar)
- Erythema
- Dry scaly raised rashes on the face and upper arm
- Fever
- Weight loss
- Joint pain
- Anemia

Diagnosis

- Increased CRP
- Increased ESR
- Positive ANA titer

Nursing Care

- Monitor the skin integrity
- Administer iron and folic acid to correct anemia
- Provide high vitamin, high iron, and high protein diet
- Apply steroids
- Provide psychological support
- Monitor for any renal impairment, check serum creatinine and BUN (Blood Urea Nitrogen)
- Administer immunoglobulins as per order.

AIDS

It is a viral disorder that destroys the T lymphocytes. The incubation period of AIDS may extend up to 10 years.

Cause

- Heterosexuals and homosexuals
- Unprotected sex
- IV drug abusers
- Health care providers
- Person receiving blood
- Babies born of infected mother

Clinical Manifestation

- Fever
- Anorexia and weight loss
- Leukopenia [decreased white blood cell (WBC)]
- Night sweats
- Neoplasm, Kaposi's sarcoma is a purplish red lesion on the skin and internal organs

Diagnosis

- ELISA (Enzyme-linked immunosorbent assay) test
- PCR 4 (polymerase chain reaction)
- Western blot test (it is the confirmatory test for AIDS)
- Decrease WBC count
- Decrease CD4 and increase CD8 lymphocytes

Nursing Care

- Administer medications (retroviral therapy), such as zidovudine, lamivudine, and stavudine
- Prevent opportunistic infection and cancer (Kaposi's sarcoma)
- Monitor for any temperature elevation and weight loss
- Monitor the respiratory status, caution for pulmonary diseases, such as pneumonia
- Monitor for fluid electrolyte imbalances
- Assess the skin daily
- Restrict the number of visitors
- Avoid enema or rectal temperature, also minimize all parenteral infections
- Provide isolation to prevent infection
- Do not allow fresh fruits and vegetables in the client's room
- Avoid contact with people with infection
- Provide emotional support

Preventive Measures

- Safe sex practices
- Do not share the razors
- Do not donate blood or semen
- Inform to the sex partner about the condition

STEVENS-JOHNSON SYNDROME

It is a common side effect of drugs, such as antibiotics, NASIDs and antiepileptic medications. Stevens-Johnson syndrome is a rare, serious disorder of your skin and mucous membranes. It begins with flu-like symptoms followed by red or purplish rashes.

Clinical Manifestation

- Rashes on the face
- Facial and tongue swelling
- Skin pain

CHAPTER 15

Pediatric Nursing

Chapter Objectives

- Keynotes in pediatric nursing
- Theories and principles of growth and development
- Common disorders in newborn
- Common disorders in pediatric neurological system
- Common disorders in pediatric respiratory system
- Common disorders in pediatric gastrointestinal system
- Common disorders in pediatric cardiovascular system
- Common disorders in pediatric genitourinary system
- Common disorders in pediatric musculoskeletal system

KEY TERMS

APGAR	TGA
RDS	COA
FAS	TOF
MAS	Pink Fallot

KEYNOTES

- Normal blood volume in a newborn is 70-80 mL per kg.
- The causative organism of rheumatic fever is group A beta hemolytic streptococci.
- The priority nursing action of a patient having neutropenia is restrict the visitors.
- Normal blood glucose level in a newborn is 40-60 mg/dL, 50-90 mg/dL in a newborn older than one day.
- The common complication of large for gestational age babies are hypoglycemia.
- In newborn hypoglycemia is blood sugar less than 40 mg/dL for first 72 hours and less than 45 mg/dL in next 3 days.
- Incomplete evacuation of fetal lung fluid may leads to transient tachypnea.
- For cardiac catheterization in pediatrics select femoral vein.
- Encourage crying in a child with respiratory disorder and discourage or avoid crying in a child with cardiac problems.
- Absence of tears while crying is a classical manifestation of dehydration.
- To treat current symptoms and prevent recurrent infections in rheumatic fever administer pencillin.
- Streptomycin cause ototoxicity.
- Normal color of stoma is pink to bright red, shining and slight swelling. Pale pink indicates low hemoglobin and low hematocrit. Black purple color indicates necrosis—notify it immediately to physician.
- Figure of eight-like appearance on chest X-ray is seen in total anomalous pulmonary venous connection.
- Endocarditis most commonly seen in mitral regurgitation.
- Infective endocarditis is most common in VSD (Ventricular Septal Defect).
- Diaphragm is the primary muscle of breathing.
- Barrel chest is seen in emphysema.
- Paradoxical chest movement is most distinctive sign of flail chest.
- Bronchopulmonary dysplasia is condition in which the newborn become passively addicted to oxygen for more than 28 days.

- Deficiency of Alpha 1 antitrypsin will result in emphysema.
- Terbutaline is the antidote of pitocin.
- In mediastinal flutter, the patient's CVP (Central venous pressure) is rising and arterial blood pressure is falling.
- A drug is to be delivered through a nebulizer, the size of droplet for its humidification is <2.5 mm.
- The term vanishing tumor is used for lobulated pleural effusion.
- The normal pulmonary artery wedge pressure is 8-12 mm Hg.
- The capacity of stomach is 1 ounce at birth.
- Blood group 'O' is more susceptible for developing peptic ulcer disease.
- Necrotizing ulcerative gingivitis is known as Vincent's angina.
- Caput medusa is the dilated veins around the umbilicus seen in liver cirrhosis.
- Rovsing's sign is seen in acute appendicitis.
- "Rat tail" appearance on barium swallow examination is seen in carcinoma of esophagus.
- "Pseudo kidney sign" on USG is seen in Ca stomach.
- "Kissing ulcers" are seen in first part of duodenum.
- Newborn receives passive immunity via the placenta through IgE.
- Newborn receives passive immunity via the colostrum, IgA.
- Elevated IgM indicates infection in utero.
- Newborn gets protection from cold by the presence of brown fat.
- In case of cold stress in newborn, there will be metabolic acidosis.

INTRODUCTION

Growth denotes to a net increase in the size, or mass of the tissue. It is largely attributed to multiplication of cells and increase in the intracellular substance. Development is concerned with growth as well as those changes in behavior which results from environmental situations.

Principles of Growth and Development

- Growth is an orderly process, occurring in systematic fashion.
- Rates and patterns of growth are specific to certain parts of the body.
- Wide individual differences exist in growth rates.
- Growth and development are influences by multiple factors.
- Development proceeds from the simple to the complex and from the general to the specific.
- Development occurs in a cephalocaudal and a proximodistal progression.
- There are critical periods for growth and development.
- Development continues throughout the individual's life span.

THEORIES OF GROWTH AND DEVELOPMENT

Theories of development provides a framework for thinking about human growth, development and learning. It provides a framework for understanding human behavior and acts as a base for the future research works. Common theories of growth and development are as follows:
- Freud's psychosexual development theory
- Erikson's psychosocial theories
- Learning theories
- Piaget's theory of cognitive development
- Carl Jung theory
- Maslow theory

FREUD'S PSYCHOSEXUAL DEVELOPMENT THEORY

Freud's Stages of Psychosexual Development

Age	Stage	Major developmental tasks
Birth–18 months	Oral stage	Relief from anxiety through mouth (sucking or bitting)
18 months–3 years	Anal stage	Learning independence and control, with focus on the excretory function.
3–6 years	Phallic stage	Identification with the parents of same sex (Oedipus complex)
6–12 years	Latency stage	Sexuality repressed' focus on relationship with same sex peers
13–20 years	Genital stage	Libido reawakened as genital organs focus on relationship with opposite sex

Oral Stage: Birth to 18 Months

During this stage, behavior is directed by the Id, and the goal is immediate gratification of needs. The focus of energy is mouth, with behavior that includes sucking, chewing, and biting. The infant feels a sense of attachment and is unable to differentiate self from who is providing mothering. With the beginning of development of the ego at age 4 to 6 months, the infant starts to view the self as separate from the mothering figure.

A sense of security and the ability to trust others is derived out of gratification from fulfilment of basic needs during this stage.

Anal Stage: 18 Months to 3 Years

The major tasks in this stage are gaining independence and control, with particular focus on the excretory function. Freud believe that the manner in which the parents and other primary care givers approach the task of toilet training may have long-term effects on the child in terms of values and personality characteristics. When the toilet training is strict and rigid, the child may choose to retain feces, becoming constipated.

Toilet training that is more permissive and accepting attaches the feeling of importance and desirability to feces production. The child becomes extroverted, productive and altruistic.

Phallic Stage: 3 to 6 Years

In this stage, the focus of energy shifts to the genital area. Discovery of differences between genders result in a heightened interest in the sexuality of self and others. This interest may be manifested in sexual self-exploratory or group exploratory play. He proposed that development of **Oedipus complex** occurred during this stage of development. Guilt feeling results with the emergence of the super ego during these years. Resolution of this internal conflict occurs when the child develops a strong identification with the parents of the same sex and internalizes that parents' attitudes, beliefs, and value system.

Latency Stage: 6 to 12 Years

During the elementary school years, the focus changes from egocentrism to one of more interest in group activities, learning and socialization with peers. The preference is homosexuality; children of this age show a distinct preference for same sex relationships, even rejecting the members of the opposite sex.

Genital Stage: 13 to 20 Years

In this stage, the reawakening of the libidinal drive with the maturation of the genital organs. The focus is on relationship of members of opposite sex and preparation for selecting mate. The development of sexual maturity evolves from self gratification to behaviors.

THEORY OF PSYCHOSOCIAL DEVELOPMENT (ERIKSON)

Age	Stage
Infancy (birth–18 months)	Trust vs mistrust
Early childhood (18 months–3 years)	Autonomy vs shame and doubt
Late childhood (3–6 years)	Initiative vs guilt
School age (6–12 years)	Industry vs inferiority
Adolescence (12–20 years)	Identity vs role confusion
Young adulthood (20–30 years)	Intimacy vs isolation
Adulthood (30–65 years)	Generativity vs stagnation
Old age (65–death)	Ego integrity vs despair

Trust *vs* Mistrust: Birth to 18 Months

- **Major developmental task:** To develop a basic trust in mothering figure and be able to generalize it to others.
- **Achievement** of task result in self-confidence, optimism, faith in the gratification of needs and desires, and hope for the future.
- **Nonachievement** results in emotional dissatisfaction with self and others, suspiciousness and difficult with interpersonal relationships. The task remains unresolved when primary caregiver fails to respond to the infant distress signal promptly and consistently.

Autonomy *vs* Shame and Doubt: 18 Months to 3 Years

- **Major developmental task:** To gain some self-control and independence within the environment.
- **Achievement** of task result in sense of self-control and ability to delay gratification, and a feeling of self-confidence in one's ability to perform. Autonomy is achieved when parents encourage and provide opportunities for independent activities.
- **Nonachievement** results in a lack of self-confidence, a lack of pride in the ability to perform, a sense of being controlled by others, and a rage against the self. The task remains unresolved when primary caregiver restrict independent behaviors both physically and verbally, or set the child up for failure with unrealistic expectations.

Initiative vs Guilt: 3 to 6 Years

- **Major developmental task:** To develop a sense of purpose and the ability to initiate and direct one's activities.
- **Achievement** of task result in the ability to exercise restraint and self-control of inappropriate social behaviors. Initiative is achieved when creativity is encouraged and performance is recognized and positively reinforced.
- **Nonachievement** results in feeling of inadequacy and a sense of defeat. Guilt is experience to an excessive degree, even to the point of accepting, liability in situations for which one is not responsible. The child may view itself as evil and deserving of punishment. The task remains unresolved when creativity is stifled and parents continually expect a higher level of achievement then the child produces.

Industry vs Inferiority: 6 to 12 Years

- **Major developmental tasks**: To achieve a sense of self-confidence by learning, competing, performing successfully and receives recognition from significant others, peers.
- **Achievement** of task result in a sense of satisfaction and pleasure in the interaction and involvement with others. The individual masters reliable work habit and develops attitude of trustworthiness. Industry is achieved when encouragement is given to activities and responsibilities in the school and community, as well as those with in the home, and recognition is given for accomplishments.
- **Nonachievement** results in difficulty in IPR (Interpersonal relationship) owing to feeling of personal inadequacy. The individual can neither cooperate nor compromise with others in group activities nor problem solve or complete tasks successfully. If this occurs the individual may manipulate or violate the rights of others to satisfy his/her own needs. This task remains unresolved when parents set unrealistic expectation for the child, when discipline is harsh and tends to impair self-esteem.

Identity vs Role Confusion: 12 to 20 Years

- **Major developmental task:** At this stage, the goal is to integrate the tasks mastered in the previous stages into a secure sense of self.
- **Achievement** of task result in a sense of confidence, emotional stability, and a view of self as a unique individual. Commitments are made to a value system, to the choice for the career, and to relationships with members of both genders. Identity is achieved when individuals are allowed to experience independence by making decisions that influence their lives. Parents should be available to offer support when needed but should gradually relinquish control to the maturing individual in an effort to encourage the development of independent sense of self.
- **Nonachievement** results in a sense of self-consciousness, doubt and confusion about one's role in life. Persons values or goals for one's life are absent. Entering adulthood, with its accompanying responsibilities, may be an underlying fear.

  This task may remain unresolved for many reasons. Example includes when independent is discouraged by the parents, when discipline within the home has been overly harsh, inconsistent, or absent.

Intimacy vs Isolation: 20 to 30 Years

- **Major developmental task:** At this stage, the objective is to form an intense, lasting relationship or a commitment to another person.
- **Achievement** of task result in a capacity for mutual love and respect between two people and an ability of an individual to pledge a total commitment to another. The intimacy goes far beyond the sexual between two people. It describes a commitment in which personal sacrifice are made for another. Intimacy is achieved when an individual as developed the capacity of giving of oneself to another.
- **Nonachievement** results in withdrawal, social isolation and aloneness. The individual is unable to perform lasting, intimate relationships, often seeking intimacy through numerous superficial sexual contacts. No career is established; he or she has a history of occupational changes.

  The task remains unresolved when love in the home is deprived. One fails to achieve the ability to give self without having been the recipient early on from primary caregivers.

Generative vs Stagnation or Self-absorption: 30 to 65 Years

- **Major developmental task:** Is to achieve the life goals established for oneself while also considering the welfare of future generations.
- **Achievement** of task results in a sense of gratification from personal and professional achievements and from meaningful contributions to others. An individual is active in the service of and to society. Generativity is achieved when the individual express satisfaction with this stage in life and demonstrates responsibility to leaving the world to better the place in which to live.

- **Nonachievement** results in lack of concern for the welfare of others and total preoccupation with self.

  The task remains unresolved when earlier developmental tasks are not fulfilled and the individual doesn't achieve the degree of maturity required to derive gratification out of a personal concern for the welfare of others.

Ego Integrity vs Despair: 65 Years to Death

- **Major developmental task.** During this stage, the goal is to review one's life and derive meaning from both positive and negative events, while achieving a positive sense of self at this stage in life.
- **Achievement** of the task results in a sense of self worth and self acceptance as one reviews life goals, accepting that some are achieved some were not. The individual derives a sense of dignity from his or her life experiences and doesn't fear death, rather viewing it as another stage of development. Ego integrity is achieved when individual have successfully completed the developmental tasks of the other stage and have little desire to make major changes in the way their life is progressed.
- **Nonachievement** results in a sense of self-contempt and disgust how life as progressed. He feels worthless and helpless to change. Anger, depression, and loneliness are evident. Impending death is feared or denied, or ideas of suicide may prevail.

  The task remain unresolved when earlier tasks are not fulfilled: self-confidence, a concern for others, and a strong sense of self identity were never achieved.

Relevance to Nursing Practice

- Erikson's theory is particularly relevant to nursing practice in that incorporates sociocultural concepts into the development of personality.
- He provides a systematic, stepwise approach and outlines specific tasks that should be completed during each stage.
- Nurses can plan care to assist these individuals in fulfilling these task and moving on to a higher developmental level.

PIAGET'S THEORY OF COGNITIVE DEVELOPMENT

Piaget concluded that there were four different stages in the cognitive development of children. They are:

Stages	Age
Sensory motor stage	Birth–2 years
Preoperational stage	2–7 years
Concrete operational stage	7–11 years
Formal operational stage	11–16 years

Sensory Motor Stage: Birth–2 Years

During this stage, the infants and toddlers acquire knowledge through sensory experiences and manipulating objects. Piaget's ideas surrounding the sensory motor stage are centered on the basis of a 'schema'. Schemas are mental representations or ideas about what things are and how we deal with them.

Preoperational Stage: 2–7 Years

During this stage, kids learn through pretend play but still struggle with logic and taking the point of view of other people.

Concrete Operational Stage: 7–11 Years

During this stage of development, child begin to think more logically, but their thinking can also be very rigid. They tend to struggle with abstract and hypothetical concepts.

Formal Operational Stage: 11–16 Years

Finally, in the formal operational stage of adolescence, the ability to use deductive reasoning and an understanding of abstract ideas increases. The structures of development become the abstract, logically organized system of adult intelligence.

CARL JUNG THEORY

Jung believed that archetypes are models of people, behaviors or personalities.

Jung suggested that the psyche was composed of three components: the ego, the personal unconscious and the collective unconscious (in which ego represents the conscious mind, personal unconscious contains memories, including those that have been suppressed and collective unconscious is a unique component in that Jung believed that this part of the psyche served as a form of psychological inheritance. It contains all of the knowledge and experiences we share as a species).

Jung identified four major archetypes:

1. **The self:** It is an archetype that represents the unification of the unconsciousness and consciousness of an individual.

2. **The shadow:** It is an archetype that consists of the sex and life instincts.
3. **The anima:** It is a feminine image in the male psyche and the animus is a male image in the female psyche.
4. **The persona:** It is how we present ourselves to the world.

NEWBORN ASSESSMENT

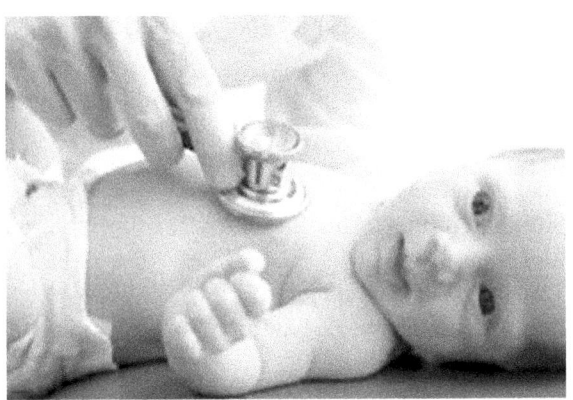

Newborn assessment is the skilled observation which is performed in the extrauterine life. It is divided into following categories:
1. Initial assessment or Apgar scoring
2. Transitional assessment or period of reactivity
3. Assessment of gestational age
4. Physical assessment

Initial Assessment

Apgar scoring is performed in the first and fifth minute after delivery.

APGAR SCORE

Sign	Score 0	Score 1	Score 2
Heart rate	Absent	Below 100 per min	Above 100 per min
Respiration	Absent	Weak, irregular	Good, crying
Muscle tone	Flaccid	Some flexion of arms and legs	Well flexion
Reflex	No	Grimace or weak cry	Good cry
Color	Blue or pale	Body pink, hands and feet blue	Pink all over

Score

- Total score: 10
- Score 8-10: No intervention is required
- Score 4-7: Gentle stimulation is required, administer oxygen
- Score 0-3: Immediate attention and care is required

Transitional Assessment (Period of Reactivity)

For 6 to 8 hours after birth, the newborn is in the first period of reactivity. During the first 30 minutes, the infant is very alert, cries vigorously, may suck his fist greedily, and appears very interested in his environment. At this time, his eyes are usually open, suggesting that this is an excellent opportunity for mother, father, and child to see each other. Then it decreases to normal.

Assessment of Gestational Age

- Normal gestational age is 37-42 weeks
- Less than 37 weeks is preterm
- Greater than 42 weeks is post-term
- Large for gestational age babies (LGA), if the fetus is more than 90% of the intrauterine growth
- Small for gestational age babies, if the fetus is less than 10% of the intrauterine growth
- In case of large for gestational age babies, there is chance to get hypoglycemia.

Physical Assessment

General Assessment

- Weight: 2.5-4.3 kg (1 kg is equal to 2.2 lbs)
- Length: 45-55 cm
- Head circumference: 33-35 cm
- Chest circumference: 30.5-33 cm

Vital Signs

- BP: 73/55 mm Hg
- Pulse: 120-160 beats per minute
- Respiration: 40-60 breaths per minute

General Appearance

- Physical activity, tone and posture is flexed
- Color is usually pink and increases after birth
- Small amount of lanugo and vernix caseosa still seen
- Mongolian spot present, a birth mark gradually fade first or second year
  - Mongolian spot is a bluish black pigmentation in the lumbar, dorsal area of buttocks
  - Mongolian spot is common in asian and dark-skinned

Head

- Anterior fontanel is diamond-shaped, 3-4 cm, close between 12 and 18 months
- Posterior fontanel is triangular shape, 0.5-1 cm, close between 2 and 3 months
- Monitor for caput succedaneum, edema of the soft scalp tissue

Ears

- Check for the symmetry
- The pinna position is horizontal line with outer canthus of eye

Eyes

- May be irritated by medication instillation
- Some discharge or edema present
- Color is slate blue

Nose

- Monitor for nasal patency
- Monitor for nasal flarring

Mouth and Throat

- Monitor for Epstein pearls, a small white epithelial cyst along the hard palate.
- Monitor for any cleft lip or cleft palate

Neck

- Check for torticollis, head held on one side
- Monitor for any abnormalities

Chest

- Check the appearance of chest, chest movements
- Anteroposterior and lateral diameter are equal (30-33 cm)

Abdomen

- Cylindrical in shape
- Umbilical cord consists of three vessels, two arteries and one vein.

Genitalia

- In females, vernix seen between labia, blood tinged mucoid vaginal discharge
- In males testes descended, rugae cover the scrotum

Back and Rectum

- Passage of meconium within 48 hours
- Monitor for any rectal atresia

REFLEXES

Moro Reflex

- Stimulated by a sudden movement or loud noise.
- A normally developing neonate will respond by throwing out the arms and legs and then pulling them towards the body.
- Emerges 8-9 weeks in utero, and is inhibited by 16 weeks (3-4 months)

Babinski's Reflex

- Stimulated by stroking the sole of the foot: toes of the foot should fan out.
- The foot itself should curl in
- Emerges at 18 weeks in utero and disappears by 6 months after birth.

Tonic Neck Reflex

- The child is placed on their back and will make fists and turn their head to the right.
- This reflex is present at 18 weeks in utero
- Disappears by 6 months after birth

Stepping Reflex

- Neonate will make walking motions with legs and feet when held in an upright position with the feet touching the ground.
- This reflex appears at birth, lasts for 3-4 months, and then reappears at 12-24 months.

Rooting Reflex

- The baby's cheek is stroked: they respond by turning their head towards the stimulus.
- They start sucking, thus allowing for breastfeeding.
- This reflex is inhibited anywhere between 6 and 12 months of age.

Palmar Grasp

- Stimulated when an object is placed into the baby's palm.
- A normally developing neonate responds by grasping the object.
- This reflex emerges 11 weeks in utero, and is inhibited 2-3 months after birth.
- A persistent palmar grasp reflex may cause issues, such as swallowing problems and delayed speech.

Plantar Grasp
- Occurs from birth and last for 10 months of age.
- Baby closes the foot when an object is placed under the sole.

Sucking Reflex
- Occurs from birth and last for 4 months of age.
- When an object is placed in the mouth baby start sucking.
- One of the baby milestones that is vital for survival.

GROWTH AND DEVELOPMENT

Stages of growth and development (Fig. 1):

Infants	0–1 year
Toddler	1–3 years
Preschooler	3–6 years
School-age	6–12 years
Adolescent	13–18 years

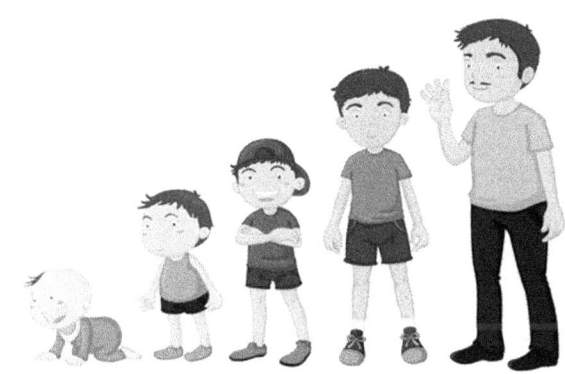

Fig. 1: Stages of growth and development

GROWTH AND DEVELOPMENT OF INFANT

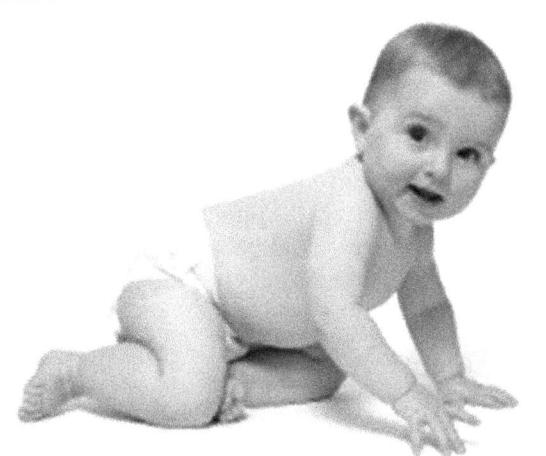

Growth

During the first year, baby will grow rapidly. By the end of the first year, your baby will have grown about 25 cm (10 inches), and will also have tripled their birth weight.

Development

Babies will reach a number of important developmental milestones during the first year:

Age	Milestones
Around 2 months	Tracking a moving object with their eyes
Around 2 to 4 months	Cooing, a soft murmuring sound
3 to 4 months	Raising head while lying on tummy
3 to 5 months	Grabbing at objects
Around 4 to 6 months	Rolling over
Around 4 to 6 months	Developing color vision
Around 5 to 6 months	Sitting alone without support
Around 6 months	Starting solid foods
Around 6 to 9 months	Pulling up and crawling
Around 6 to 9 months	Laughing, babbling, and making "raspberry" sounds
Around 9 to 12 months	Imitating sounds (and perhaps saying "Mama" and "Dada" without knowing what they mean)
Around 9 to 12 months (may be later)	Trying to walk or taking their first steps
Around 12 months	Understanding several words

GROWTH AND DEVELOPMENT OF TODDLER

Growth

During the second year, child's growth in length will begin to slow down. On average, a child will grow 8 cm to 13 cm (3 to 5 inches) in length and gain 1.4 kg to 2.3 kg (3 lbs to 5 lbs) between 12 and 24 months of age. During the third year of life (from age 2 to 3), your child will probably grow about 5 cm to 8 cm (2 to 3 inches) in height and gain about 1.8 kg (4 lbs).

Developments

At 18 Months

- Walking well with feet slightly apart
- Climbing, managing corners and obstacles well
- Saying six to 12 recognisable words
- Repeating last words of sentences

- Wanting to be more independent and do things without help
- Showing personality traits
- Playing alone, but still liking to be near adults
- Easily frustrated and throwing temper tantrums
- Using objects and routines for comfort and security.

At Two Years

- Walking up stairs and maybe walking backward
- Squatting and standing without using hands
- Kicking a ball and throwing over arm
- Saying 50 or more recognizable words and understanding more
- Becoming increasingly independent but still constantly demanding parents' attention
- Clinging tightly in affection, fear or fatigue
- Throwing temper tantrums when frustrated
- Starting to develop an imagination.

At 3 Years

- Identifying some pictures by naming them
- Balancing on one foot, walking on tiptoes and walking upstairs
- Constantly asking questions
- Listening to and telling stories
- Washing and drying hands
- Identifying a friend by name
- Using less 'baby talk' in speech
- Speaking in ways that can be understood half the time
- Decreasing temper tantrums
- Developing fears of the dark or animals.

GROWTH AND DEVELOPMENT OF PRESCHOOLER

Preschooler is also known as early childhood. It starts from 3 to 5 years.

Growth

During this period of life (3 to 6 years), the weight increases from 13.5 to 21.5 kg by the end of five years.

Developments

- Walk straight
- Walk backward and walk on tiptoes
- Runs without looking at feet
- Catches ball with extending arms, kicks a ball
- Jumps from heights of several inches
- Run on tiptoes
- Pedals a tricycle quickly
- Climbs on ladders, trees, playground
- Imitate dance step if taught
- Build a tower of 9-10 blocks
- Can help with simple house hold task
- Copies a square, draws a simple face and cut around pictures with scissors
- Can put coats without assistance
- Can undress self in most instances and can put pants up and down
- Can go for toilet alone and flushes toilet after each use
- Brush teeth with help
- Can be able to lace shoes
- Baths self and combs hair with help
- Can blow nose when asked

GROWTH AND DEVELOPMENT OF SCHOOL-AGE

Growth

During this age group (6 to 12 years), child may be 43 inches tall and weigh about 43 pounds. As puberty starts, child's height and weight will increase quickly. The child may reach 59 inches height and weigh about 90 lbs (40 kg) by age 12 (1 kg is equal to 2.2 lbs and 1 inch is 2.5 cm).

Developments

- Writing skills improve
- Fine motor is refined
- Fine motor with more focus
- Building: Models—legos, sewing, musical instrument, painting, typing skills
- Between 8 and 10 years develop team sports for the physical and emotional development
- Greater ability to concentrate and participate in self-initiating quiet activities that challenge cognitive skills, such as reading, playing computer and board games.

GROWTH AND DEVELOPMENT OF ADOLESCENCE

Growth

During this age group (12-18 years), boys grow about 4 inches per year during this timeframe. Girls grow about 3½ inches per year. Boys gain about 20 pounds per year. Girls gain about 18 pounds per year. The teenage years are also called adolescence.

Developments

- Develops the ability to think abstractly
- Is concerned with philosophy, politics, and social issues

- Thinks long-term and setting goals
- Compares one's self to one's peers
- May be in love
- Has long-term commitment in relationship
- Child become more independent
- Child is more influenced by friends and peer pressure
- Child learns to think in new ways and understand complex ideas.
- Child will develop his self-image and plan for the future.

NEWBORN CONDITIONS (DISORDERS)

RESPIRATORY DISTRESS SYNDROME (RDS)

It is a serious lung disorder caused by lung maturity and inability of the lung to produce surfactant. Surfactant is a surface active agent, a group of phospholipids which decreases the surface tension in the lungs and thereby air from the atmosphere enters to the lungs.

Clinical Manifestations

- Nasal flaring or flaring of nares
- Respiratory distress
- Increased apical pulse
- Diminished breath sounds
- Chest retractions

Nursing Care

- Monitor the color and respiratory rate of the child
- Monitor ABG report, it shows metabolic acidosis
- Prepare to administer surfactant therapy

MECONIUM ASPIRATION SYNDROME (MAS)

It is seen in term and post-term newborns.

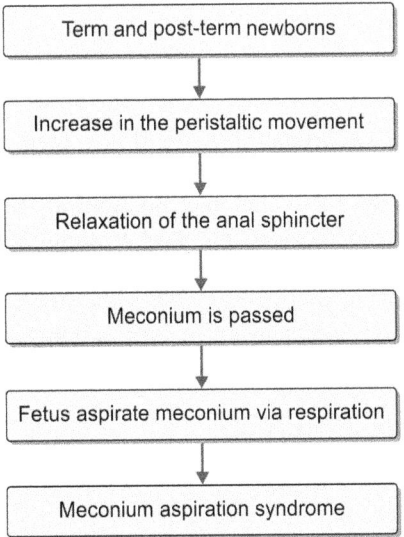

Clinical Manifestations

- Tachycardia
- Tachypnea
- Cyanosis
- Chest retractions
- Umbilical cord and nails are stained with green color.

Nursing Care

- Suction the mouth soon after the delivery of head
- In case of severe MAS, connect the child to an extra-corporeal circulation.

ERYTHROBLASTOSIS FETALIS (Rh INCOMPATIBILITY)

It is the destuction of RBC in the fetus that results from antigen antibody reaction. It leads to hemolytic anemia and hyperbilirubinemia. It is manifested as pathological jaundice.

Clinical Manifestation

- Anemia
- Jaundice in the fetus before 24 hours after delivery (pathological jaundice)
- Edema

Pathology

- Rh negative—absence of antigen
- Rh positive—presence of antigen
- When an Rh negative mother gives birth to Rh negative child—there is no problem
- When an Rh positive mother gives birth to Rh negative child—there is no problem
- When an Rh negative mother gives birth to Rh positive child—erythroblastosis fetalis.

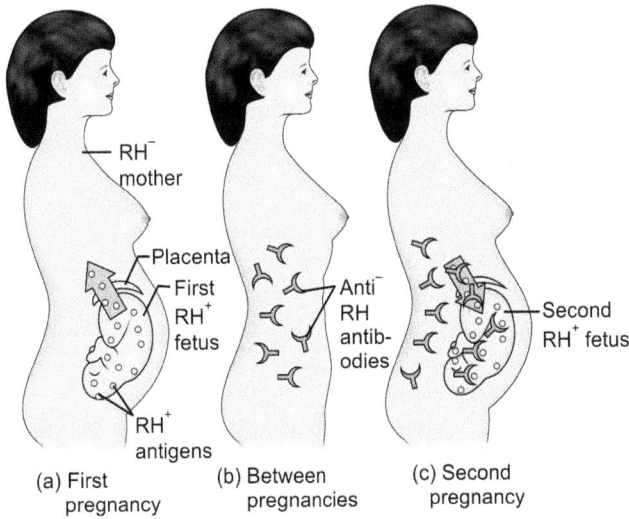

When an Rh negative mother gives birth to Rh positive child, the positive antigen present in the fetus enters to the maternal blood and react with maternal antibody to form antigen antibody complex (anti-Rh antibodies). This will take some time and by that time the first child is delivered with no problem. During the second pregnacny if the mother is giving birth to the Rh positive child the anti-Rh antibodies present in the maternal blood enters to the fetus body and destroy the fetal RBC. This process is called as erythroblastosis fetalis (destruction of erthrocytes in the fetus).

Nursing Care

- Administer RhD immunoglobulin or RhoGAM within 72 hours after the delivery of first fetus.
- Assist with exchange transfusion, fetal blood is replaced by maternal blood.

HYPERBILIRUBINEMIA

It is characterized by increase in the serum bilirubin level (greater than 12 mg/dL) in the newborn. The treatment is aimed to prevent kernicterus, a permanent neurological damage due to the invasion of bilirubin in the brain cells.

Types

- Physiological jaundice: Jaundice occurs after 24 hours of delivery
- Pathological jaundice: Jaundice occurs before 24 hours after delivery or at the time of birth. Pathological jaundice occurs as a result of hemolytic anemia.

Clinical Manifestation

- Increased serum bilirubin level
- Jaundice
- Enlarged liver
- Poor sucking and swallowing reflex
- Dark concentrated urine (urobilin)

Nursing Care

- Monitor for the presence of jaundice
- Assess the level of jaundice
- Prepare the child for phototherapy
  - Expose the newborn skin as much as possible
  - Provide adequate hydration
  - Cover the eyes with eye shield
  - Expect watery stool when the child is on phototherapy
  - Reposition every two hours
  - Monitor for bronze baby syndrome (grayish discoloration of the skin)
  - While collecting the blood sample turn off the phototherapy light
  - Do not leave the specimen under light for prolonged time because it may leads to bilirubin breakdown.

FETAL ALCOHOLIC SYNDROME (FAS)

It is caused due to maternal alcohol use during pregnancy.

Clinical Manifestation

- Unturned nostril
- Hypotonia
- Abnormal palmar creases
- Tremor or seizures

Nursing Care

- Monitor for respiratory distress
- Assess the sucking and swallowing reflex
- Provide psychological support

ADDICTED NEWBORN

A newborn become passively addicted to drug that has passed through the placenta.

Clinical Manifestation

- High pitch cry
- Respiratory distress
- Tremors

Nursing Care

- Monitor the respiratory and cardiac status
- Initiate seizure precautions

RETINOPATHY OF PREMATURITY

Retinopathy of prematurity (ROP) or Terry syndrome, previously known as retrolental fibroplasia (RLF), is a disease of the eye affecting prematurely-born babies generally having received intensive neonatal care, in which oxygen therapy is used on them due to the premature development of their lungs. If a newborn is on oxygen dependent for more than 30 days, it may damage the retinal cells. The treatment for ROP is laser photocoagulation.

Clinical Manifestation

- Vitreous hemorrhage
- Blindness

NECROTIZING ENTEROCOLITIS

Necrotizing enterocolitis (NEC) is a medical condition primarily seen in premature infants, where portions of the bowel undergo necrosis.

Clinical Manifestation

- Hyponatremia
- Thrombocytopenia
- Metabolic acidosis

PERIVENTRICULAR INTRAVENTRICULAR HEMORRHAGE (PIVH)

It is the bleeding into the ventricles. If a newborn delivered with less than 1500 gm or before 32 weeks of gestation may cause bleeding into the ventricles of the brain.

Clinical Manifestation

- Absent moro reflex
- Bulging fontanel
- High pitch cry
- Loss of consciousness

NEUROLOGICAL SYSTEM

HYDROCEPHALUS

Increase amount of CSF in the ventricles of brain.

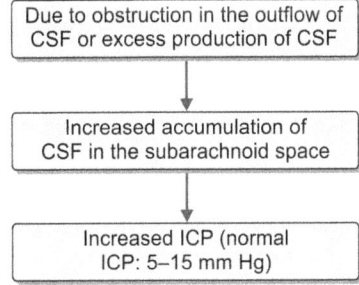

Clinical Manifestation

- High pitched cry
- Vomiting
- Enlarged head
- Bulging fontanel
- Macewen sign (a dull sound or pot sound while percussion).

Nursing care

- Provide VP (ventriculoperitoneal) or VA (ventriculoatrial) shunt to transfer the CSF.
- A siliconized catheter is connected to the ventricles and end portion in to peritoneum.
- Position the child to unoperated side
- Slightly elevate the head of bed
- Teach the signs and symptoms of increased ICP.

REYE'S SYNDROME

Reye's syndrome is a rare but serious condition that causes swelling in the liver and brain. Reye's syndrome most often affects children and teenagers recovering from a viral infection, most commonly the flu or chickenpox.

It is an acute encephalopathy with fatty degeneration of liver cells. It occurs as a complication of aspirin therapy associated with the illness.

Clinical Manifestation

- Child appears to be recovering from viral infection
- Decreased blood sugar level
- Increased level of ammonia in blood due to the fatty generation of liver
- Seizures, convulsions
- Abnormal posturing
- Diarrhea
- Rapid breathing

Nursing Care

- The priority nursing care of the child with Reye's syndrome is provide a quiet environment
- Administer tylenol (acetaminophen)
- Monitor for any seizures
- Provide side rails
- Provide low protein diet
- Assess the circulatory status.

SPINA BIFIDA

It is birth defect in which there is failure of the post vertebral arch to fuse during the embryonic development. It is also called as neural tube defect. Low levels of folic acid during pregnancy is a risk for developing spina bifida.

Types

- **Spina bifida occulta:** A defect in the bony structure without protrusion of cord or meninges.
- **Spina bifida cystica:** A cystic swelling through the protrusion involving meninges and spinal cord.
- **Meningocele:** A type of spina bifida cystica characterized by herniation of meninges through an abnormal opening in the backbone or skull.

- **Myelomeningocele:** A type of spina bifida cystica characterized by the herniation of spinal cord contents and meninges through an abnormal defect in the backbone.

Clinical Manifestation

- Muscle weakness of the legs, sometimes involving paralysis
- Bowel and bladder problems
- Paralysis of lower extremities
- Seizures

Nursing Care

- Closure of the sac should be done between 24 and 48 hours to prevent further complication
- Cover the sac with a sterile dressing soaked with normal saline
- Position the infant in prone or side lying position
- Monitor for any complication
- Provide emotional support

CEREBRAL PALSY

Cerebral palsy refers to a range of disabilities relating to movement and posture which is not hereditary. It is caused by damage to the brain. One of the main causes of cerebral palsy is falling of child from the crib.

Types

- **Spastic cerebral palsy:** Most common type, Spasticity means stiffness or tightness of muscles.
- **Athetoid cerebral palsy:** Athetosis means uncontrolled movements, which often lead to erratic movements.
- **Ataxic cerebral palsy:** Ataxia means a lack of balance and coordination. It often presents as unsteady, shaky movements called tremors.
- **Mixed type cerebral palsy:** May involve a combination of types of cerebral palsy.

Clinical Manifestation

- Feeding difficulties
- Delayed development
- Poor muscle control
- Muscle spasms
- Lack of coordination

Nursing Care

- Provide a safe environment
- Provide side rails or padded crib
- Observe the child's behavior

TAY-SACHS DISEASE

Tay-Sachs disease (also known as GM2 gangliosidosis or hexosaminidase A deficiency) is a rare autosomal recessive genetic disorder.

The cells of the nervous system (neurones), including the brain and spinal cord, need an enzyme called B-hexosaminidase A (Hex A) to regularly breakdown a particular fatty substance called GN12 ganglioside that is normally present.

Clinical Manifestation

- Loss of development
- Immobility
- Loss of vision
- Hyperreflexia

Nursing Care

- Provide genetic counseling.

RESPIRATORY SYSTEM

TONSILLITIS

Inflammation of the tonsils caused by group A beta hemolytic streptococci.

Clinical Manifestation

- Enlarged red tonsils
- Fever
- Difficulty in swallowing
- Snoring
- White patches on the tonsils

Nursing Care

- Administer pain medications
- Administer antibiotics as ordered
- Administer lozenges and salt water gargle
- Prepare the patient for tonsillectomy
- After tonsillectomy position the patient on abdomen or prone or side lying to facilitate drainage
- Avoid suctioning after tonsillectomy
- Check for frequent swallowing, it indicates bleeding
- Monitor for increase in pulse and vomiting red blood, indicates arterial bleeding
- Avoid spicy foods after tonsillectomy

EPIGLOTTITIS

Epiglottitis is a life-threatening bacterial infection of the epiglottis. The causative agent is hemophilus influenza type B. It is a bacterial form of croup seen between 3 and 7 years of age.

Clinical Manifestation

- High fever
- Diminished cough
- Tachycardia and tachypnea
- Lateral neck X-ray shows a mass

Nursing Care

- Administer oxygen
- Avoid direct examination of epiglottis, because it may cause spasm of the epiglotis and leads to complete obstruction

CROUP SYNDROME

It is also called as acute spasmodic laryngitis. It is common in children between 1 and 3 years of age. The attack is most common in the night time.

Clinical Manifestation

- Inspiratory stridor
- Barking cough
- Chest retractions
- Nasal flaring

Nursing Care

- Provide warmth to the child
- Instruct the parents to take the child to bathroom, close the door and turn the hot water bath on, sit on the floor of the steamy bathroom with the child
- Provide cold mist vaporizer
- Assure the parents that it is a self-limiting condition

BRONCHIOLITIS

Bronchiolitis is the inflammation of bronchioles, the smallest airways in the lungs. It is most common around six months of age and is rarely seen after age two. It is usually caused by the respiratory syncytial virus (RSV, which is present in the winter and spring months).

Clinical Manifestation

- Wheezing
- Breathing difficulty
- Cold

Nursing Care

- Monitor for any complications (ear infection)
- Provide suctioning to clear the secretion (bulb suction should be used on infants to help clear nasal passages, especially before feedings)
- Provide vaporizer in the bedroom.

CARDIOVASCULAR SYSTEM

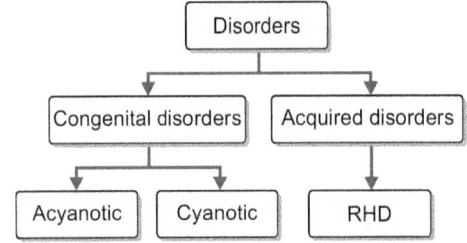

ACYANOTIC HEART DISORDERS

These are disorders in which the blood flows from the left to right (oxygenated blood flows toward deoxygenated blood as seen in Figure 2). There is no cyanosis.

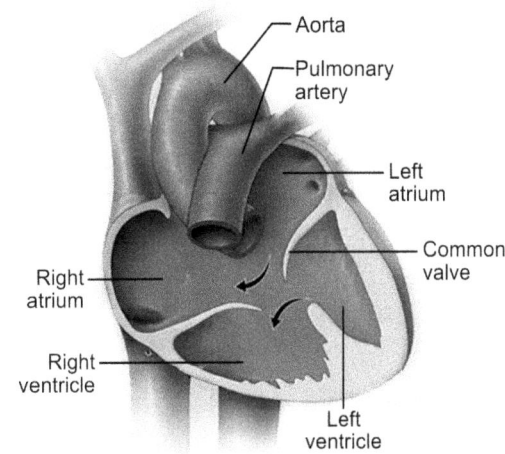

Fig. 2: Acyanotic heart disorders

Acyanotic heart disorders are disorders which causes increased pulmonary blood flow or disorders which causes decreased cardiac output. The common acyanotic heart disorders are:

Atrial Septal Defect (ASD)

Abnormal connection between the right and left atrium. The blood flows from the left atrium to right atrium. Surgical correction between 2 and 4 years.

Ventricular Septal Defect (VSD)

Abnormal connection between the right and left ventricle. The blood flows from the left ventricle to right ventricle. Surgical correction between 3 and 4 years.

Atrioventricular Septal Defect (AVSD)

AVSD is also known as atrioventricular canal defect (AVCD), previously known as "common atrioventricular canal"

(CAVC) or "endocardial cushion defect", is characterized by a deficiency of the atrioventricular septum of the heart. The main complication of AVSD is pulmonary hypertension and pneumonia.

Patent Ductus Arteriosus (PDA)

Ductus arteriosus fails to close at birth. Ductus arteriosus is a blood vessel connecting pulmonary artery and aorta which is seen in fetus. Usually, it will close at the time of birth. In premature newborn treat with indomethacin to close. We can hear a machinery type of murmur at the middle to upper left sternal border. Surgical correction after 4 years.

Coarctation of Aorta (COA)

Narrowing of aorta below the left subclavian area. In COA, the upper extremities will be warm and lower extremities will be cool. Increased pulse and BP in the upper extremities and decreased BP and pulse in the lower extremities.

Pulmonary Stenosis

Narrowing or obstruction of the pulmonary valve. It results in right ventricular hypertrophy.

Aortic Stenosis

Narrowing or obstruction of the aortic valve.

Clinical Manifestation of Acyanotic Heart Disorders

- FTT (failure to thrive)
- Poor weight gain
- Tachycardia
- Tachypnea
- Respiratory distress and irritability
- Congested cough
- Diaphoresis
- Fatigue
- Frequent respiratory infections
- Machine-like heart murmur
- Delayed growth and development

Nursing Care

- Administer medications, such as digoxin or lanoxin
- Administer diuretics
- Avoid crying
- Provide semi erect position in the caregivers arm
- Prepare the patient for intracardiac repair

CYANOTIC HEART DISORDERS

These are disorders in which the blood flow from the right to left as seen in Figure 3. So, there will be manifestations of cyanosis or TET spell.

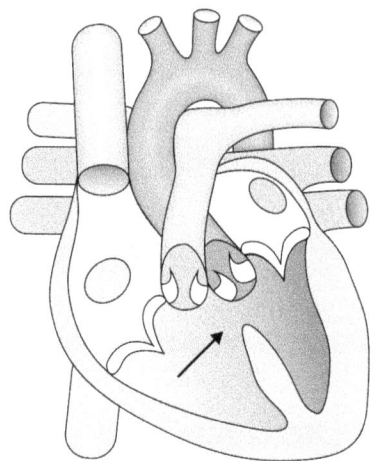

Fig. 3: Cyanotic heart disorders

Common cyanotic heart disorders are:

Tetralogy of Fallot (TOF)

A rare condition caused by the combination of 4 heart defects at birth. Tetralogy of fallot is associated with maternal rubella infection (German measles), poor nutrition, maternal alcohol use, etc.
1. Ventricular septal defect
2. Pulmonary stenosis
3. Right ventricular hypertrophy
4. Overriding of aorta (the aorta is located between the left and right ventricles)

Clinical Manifestation of TOF

- TET spell, hypoxic episodes to some activities such as crying, feeding, defecation. It is manifested as cyanosis. The management of TET spell is oxygen administration, knee chest position, administer morphine and propranolol.
- Polycythemia
- Breathing difficulty
- Heart murmurs
- Clubbing of digits.

Pentalogy of fallot = TOF + ASD
Pink fallot = no cyanosis in tetralogy of fallot

Transposition of Great Arteries (TGA)

Aorta originates from the right ventricle and pulmonary artery originates from the left ventricle.

Truncus Arteriosus

Only one vessel from the right and left ventricle instead of two (pulmonary artery and aorta).

Clinical Manifestations of Cyanotic Heart Disorders

- Cyanosis
- Polycythemia
- Clubbing of digits
- Poor feeding
- Squating position or frog-like position

Nursing Care

- Avoid crying
- Do not interfere the child when the child is in squating position (in order to decrease the venous return and to reduce the workload of the heart they themselves maintain squating or frog-like position).
- Organize the care to decrease the child's expenditure of energy.
- Use soft nipples for feeding.

RHEUMATIC HEART DISEASE

Rheumatic heart disease (RHD) is an acquired heart disorder caused due to rheumatic fever. An inflammatory disorder involves the heart, joints, connective tissues and central nervous system. It is peak in school age.

The causative agent of rheumatic fever is group A hemolytic streptococci. It is thought to be an autoimmune disorder.

Clinical Manifestation

- Chest pain
- Heart palpitations
- Breathlessness on exertion
- Breathing problems when lying down (orthopnea)
- Waking from sleep with the need to sit or stand up (paroxysmal nocturnal dyspnea)
- Swelling (edema)
- Fainting (syncope)
- Stroke
- Fever associated with infection of damaged heart valves.

Diagnosis

Modified Jones criteria are used to diagnose RHD along with increased ESR, elevated or rising antistreptolysin O titer. According to revised Jones criteria, the diagnosis of rheumatic fever can be made when two of the major criteria, or one major criterion plus two minor criteria, are present along with evidence of streptococcal infection.

Major Criteria

- **Carditis:** Seen in 50% clients, inflammation of the heart muscle
- **Polyarthritis:** Multiple joint inflammation, joints become swollen and painful
- **Chorea (Sydenham's chorea):** Abnormal purposeless movements of face and arms
- **Subcutaneous nodules:** Painless collection of collagen fibers or nodules over bones or tendon
- **Erythema marginatum:** Reddish rashes over the trunk or arms.

Minor Criteria

- Fever of 38.2–38.9°C (100.8–102.0°F)
- Arthralgia: Joint pain without
- Raised erythrocyte sedimentation rate or C-reactive protein
- Leukocytosis
- ECG showing features of heart block, such as a prolonged PR interval
- Previous episode of rheumatic fever or inactive heart disease.

Nursing Care

- Administer antibiotics as ordered, pencillin or penidure used in acute stage
- Administer pencillin until the age of 20 years or 5 years after the attack to prevent further attack.
- Provide safe environment
- Erythromycin is a substitute for pencillin in case of allergy
- Administer salicylates for anti-inflammatory effect
- Administer steroids.

GASTROINTESTINAL SYSTEM

VOMITING

It is the backflow of gastric contents toward the mouth. It extends from mild regurgitation to projectile vomiting.

Clinical Manifestation

- Signs of dehydration
- Bulging fontanelles
- Absence of tears while crying
- Decreased skin turgor
- Metabolic alkalosis

Nursing Care

- Monitor for dehydration
- Provide oral rehydration therapy
- Assess the severity of vomiting, projectile vomiting is seen in pyloric stenosis and increased ICP.

DIARRHEA

Acute diarrhea is seen in children less than 5 years of age. It is due to food allergy. Chronic diarrhea is due to rotaviral infection.

Clinical Manifestations

- Signs of dehydration
- Absence of tears while crying
- Decrease skin turgor
- Sunken fontanelles
- Metabolic acidosis

Nursing Care

- Obtain a history of gastroenteritis (priority nursing care)
- Provide oral rehydration therapy
- Monitor the electrolyte levels, in case of acute diarrhea
- Monitor renal function test while administering potassium.

CLEFT LIP AND CLEFT PALATE

Failure to fuse the soft tissue and bony prominence during the embryonic development. It is associated with maternal rubella infection or due to chromosomal abnormalities.

Nursing Care

- Monitor for any complications (otitis media in case of cleft palate infection)
- Teach ESSR method of feeding
  - E—enlarged nipple
  - S—sucking reflex
  - S—swallowing
  - R—rest
- Provide soft and large nipples
- Teach Haberman feeder method
- Monitor the risk of infection after surgical correction
- Surgical correction of cleft lip should be performed between 3 and 6 months
- Surgical correction of cleft lip should be performed between 6 and 24 months.

CELIAC DISEASE

It is also called as gluten enteropathy, a congenital anomaly in which there will be inability to digest gluten rich diet. Gluten is a type of protein which is seen in BROW:
- B: Barley
- R: Rye
- O: Oats
- W: Wheat

Clinical Manifestation

- Diarrhea
- Weight loss
- Large undigested fecal matter
- Anemia
- Damage to the dental enamel

Nursing Care

- Avoid gluten rich diet (provide gluten free diet)
- Administer vitamins and minerals
- Administer steroids

INTUSSUSCEPTION

Telescoping of the bowel, commonly at the ileocecal junction.

Clinical Manifestation

- Abdominal pain
- Currant jelly-like stool
- Sausage-shaped mass while palpating abdomen
- X-ray shows staircase pattern

Nursing Care

- Monitor for signs of perforation and shock
- Administer IV fluids
- Prepare for hydrostatic reduction

HIRSCHSPRUNG'S DISEASE

It is a condition that affects the large intestine (colon) and causes problems with passing stool. It is also called as congenital aganglionic megacolon.

Clinical Manifestation

- Ribbon-like stool
- Failure to have a bowel movement within 48 hours after birth.
- Swollen belly

- Vomiting, including vomiting a green or brown substance
- Constipation or gas, which might make a newborn fussy
- Diarrhea

Nursing Care

- Maintain low fiber, high calorie and high protein diet
- Prepare the child for surgery
- Remove the aganglionic colon or diseased colon and create an ostomy
- Provide ostomy care and monitor the site for any infections

ESOPHAGEAL ATRESIA OR TRACHEOESOPHAGEAL ATRESIA (TEF)

A congenital anomaly in which the esophagus (food pipe) terminates before reaching the stomach. Tracheoesophageal fistula is an abnormal connection between trachea and esophagus.

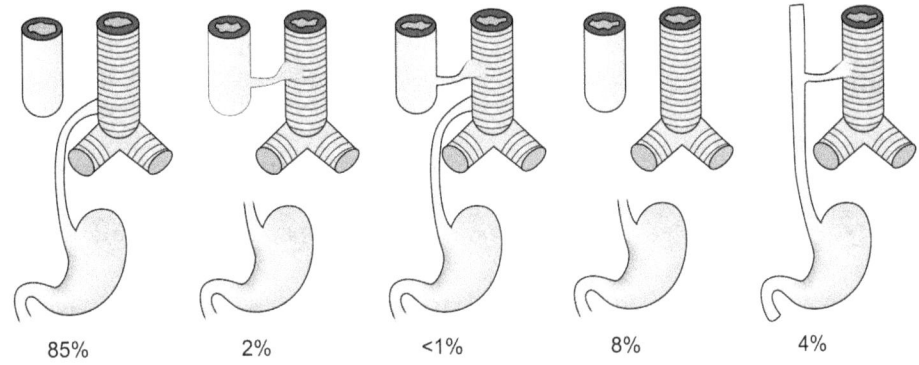

Anatomical variations of esophageal atresia and tracheoesophageal fistula, indicating relative frequency

Types of TEF

- **Type A: Esophageal atresia with distal tracheoesophageal fistula**—upper end of esophagus ends in a blind pouch and lower end connects to the trachea, seen in 85% of cases, gastric contents and acids can enter directly into lungs.
- **Type B: Esophageal atresia with proximal tracheoesophageal fistula**—upper end of esophagus ends in a blind pouch and connects to the trachea, seen in 2% of cases, food and saliva can travel into lungs.
- **Type C: Esophageal atresia with dual tracheoesophageal fistula**—both the upper and lower end of esophagus connect to the trachea, seen in less than 1% of cases.
- **Type D: Esophageal atresia with no tracheoesophageal fistula**—both the upper and lower end of esophagus ends in a blind pouch, seen in 8% cases.
- **Type E: H-type tracheoesophageal fistula**—there is no esophageal atresia but there is a fistula connection between the esophagus and trachea, seen in 4% of cases.

Clinical Manifestation

- Excessive drooling or salivation from mouth
- 3Cs (coughing, cyanosis and choking)
- Vomiting and aspiration
- Regurgitation
- Abdominal distension
- Respiratory distress

Nursing Care

- Maintain NPO
- Prepare the child for surgical corrections
- Maintain supine or upright position (30 degree) to facilitate drainage and to prevent aspiration
- If a gastrostomy tube is inserted, it may left open to escape the air in the GI tract.
- Prepare the child for parenteral nutrition

LACTOSE INTOLERANCE

A congenital anomaly in which there is deficiency of lactase, an enzyme required for the metabolism of lactose. Lactose is a sugar found in milk. So, the symptoms will appear after the ingestion of milk.

Clinical Manifestation

- Abdominal pain and bloating
- Diarrhea and gas formation

Nursing Care

- Instruct the mother don't give up milk products entirely. They are an important source of nutrients, especially calcium.

- Substitute milk with soya-based powder, a lactose free and good source for calcium
- Provide yogurt and hard cheese, such as cheddar, edam which contain inactivate form of lactose
- Avoid low-fat or non-fat milks, drink full-fat milk because the fats slow the journey of the milk through the intestines and allow the lactase enzymes more time to breakdown the sugars.

PYLORIC STENOSIS

Hypertrophy of the circular muscles of the pyloric canal (pylorus is the opening between stomach and duodenum).

Clinical Manifestation

- Projectile vomiting
- Dehydration
- Changes in the bowel movement
- Weight loss

Nursing Care

- Prepare child for surgery (pyloromyotomy), an opening created in the pylorus.

APPENDICITIS

It is the inflammation of the appendix. Appendix is a finger-like projection protruded from the junction of small intestine and large intestine (ileum and cecum).

Clinical Manifestation

- Pain in the periumbilical area and radiate to the right lower quadrant
- Rebound tenderness or Blumberg sign
- Pain in the McBurney's point
- Rovsing's sign (palpation of the left lower quadrant of a person's abdomen increases the pain felt in the right lower quadrant)
- Loss of appetite and low grade fever

Nursing Care

- Provide right side or semi Fowler's position for the comfort of patient
- Monitor the severity of pain, sudden absence of pain indicates rupture
- Do not apply hot over the area because it may cause rupture
- Monitor for the signs of peritonitis, tachycardia, fever, chills, etc.
- Prepare the patient for appendectomy

Appendicectomy (Appendectomy)

Appendectomy can be performed as open surgery using one abdominal incision about 2 to 4 inches (5 to 10 centimetres) long (laparotomy). Or the surgery can be done through a few small abdominal incisions (laparoscopic surgery). During a laparoscopic appendectomy, the surgeon inserts special surgical tools and a video camera into your abdomen to remove your appendix. In general, laparoscopic surgery allows you to recover faster and heal with less pain and scarring. It may be better for people who are elderly or obese. But laparoscopic surgery isn't appropriate for everyone. If your appendix has ruptured and infection has spread beyond the appendix or you have an abscess, you may need an open appendectomy, which allows your surgeon to clean the abdominal cavity.

Expect to spend one or two days in the hospital after your appendectomy. If your appendectomy was done laparoscopically, limit your activity for three to five days. If you had an open appendectomy, limit your activity for 10 to 14 days.

IRRITABLE BOWEL SYNDROME

It is a common disorder affecting the large intestine. It results form increase in the gastric motility. It is a psychosomatic disorder.

Clinical Manifestation

- Alternate diarrhea and constipation
- Abdominal pain
- Bloating
- A sensation that the bowels are not fully emptied after passing a motion.

Nursing Care

- Increase in the dietary fiber and fluid
- Administer antidepressant
- Administer anticholinergics
- Provide psychological support and teach stress management techniques.

RECTAL ATRESIA

It is also called as imperforate anus, absence of rectal opening at the time of birth.

Clinical Manifestation

- Inability to insert a rectal thermometer
- Failure to pass meconium after birth
- Swollen abdomen
- Stool passing through the wrong place (urethra, scrotum, vagina)

Nursing Care

Prepare the child for surgical correction, before the surgery a temporary colostomy is used to allow the infant to grow before surgery. For a colostomy, the surgeon creates two small openings (stoma) in the abdomen. The lower part of the intestines is attached to one and the upper part of the intestines to the other. A pouch attached to the outside of the body catches waste products.

GENITOURINARY SYSTEM

NEPHROTIC SYNDROME

It is an autoimmune disorder characterized by proteinuria, hypoalbuminemia and edema.

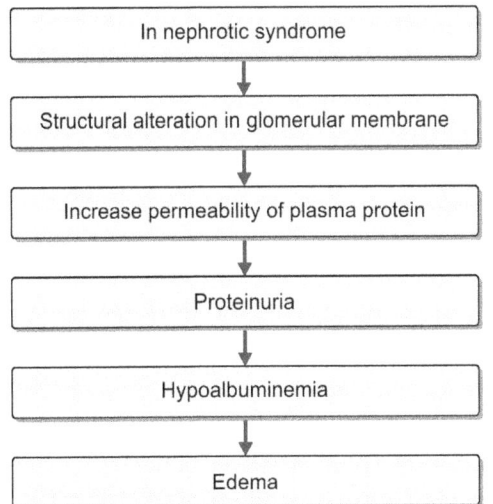

Clinical Manifestation

- Proteinuria (loss of protein through urine)
- Hypoalbuminemia (decreased protein in blood due to proteinuria)
- Dependent edema (due to vascular volume depletion and fluid shift)
- Scrotal edema
- Puffiness around the face.

Nursing Care

- Administer corticosteroids
- Administer diuretics (Lasix and spironolactone)
- Administer antihypertensive medications (captopril or losartan)
- Provide high protein and low sodium diet
- Avoid IM injections in nephrotic syndrome (IM injection is contraindicated in MI (Myocardial infarction), ITP (Idiopathic thrombocytopenic purpura), DIC (Disseminated intravascular coagulation), NMS (Neuroleptic malignant syndrome)]
- Provide scrotal support.

GLOMERULONEPHRITIS

Acute glomerulonephritis is an inflammation of the glomeruli occurs as a complication of antigen-antibody reaction secondary to group A beta hemolytic streptococci infection. It is common in boys 6–7 years.

Clinical Manifestation

- Pink or cola-colored urine or tobacco-colored urine from red blood cells in your urine (hematuria)
- Foamy urine due to excess protein (proteinuria)
- Increased WBC, ESR
- Increased urine specific gravity
- Decreased hemoglobin and HCT
- High blood pressure (hypertension)
- Fluid retention (edema) with swelling evident in your face, hands, feet and abdomen
- Fatigue from anemia or kidney failure

Nursing Care

- In acute nephritis, electrolyte replacement is magnesium sulphate to prevent toxemia and seizure
- Initiate seizure precaution
- Administer digoxin in case of circulatory overload
- Administer antihypertensive medications
- Administer diuretics
- Monitor for complications, such as renal failure, pulmonary edema, encephalopathy, etc.

ENURESIS

It is the inability to control urination. Involuntary passage of urine after the age of 5 years, it is also called as bedwetting (nocturnal enuresis).

Nursing Care

- Assess the age of the child, exclude child less than 5–7 years
- Assess the history of child regarding fluid intake, bladder emptying
- Encourage the parents regarding good fluid intake (7 drinks of clear fluid a day)
- Encourage bladder emptying at bedtime
- Give information to parents about waterproof bed protection and night-time nappies
- Encourage confidence building and positive thinking.

HYPOSPADIAS AND EPISPADIAS

Hypospadias is a congenital defect of males in which the opening of urethra on the underside (ventral side) of penis. Epispadias is a congenital defect of male in which the opening of urethra on the upper surface (dorsal side) of the penis. In a male, the external opening of the urinary tract (external meatus) is normally located at the tip of the penis. Circumcision is not performed for a newborn with epispadias and hypospadias because the foreskin is used for the surgical reconstruction later.

CRYPTORCHIDISM

It is also known as undescended testis. It is a congenital anomaly seen in premature newborn in which the testicles not moved or descended into the scrotum.

Clinical Manifestations

- Absence of one or both testicles in the scrotum

Nursing Care

- Prepare the child for orchiopexy
- Monitor for complications, such as testicular cancer and infertility
- Testicular cancer is more associated with undescended testis.

BLADDER EXSTROPHY

A congenital anomaly in which the bladder opens to the abdominal wall, associated with epispadias.

Cover the area with non-adherent film to prevent infection. Do not apply any white petroleum jelly into the bladder mucosa because it may damage the tissues.

MUSCULOSKELETAL SYSTEM

CONGENITAL HIP DISLOCATION

Congenital hip dislocation is also known as developmental dysplasia in which the displacement of the head of femur from the acetabulum. It may be unilateral or bilateral.

Clinical Manifestation

- Limited range of motion
- Folds on legs and buttocks are uneven when legs are extended and examined side by side
- Skin folds with the knees bent
- When lying on abdomen or prone position the buttocks of the affected extremity will be flat
- Positive trendelenburg test, if the child is able to walk or stand, make the child to stand on affected leg, the pelvis will dip to normal side
- Ortolani's sign or Ortolani's click

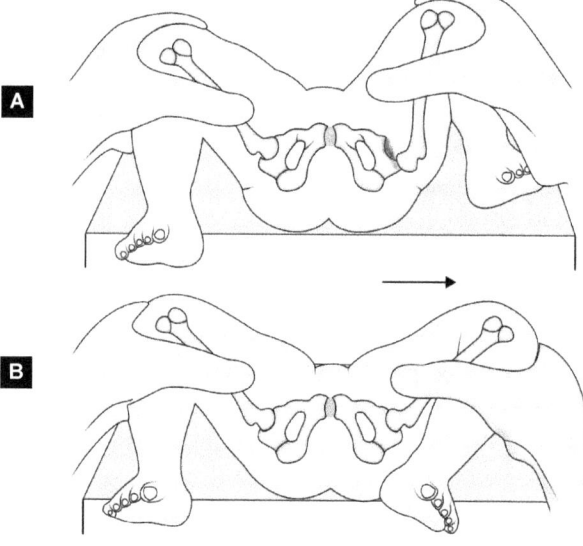

Figs 4A and B: Ortolani's sign

- Place the infant in supine position
- Bend the knees and place thumb on internal side of thigh (lesser trochanter) and fingers at the hip joint (greater trochanter) as seen in the above picture (Fig. 4A)
- Bring the femur 90 degree to the hip
- Abduct the legs apart (as seen in Fig. 4B), in case of hip dislocation a click sound is heard. In normal case there is no sound.
- A clicking or clunking sound is a positive Ortolani's sign and it happens when the femoral head is reentering or snaps with the acetabulum.
- Barlow's sign or Barlow's test
  - Place the infant in supine position
  - Bend the knees and place thumb on internal side of thigh (lesser trochanter) and fingers at the hip joint (greater trochanter) as seen in the above picture (Fig. 5A)
  - Bring the femur 90 degree flexion while exerting a backward pressure (down and laterally)
  - Adduct the hip slowly and gently (bringing the thigh toward the midline as seen in Fig. 5B).
  - Note any feeling of the femoral head slipping. Normally, the hip joint is stable.
  - The feeling of the femoral head slipping out of the socket postolaterally is a positive Barlow's sign. The affected knee will be little lower than unaffected extremity.

Pediatric Nursing

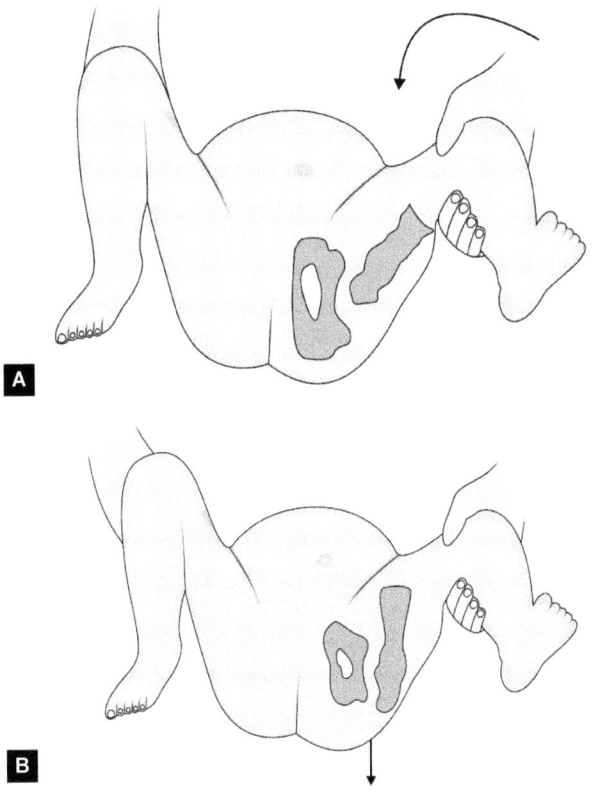

Figs 5A and B: Barlow's test

Nursing Care

- Maintain proper position of the legs
- Use triple diapering
- Place the child in a frog position and immobilize the child
- Provide Bryant's traction (Fig. 6)

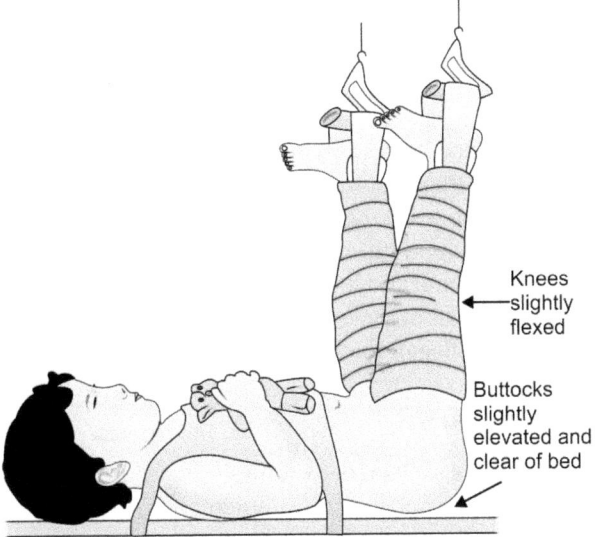

Fig. 6: Bryant's traction

Bryant's traction is an orthopedic mechanism used to immobilize both lower extremities in the treatment of a fractured femur or in the correction of a congenital hip dislocation. The mechanism consists of a traction frame supporting weights, which are connected by ropes that run through pulleys to traction foot plates. The weight applied to the traction mechanism is usually less than 35 pounds.

   Place the child in supine position

   Elevate both the legs 90 degree angle to bed

   Buttocks slightly off from the mattress, the traction pull elevates the lower extremities to a vertical position with the patient supine, the trunk and the lower extremities forming a right angle.

TIBIAL TORSION

It is the rotational deformity of the tibia, inward twisting showing the appearance of pigeon-toed appearance. It is commonly seen in toddlers. It may be:
- Inward rotation (knees forward and foot inward)
- Upward rotation (knees forward and foot outward)

Clinical Manifestation

- Straight line between tibial tuberosity and second toe is seen in normal case; in case of tibial torsion, line passes through the fourth or fifth toe.

Nursing Care

- Teach stretching exercises.

SCOLIOSIS

Abnormal lateral curvature of the spine.

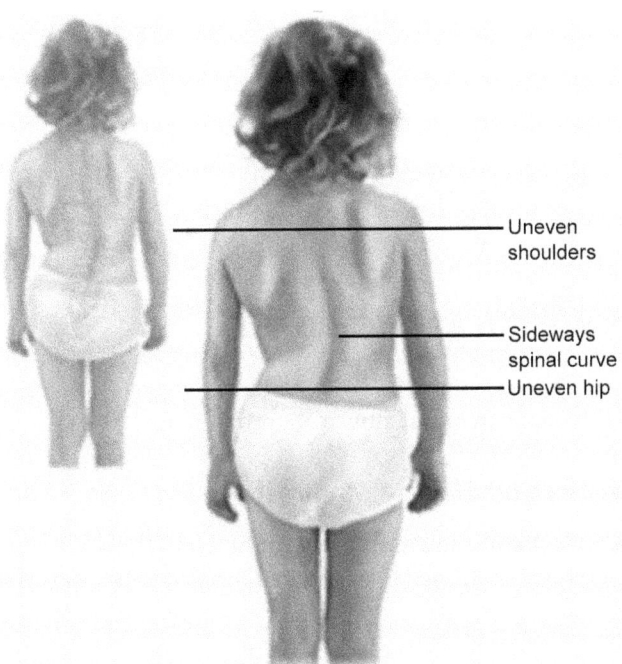

Clinical Manifestation

- Uneven shoulder height and hip height
- One shoulder blade that appears more prominent than the other
- Uneven waist
- One hip higher than the other

Nursing Care

- Teach the stretching exercises
- Monitor for the asymmetry in rib cage
- Apply Milwaukee brace, worn on 23 hours per day for 3 years.
- Apply braces; braces are of two main types:
  - Underarm or low-profile brace: Also called a thoracolumbosacral orthosis, this close-fitting brace is almost invisible under the clothes, as it fits under the arms and around the rib cage, lower back and hips.
  - Milwaukee brace: It extends from the chin cup and neck pad to pelvis. The brace has a flat bar in the front and two flat bars in the back.

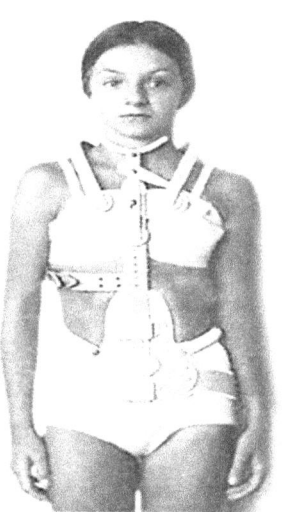
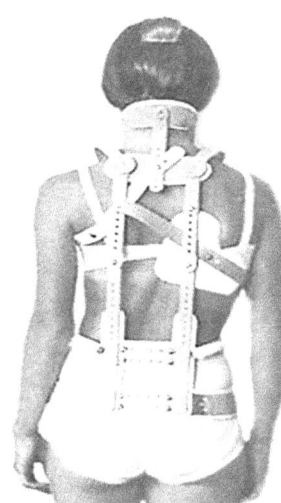

MUSCULAR DYSTROPHY

It is a group of disorder characterized by muscle weakness. It is genetic in origin, due to abnormal genes.

Types and Clinical Manifestation

- **Duchenne muscular dystrophy (DMD):** In this, the child is confined to wheelchair by the 8 to 10 years. It is manifested as pelvic gridle weakness, child uses hands to push up from the floor, known as Gowers' sign, frequent falls, difficulty getting up from a lying or sitting position, etc.
- **Becker muscular dystrophy:** Signs and symptoms are similar to those of Duchenne muscular dystrophy, but typically are milder and progress more slowly. Symptoms generally begin in the teens but may not occur until the mid-20s or even later.
- **Myotonic:** Also known as Steinert's disease, this form is characterized by an inability to relax muscles at will following contractions.
- **Facioscapulohumeral (FSHD):** Muscle weakness typically begins in the face and shoulders.
- **Congenital:** This type affects boys and girls and is apparent at birth or before age 2. Some forms progress slowly and cause only mild disability, while others progress rapidly and cause severe impairment.
- **Limb-girdle:** Hip and shoulder muscles are usually the first affected. People with this type of muscular dystrophy may have difficulty lifting the front part of the foot and so may trip frequently.

Nursing Care

- Assess the activities of daily-living
- Provide genetic counseling
- Prepare the child for electromyelography and muscle biopsy

OSTEOGENESIS IMPERFECTA

Osteogenesis imperfecta means imperfect bone formation, a group of genetic disorder affecting the collagen fibers resulting in pathological fractures.

Clinical Manifestation

- Malformed bones and loose joints
- Soft and fragile bones, muscle weakness
- Sclera (whites of the eyes) that look blue, purple, or gray
- Barrel-shaped rib cage
- Curved spine and brittle teeth
- Hearing loss or otosclerosis (often starting in 20s or 30s)
- Type 1 collagen that does not work well

Nursing Care

- Assess the skeletal deformities
- Administer magnesium supplements

- Reduction and immobilization
- Proper genetic counseling

CLUB FOOT

Abnormal rotation of the foot at the ankle, it may be mild or severe. Club foot is also known as Talipes.
- Varus: Inward rotation
- Valgus: Outward rotation
- Calcaneous: Upward rotation (walk on heals)
- Equina: Downward rotation (walk on toes)
- Talipes equinovarus: The most common form
- Talipes equinovalgus: Where the foot points outward and down
- Talipes calcaneovarus: Where the foot points inward and up
- Talipes calcaneovalgus: Where the foot points inward and down

Nursing Care

- Perform exercise as ordered
- Cast application and immobilization.

CHAPTER 16

Psychiatric Nursing

Chapter Objectives

- Keynotes in the psychiatric nursing
- Theories of personality
- Psychotherapy and ECT
- Classification of disorders

KEY TERMS

Psychotherapy   PTSD
Mania   Depression
OCD   Suicide
ADHD   MR

KEYNOTES

- The manageable side effects of neuroleptics is tremor.
- An appropriate activity for the nurse to recommend the client who is extremely agitated in daily walks.
- The ability to tolerate frustration is due to the ego state of development.
- The other name of super ego is consciousness.
- The priority nursing care of a patient with alcohol withdrawal is administer diazepam.
- Sleep disorders are also called as parasomnias.
- The first stage of sleep is NREM (Non-rapid eye movement sleep).
- Conversion is an example of a defense mechanism in which the anxiety converted into physical symptoms.
- Parent-child relationship is required for the child for the development of personality.
- Medication used for aversion therapy is disulfiram.
- The triad symptoms of depression are hopelessness, powerlessness and worthlessness.
- The classical manifestation of a patient with eating disorder is lanugo, hypothermia and hypotension.
- Hypnosis is contraindicated in phobia.

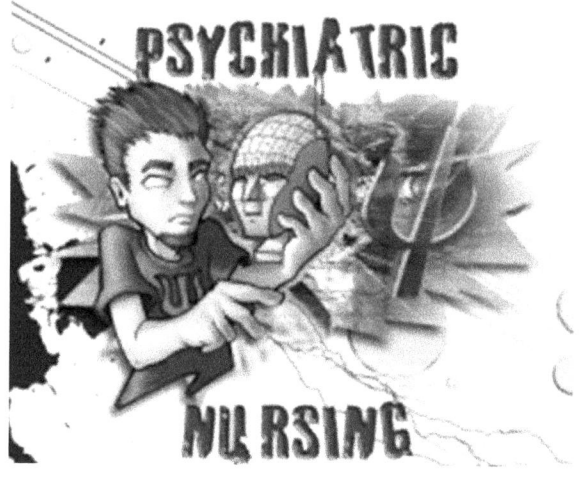

INTRODUCTION

Psychiatry is a medical specialty devoted to the study, diagnosis, treatment, and prevention of mental disorders. These include various affective, behavioral, cognitive and perceptual abnormalities. Psychiatric nursing or mental health nursing is the specialty of nursing that cares for people of all ages with mental illness or mental distress, such as schizophrenia, bipolar disorder, psychosis, depression or dementia.

- Psychology: Study of mind
- Psychiatry: Study of deviations of mind
- Founding father of Psychiatry: Sigmund Freud
- Father of American Psychiatry: Benjamin Rush

- Father of Modern Psychiatry: Robert Spitzer
- First psychiatric nurse: Linda Richards

MENTAL HEALTH

A state of equilibrium between cognition (thinking), conation (action) and affection.

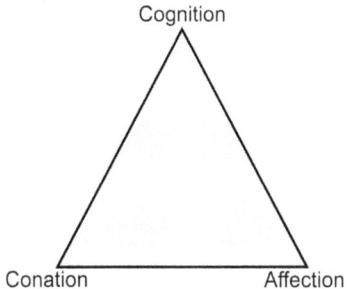

MENTAL ILLNESS

A state of disequilibrium between cognition (thinking), conation (action) and affection.

REVOLUTIONS IN THE FIELD OF PSYCHIATRY

There are mainly four revolutions in the field of psychiatry, they are:

First	Philippe pinel revolution	17th century
Second	Sigmund Freud revolution	1856–1939
Third	Community psychiatry	1962–1985
Fourth	Psychopharmacology	1985 onward

THEORIES OF PERSONALITY

Psychoanalytical Theory

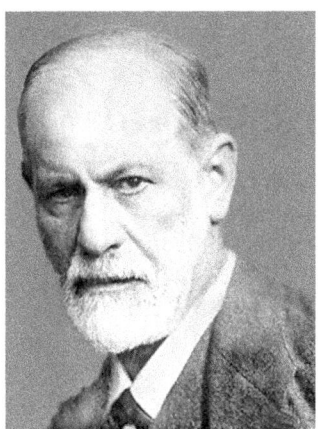

Sigmund Freud

According to Freud, almost the entire mental life is directed from the unconscious forces. The conscious level is very small part of the unconscious mind. Accordingly, only 1/10th part of an iceberg remains above the water, while the 9/10th is concealed below the water; similarly, the conscious level of the man's mind is very small part of the unconscious. Thus most of the human activities are motivated from the unconscious. Freud devised many methods to explain the unconscious, the techniques used which is known as **"Psychoanalysis"**.

Father of psychoanalytical theory is Sigmund Freud. The entire theory is conceptualized into four parts:
1. Structure of personality
2. Stages of mind (topology of mind)
3. Dynamics of mind
4. Stages of psychosexual development

Structure of Personality

It consists of:
- **Id**: Pleasure principle, immediate satisfaction of the need. The child will not wait for any moment to achieve the need.
- **Ego:** Reality principle. He will wait for a moment to achieve the need. The ability to tolerate frustration is due to the ego state of development.
- **Super ego**: Perfection principle. The other name of super ego is consciousness. The super ego is important in the socialization of an individual as it assists the ego in the control of id impulses. When the superego becomes rigid and punitive, problems with low confidence and low self esteem arise.

Stages of Mind (Topology of Mind)

It includes:
- **Consciousness:** All the memories remain with the individual's awareness. Well oriented to time, place and person.
- **Unconsciousness:** All the memories those are unable to bring to the conscious awareness. Not oriented to time, place and person.
- **Precociousness:** Certain memories are suppressed into the inner mind that he does not want to remember, e.g. death of a friend, telephone number, etc.

Dynamics of Personality

Freud used the term *cathexis and anticathexis* to describe the force within the Id, ego and superego that are used to invest psychic energy, a force required for mental functioning.
- **Cathexis:** The concentration of mental energy on one particular person, idea, or object. An example is the individual who instinctively turn to alcohol to relieve stress.

- **Anticathexis:** The use of psychic energy by the ego and the superego to control id impulses. For example, the ego attempt to control the use of alcohol with rational thinking to control the use of alcohol with rational thinking, such as, 'I already have ulcers from drinking too much'. The superego would exert control with, 'I shouldn't drink. If I drink, my family will be hurt and angry'.

Freud believes that an imbalance between cathexis and anticathexis resulted in internal conflicts, producing tension and anxiety in an individual.

Stages of Psychosexual Development

There are five stages of psychosexual development, they are:

Oral Stage (Birth–18 Months)

Achieves pleasure through mouth by sucking.

Anal Stage (18 Months–3 Years)

Achieves pleasure through bowel and bladder control and elimination.

Phallic Stage (3–6 Years)

Identification with the parents of same sex; development of sexual identity; focus on genital organ. Development of oedipus complex. Attachment to parents of opposite sex.

Latency Stage (6–12 Years)

Sexuality repressed, focus on relationship with same sex peers.

Genital Stage (12–20 Years)

Attached to the opposite sex, libido reawakened as genital organs focus on relationship with opposite sex.

THEORY OF PSYCHOSOCIAL DEVELOPMENT

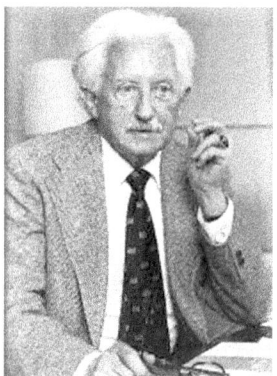

Erik Erikson

Erikson studied the influence of social process on the development of the personality. He described 8 stages of the life cycle during which an individual struggles with developmental "crises". Specific task associated with each stage must be completed for resolution of the crises and the emotional growth to occur.

Age	Stage	Major developmental task
Infancy (birth–18 months)	Trust vs Mistrust	To develop a basic trust in the mothering figure and be able to generalize to others
Early childhood (18 months–3 years)	Autonomy vs shame and doubt	To gain some self-control and independence with the environment
Late childhood (3–6 years)	Initiative vs guilt	To develop sense of purpose and the ability to initiate and direct own activities.
School age (6–12 years)	Industry vs inferiority	To achieve a sense of self-confidence by learning, competing, performing successfully.
Adolescence (12–20 years)	Identity vs role confusion	To integrate the tasks mastered in the previous stages in to a secure sense of self.
Young adulthood (20–30 years)	Intimacy vs isolation	To form an intense, lasting relationship or a commitment to another person, cause, institution or creative efforts.
Adulthood (30–65 years)	Generativity vs stagnation	To achieve the life goals established for oneself, while also considering the welfare of future generations.
Old age (65–death)	Ego integrity vs despair	To review one's life and derive meaning from both positive and negative events, while achieving a positive sense of self-worth.

INTERPERSONAL THEORY

Father of interpersonal theory is sullivan. Sullivan (1953) believed that individual behavior and development are the direct result of interpersonal relationships. Prior to the development of his own theoretical framework, Sullivan embraced the concepts of Freud. Later, he changed the focus of his work from the intrapersonal view of Freud to one with more interpersonal flavor in which human behavior could be observed in social interactions with others.

Age	Stage	Major developmental tasks
Birth–18 months	Infancy	Relief from anxiety through oral gratification of needs
18 months–6 years	Childhood	Learning to experience a delay in personal gratification without undue anxiety
6–9 years	Juvenile	Learning to form satisfactory peer relationships
9–12 years	Preadolescence	Learning to form satisfactory relationship with persons of same sex; initiating feelings of affection for another person
12–14 years	Early adolescence	Learning to form satisfactory relationship with persons of opposite sex; developing a sense of identity
14–21 years	Late adolescence	Establishing self-identity; experiencing satisfying relationships; working to develop a lasting, intimate opposite-sex relationship

MASLOW'S HIERARCHY OF NEEDS

Maslow's hierarchy of needs is a theory in psychology proposed by Abraham Maslow in his 1943. Hierarchy of needs in the order of importance.

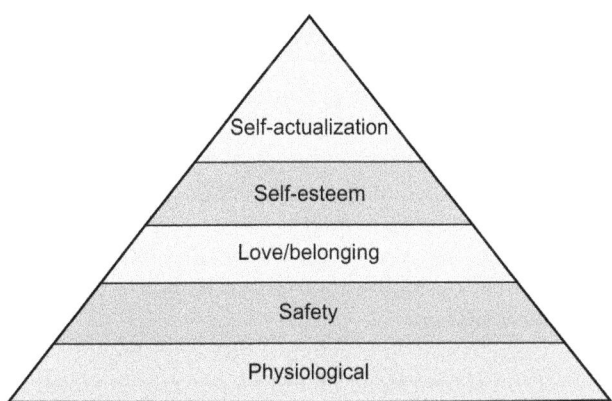

- Physiological needs: Food, air, oxygen, water, etc.
- Safety needs: Protection, freedom from harm
- Love and belonging: Freedom from loneliness
- Self-esteem: Freedom from inferiority and helplessness
- Self-actualization: Esthetic need, self-fulfilment.

THERAPEUTIC RELATIONSHIP

Therapeutic relationship is one to one interaction between a nurse and a patient, in which the nurse use various measures to change the maladaptive behavior of the patient to become adaptive behavior.

Therapeutic relationship is defined as a nurse-patient relationship "as an interaction process in which the nurse fulfills her role by using her professional knowledge and skill in such a way that she/he is able to help the patient physically, socially and emotionally."

Phases of Therapeutic Relationship

There are four phases:
- Preorientation or preinteraction phase
- Orientation phase
- Working phase
- Termination phase

Preinteraction Phase

The phase begins when the nurse is assigned to initiate a therapeutic relationship and includes all that the nurse thinks, feels or does immediately prior to the first interaction with the patient. The nurse should also explore the feelings of inferiority, insecurity, approval seeking behaviors, etc.

Nurse's Task

- Self-exploration
- Create the setting—comfortable, safe
- Prepare for the interaction/relationship—review patient's history, diagnosis, review nursing theory
- Anticipate obstacles, difficulties

Orientation or Introductory Phase

It is during the introductory phase that the nurse and the patient meet for the first time. One of the nurse's primary concerns is to find out why the patient sought help. This forms the basis of the nursing assessment and helps the nurse to focus on the patient's problems and to determine patient level of motivation.

Nurse's Task

- Introduction
- Discuss nurse's role
- Gives patient information about the purpose, possible goals, and the timeframe of the relationship
- Include the patient as a partner in the relationship.

Working Phase

Most of the therapeutic work is carried out during the working phase. The nurse and the patient explore relevant stressors and promote the development of insight in the patient. By linking perceptions, thoughts, feelings and actions, the nurse help the patient to master the anxieties, increase independence and coping mechanisms. Actual behavioral change is focus of attention in this phase of relationship.

Nurse's Task

- Implement the plan of care
- Evaluate intermediate outcomes
- Re-plan if necessary; think of alternative solutions
- Implement alternative solutions
- Refer patient, if necessary.

Termination Phase

This is most difficult, but most important phase in the therapeutic nurse patient relationship. The goal of this phase is to bring a therapeutic end to the relationship:
- Begins during the first interaction with the patient
- Occurs when goals have been reached or referral is advisable.
- Nurse and patient examine meaning and value of the relationship.

THERAPEUTIC IMPASSES

The term therapeutic impasses may be used to describe a number of situations that can arise in psychotherapy. Impasses can occur as a result of disagreement between the therapist and client, A few examples include:
- A client who becomes resistant to exploring vulnerable feelings or experiences to such a degree that he or she is also unwilling to explore the resistance.
- A disagreement between the therapist and client about the proper way to resolve a conflict.
- Unresolved sexual feelings between the therapist and client.
- An unhealthy relationship between the therapist and client.
- An unsuccessful therapeutic intervention or modality.

The common therapeutic impasses are:

Transference

The feeling of patient toward the nurse, e.g. the patient considers the nurse as previous lover.

Counter Transference

The feeling of nurse toward the patient, e.g. the nurse considers the patient as father.

IMPAIRED NURSE SYNDROME

The drug addition, alcoholism and other substance abuse disorders which is commonly seen among the nurses.

Signs and Symptoms

- Frequent toilet visiting of the nurses
- Frequent absenteeism
- Frequent lateness
- Patient is not getting any relief from the pain medications

Management

- Strengthen about the code of ethics
- Report to the higher authorities.

HISTORY COLLECTION AND MENTAL STATUS EXAMINATION (MSE)

Psychiatric History

- **Identifying information:** Age, sex, marital status, race, referral source
- **Chief complaint (CC):** Reason for consultation; the reason is usually a direct quote from the patient.
- **History of present illness (HPI)**
  - Current symptoms: Date of onset, duration and course of symptoms.
  - Previous psychiatric symptoms and treatment.
  - Recent psychosocial stressors: Stressful life events that may have contributed to present condition.
  - Reason the patient is presenting now.
  - This section provides evidence that supports or rules out relevant diagnoses. Therefore, documenting the absence of pertinent symptoms is also important.
  - Historical evidence in this section should be relevant to the current presentation.
- **Psychiatric history**
  - Previous and current psychiatric diagnoses.
  - History of psychiatric treatment, including outpatient and inpatient treatment.
  - History of psychotropic medication use.
  - History of suicide attempts and potential lethality.
- **Medical history**
  - Current and/or previous medical problems.
  - Type of treatment, including prescription, over the counter medications, home remedies.
- **Family history**
  - Relatives with history of psychiatric disorders, suicide or suicide attempts, alcohol or substance abuse.
- **Social history**
  - Source of income
  - Level of education
  - Relationship history (including marriages, sexual orientation, number of children, individuals who currently live with patient)
  - Support network

- Current alcohol or illicit-drug usage
- Occupational history
- **Developmental history**
  - Family structure during childhood, relationships with parental figures and siblings; developmental milestones, peer relationships, school performance.

Mental Status Examination

The mental status examination or mental state examination, abbreviated MSE, is an important part of the clinical assessment process in psychiatric practice. It is a structured way of observing and describing a patient's current state of mind, under the domains of appearance, attitude, behavior, mood and affect, speech, thought process, thought content, perception, cognition, insight and judgment.

The mental status exam is an assessment of the patient at the present time. Historical information should not be included in this section.

- **General appearance and behavior**
  - Grooming, level of hygiene, characteristics of clothing.
  - Unusual physical characteristics or movements.
  - Attitude. Ability to interact with the interviewer.
  - Psychomotor activity. Agitation or retardation.
  - Degree of eye contact.
- **Affect**
  - **Definition:** External range of expression, described in terms of quality, range and appropriateness
  - **Types of affect**
    - **Flat:** Absence of all or most affect.
    - **Blunted or restricted:** Moderately reduced range of affect.
    - **Labile:** Multiple abrupt changes in affect.
    - **Full or wide range of affect:** Generally appropriate.
- **Mood**
  - Internal emotional tone of the patient (i.e. dysphoric, euphoric, angry, euthymic, anxious).
- **Thought processes**
  - **Use of language:** Quality and quantity of speech. The tone, associations and fluency of speech should be noted.
  - **Common thought disorders**
    - **Pressured speech:** Rapid speech, which is typical of patients with manic disorder.
    - **Poverty of speech:** Minimal responses, such as answering just "yes or no."
    - **Blocking:** Sudden cessation of speech, often in the middle of a statement.
    - **Flight of ideas:** Accelerated thoughts that jump from idea to idea, typical of mania.
    - **Loosening of associations:** Illogical shifting between unrelated topics.
    - **Tangentiality:** Thought that wanders from the original point.
    - **Circumstantiality:** Unnecessary digression, which eventually reaches the point.
    - **Echolalia:** Echoing of words and phrases.
    - **Neologisms:** Invention of new words by the patient.
    - **Clanging:** Speech based on sound, such as rhyming and punning rather than logical connections.
    - **Perseveration:** Repetition of phrases or words in the flow of speech.
    - **Ideas of reference:** Interpreting unrelated events as having direct reference to the patient, such as believing that the television is talking specifically to them.
- **Thought content**
  - **Hallucinations:** False sensory perceptions, which may be auditory, visual, tactile, gustatory or olfactory
  - **Delusions:** Fixed, false beliefs firmly held in spite of contradictory evidence.
    - **Persecutory delusions:** False belief that others are trying to cause harm, or are spying with intent to cause harm.
    - **Erotomanic delusions:** False belief that a person, usually of higher status, is in love with the patient.
    - **Grandiose delusions:** False belief of an inflated sense of self-worth, power, knowledge, or wealth.
    - **Somatic delusions:** False belief that the patient has a physical disorder or defect.
  - **Illusions:** Misinterpretations of reality.
  - **Derealization:** Feelings of unrealness involving the outer environment.
  - **Depersonalization:** Feelings of unrealness, such as if one is "outside" of the body and observing his own activities.
  - **Suicidal and homicidal ideation:** Suicidal and homicidal ideation requires further elaboration with comments about intent and planning (including means to carry out plan).
- **Cognitive evaluation**
  - **Level of consciousness.**
  - **Orientation:** Person, place and date.
  - **Attention and concentration:** Repeat five digits forwards and backwards or spell a five letter word ("world") forwards and backward.
  - **Short-term memory:** Ability to recall three objects after five minutes.

- **Fund of knowledge:** Ability to name past five presidents, five large cities, or historical dates.
- **Calculations:** Subtraction of serial 7s, simple math problems.
- **Abstraction:** Proverb interpretation and similarities.
- **Insight:** Ability of the patient to display an understanding of his current problems, and the ability to understand the implication of these problems.
- **Judgment:** Ability to make sound decisions regarding everyday activities. Judgment is best evaluated by assessing a patient's history of decision-making, rather than by asking hypothetical questions.

THERAPEUTIC COMMUNICATION

Therapeutic communication is the art of transferring or exchanging information ideas or thoughts easily and correctly through verbal or nonverbal language. The purpose of therapeutic communication is:
- Establishing a therapeutic provider-client relationship
- Identify client's concerns and problem.
- Assess client's perception of the problem.
- Recognize client's needs.
- Guide client toward a satisfying and socially acceptable solution.

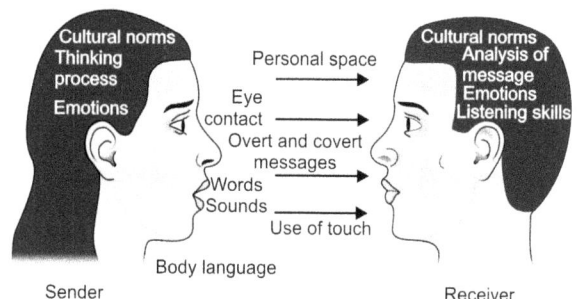

Therapeutic Communication Techniques

- **Use silence:**
  - Utilizing absence of verbal communication
  - Silence encourages conversation
  - Other words expected silence
  - It gives patient opportunity to collect and organize thoughts.
- **Giving recognition:**
  - Acknowledging, indicating awareness, to greet patient by name.
- **Offering self:**
  - Making oneself available unconditionally—nurse who is always conditional.
- **Giving broad opening:**
  - Allow your patient to take the initiation to introducing the topic.
- **Offering general leads:**
  - Giving encouragement to continue
- **Placing the event in time or in sequence**
  - Clarifying the relationship of events in time
- **Making observations:** Verbalizing what is perceived.
- **Encouraging comparison:** Asking the similarities and differences be noted.
- **Encouraging description of perception:** Asking patient to verbalize what he perceives.
- **Restating:** Repeating the main idea expressed.
- **Reflecting:** Directing back to the patients questions, feelings, ideas.
- **Focusing:** Concentrating on a single point "this point seems worth looking at more closely".
- **Seeking clarification:** Seeking to make clear that which is not meaningful or that what is vague.
- **Rejecting**
- **Agreeing**

Nontherapeutic Communication Techniques

- **Reassuring:** Do not give false reassurance, e.g. in medical condition, such as fever, we can give reassurance that take this paracetamol your fever will subside, but it is not applicable in psychiatric aspect.
- **Advising:** Do not give advice
- **Requesting explanation:** Asking client to provide the reason for his feeling.
- **Stereotypical response:** Do not give stereotypical response (don't focus on two aspects), e.g. patient: I hate being in hospital. Nurse: There are good and bad about staying in hospital.
- **Defending**
- **Changing the topic**
- **Approving**
- **Disapproving**
- **Agreeing**
- **Disagreeing**

COMMUNITY MENTAL HEALTH

The community mental health services were focused to render the care services in the familiar home environment. The client will develop adaptive coping strategies very easily to overcome the stressors related to mental illness. "Community mental health means all activities undertaken in the community in the name of mental health".

Public Health Model

Caplan (1964) developed the guiding principles for community mental health nursing in the early years. In this model the client is the community rather than the individual and the focus of practice is the factors that promote or inhibit mental health. Caplan focused on preventive psychiatry and introduced three important terms; primary prevention, secondary prevention, tertiary prevention.

- Primary prevention refers to the activities directed at reducing the incidence of mental disorders with in a population.
- Secondary prevention refers to the activities directed at reducing the prevalence of mental disorders by shortening the duration of a sufficient number of established cases.
- Tertiary prevention refers to the activities directed at reducing the defects that are associated with mental disorders.

Primary Prevention

Primary prevention aims at promotion of mental health and prevention of mental disorders, i.e reduction of occurrence of new cases of mental disorders. The nurse could play a major role in identifying high-risk groups and prevent the occurrence of mental illness in them. Some of them are as follows:

- Antenatal care to mother and educating her regarding the adverse effect of radiation, certain drugs and prematurity.
- Ensuring timely, efficient, obstetrical assistance to guard against the ill effects of anoxia and injury to new-born at birth.
- Providing dietary corrections to those infants suffering from metabolic disorders.
- Correction of endocrine disorders.
- Rendering crisis counseling to the parents of physically and mentally handicapped children.
- Training programs for mentally and physically handicapped children like blind, deaf and mute.
- Identifying the problems of scholastic performance and emotional disturbances among school going children's and giving timely interventions. School teachers could be taught to recognize the beginning symptoms of mental health problems and substance use disorders.
- Ensuring harmonious relationship among the members of the family and teaching healthy adaptive techniques at the time of stress producing events.
- Extending the mental health education services at child guidance clinic regarding healthy child rearing practice; at the parent teachers association regarding the triad relationship between teacher, child and parent, and at various extramural health agencies regarding integration of mental health into general health practice.
- Providing counseling services to adolescents and retired persons to pass through transitional crisis, to the members of bereavement family to accept to loss.
- Corrective suggestions and guidance to the culturally deprived groups to secure biopsychosocial supplies (food, love, shelter, health, recreation, etc.) otherwise the deprivation of it leads to alcoholism, crime and mental illness.
- Strengthening the social support to frustrated group and helping them to retain their usefulness.

Secondary Prevention

It focuses on early identification and effective treatment for those suffering with mental disorders.

- Early detection of mental disorders in the community
- Early referral
- Early diagnosis and effective (prompt) treatment
- Consultation service

Tertiary Prevention

Tertiary prevention aims to reduce the rate of disabilities due to longer duration of suffering from mental disorders. It aims to help the patient in the readjustment with the family and community from where he comes through-rehabilitation program.

- Social reintegration of discharged chronic mentally ill back into to community.
- Finding vocational rehabilitation and job placement for the mentally restored for self dependency.
- Re-equipping the mentally restored with daily living care abilities.
- Extending psychiatric rehabilitation and administration of medication at the door step of the mentally ill.

CRISIS INTERVENTION

A crisis is an internal disturbances caused by a stressful event or a perceived threat to self. It is a sudden or unexpected event that occurs in one's life.

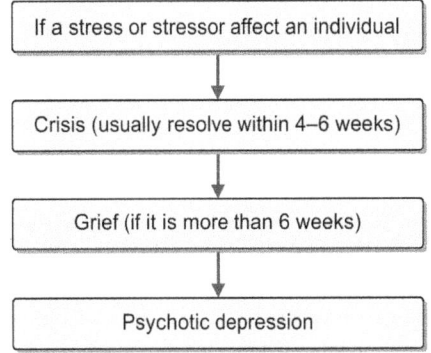

Grief is a multifaceted response to loss, particularly to the loss of someone or something that has died, to which a bond or affection was formed. In grief there are different phases of grief reaction. The grief reaction model is put forward by Kubler-Ross and the model is called as DABDA model.

Kubler-Ross Model

It is a 5-staged model of dying postulated by Kubler-Ross (1975), a psychiatrist who was significantly influenced by Sigmund Freud.

1. *Denial:* A state of unacceptance (lack of acceptance), a patient in the state of denial starts crying, e.g. the state which is seen in a patient who is first diagnosed as a case of cancer or MI.
2. *Anger:* The dying person anger is directed to self, god and others.
3. *Bargaining:* Through this person attempts to postpone or reverse death.
4. *Depression:* This aids the client to detach himself from life and living and thereby accept death.
5. *Acceptance:* Accepting the condition. Person comprehends the reality of the ensuring loss and feels at peace about the outcome.

DEFENSE MECHANISM

These are mental mechanism or coping mechanism used to reduce the stress or anxiety developed from an unexpected situation. Common defense mechanisms are:

- **Denial:** It is the refusal to accept reality or fact. For example, an MI patient cannot accept the diagnosis in the first stage.
- **Regression:** Childish behaviors, such as bedwetting, nail biting, etc. Reversion to the earlier stage of development in the face of unacceptable thoughts or impulses, e.g. An adult may regress when under a great deal of stress, refusing to leave their bed and engage in normal, everyday activities.
- **Acting out:** Performing an extreme behavior in order to express thoughts or feelings the person feels incapable.
- **Dissociation:** Dissociation is when a person loses track of time, a person who dissociates often loses track of time or themselves and their usual thought process and memory.
- **Projection:** Placing own undesirable trait onto another, blaming others for own difficulty.
- **Reaction formation:** Converting of unwanted or dangerous thoughts, feeling or impulses into their opposites. Engaging in behavior that is opposite of true desires.
- **Repression:** Repression is the unconscious blocking of unacceptable thoughts, feelings and impulses. "Repressed memories" are memories that have been unconsciously blocked from access or view.
- **Displacement:** Displacement is the redirecting of thoughts feelings and impulses directed at one person or object, but taken out upon another person or object, e.g. a husband starts firing her wife and she can't express her anger against husband due to fear of being fired. So she scolded the children and children show anger towards the dog.
- **Intellectualization:** Intellectualization is the overemphasis on thinking when confronted with an unacceptable impulse, situation or behavior without employing any emotions.
- **Rationalization: Developing an acceptable and justifiable reason for the behavior:** Rationalization is putting something into a different light or offering a different explanation for one's perceptions or behaviors in the face of a changing reality.
- **Undoing:** Undoing is the attempt to take back an unconscious behavior or thought that is unacceptable or hurtful. For instance, after realizing you just insulted your significant other unintentionally, you might spend the next hour praising their beauty, charm and intellect.
- **Sublimation:** Sublimation is simply the channelling of unacceptable impulses, thoughts and emotions into more acceptable ones. Anxiety channelled into socially acceptable behavior.
- **Compensation:** Compensation is a process of psychologically counterbalancing perceived weaknesses by emphasizing strength in other areas. A student who is weak in studies but he is bright in sports.
- **Conversion:** Anxiety converted into a physical symptom that is motor or sensory in nature.

TREATMENTS IN PSYCHIATRY

- Psychotherapy
- Drug therapy
- Hospitalization
- ECT

PSYCHOTHERAPY

A form of treatment in which a trained person deliberately establishes a professional relationship with the client, with the objective of removing or modifying existing symptoms and promoting positive personality, growth and development.

Role of Nurse in Psychotherapy

- Explain the purpose and rules of psychotherapy
- Introduce the group members
- Promote group cohesiveness

- Encourage participation of group members
- Set the limit

Types of Psychotherapy

Individual Psychotherapy

Psychotherapy between one patient and one psychotherapist.

Group Psychotherapy

Psychotherapy between a group of patient and psychotherapist, It may be homogenous group therapy (same group of patient such as alcoholic groups) and heterogeneous group therapy (different group of patient).

Behavior Therapy

The principles of behavioral therapy as we know it today are based on the early studies of classical conditioning by Pavlov (1927), and operant conditioning by Skinner (1938).

Classical Conditioning

It is a process of learning that was introduced by Russian Physiologist Pavlov. In his trials he found that, as expected that the dog salivated when they began to eat the food that was offered to them. This was the reflective response that Pavlov called as unconditioned response. However, he also noticed that with time, the dogs began to salivate when the food came to the range of view, before it was even presented to them for consumption. Concluding that this response was not reflexive but had been learned. Pavlov called it a conditioned response. He carried the experiments even further by introducing a unrelated stimulus, one that had no previous connection to the animal food. The animal responded with the expected reflexive salivation to the food. After a number of trials with the combined stimuli (food and bell), Pavlov found that the reflexive salivation began to occur when the dog was presented with the sound of the bell in the absence of food.

This was an important discovery in terms of how learning can occur. Pavlov found that unconditioned responses (salivation) occur in response to unconditioned stimuli (eating food). He also found that, overtime, an unrelated stimulus (sound of the bell) introduced with the unconditioned stimulus could elicit the same response alone, i.e. conditioned response. The unrelated stimulus is called the conditioned stimulus.

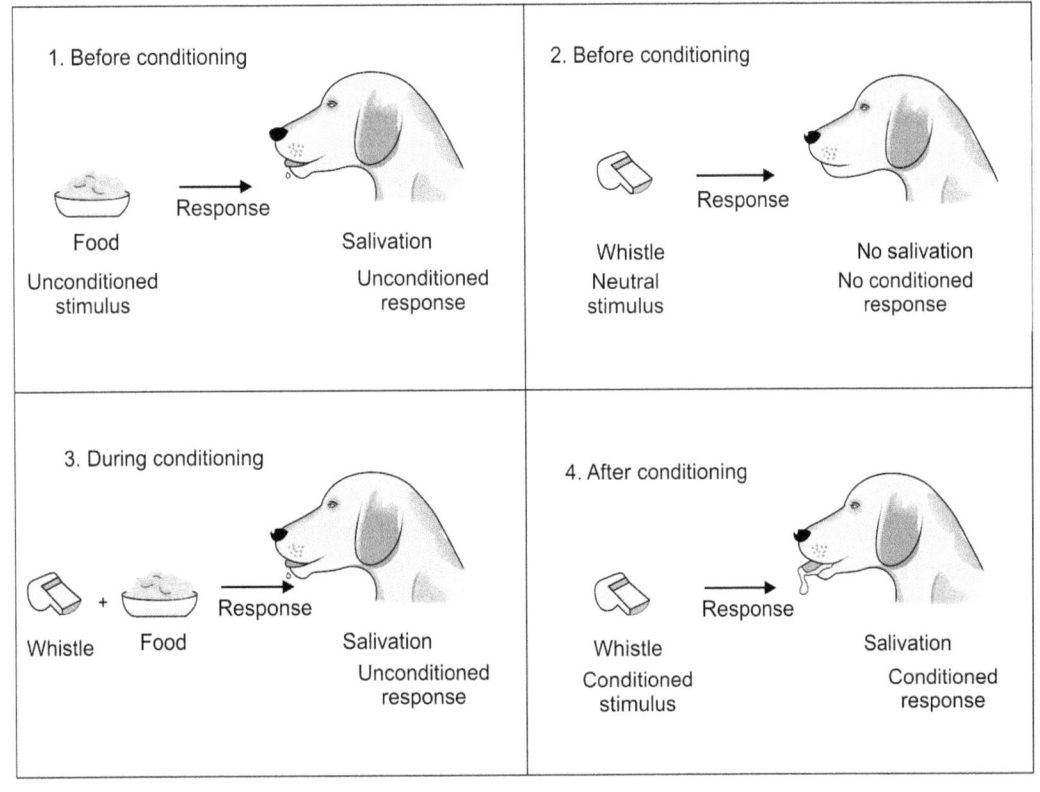

Operant Conditioning

It is a process of learning that was introduced by BF Skinner in 1953. In this theory, he mentioned about reinforcement. There are two types of reinforcement, positive reinforcement and negative reinforcement. Positive reinforcement helps to learn adaptive behavior and negative reinforcement is used to remove the maladaptive behavior.

Operant conditioning	Reinforcement Increase behavior	Punishment Decrease behavior
Positive stimulus (something added)	Positive reinforcement Add something to increase behavior	Positive punishment Add something to decrease behavior
Negative stimulus (something removed)	Negative reinforcement Remove something to increase behavior	Negative punishment Remove something to decrease behavior

Techniques used are:
- **Systematic desensitization:** It is used for the treatment of phobia. Patient is exposed to stimuli by step by step manner.
- **Hypnosis:** It is contraindicated in patient with phobia.
- **Token economy:** A token economy is a form of behavior modification designed to increase desirable behavior and decrease undesirable behavior with the use of tokens. Individuals receive tokens immediately after displaying desirable behavior. The tokens are collected and later exchanged for a meaningful object or privilege.
- **Flooding:** Sometimes called implosive therapy is also used to desensitize individuals to phobic stimuli.

Milieu Therapy

Also called *therapeutic community*, or *therapeutic environment*, this type of therapy consists of a scientific structuring of the environment in order to effect behavioral changes and to improve the individual's psychological health and functioning.

Electroconvulsive Therapy

Electroconvulsive therapy (ECT) is a physical/somatic therapy in which an electric current is passed with the help of two electrodes, through the temporal region in between the two hemispheres on the brain, to produce a grandmal type of seizures.

It is introduced in 1938 by Cerletti and Bini.

Indication
- Mania
- Schizophrenia
- Schizoaffective disorder
- Postpartum psychosis
- Severe catatonic stupor
- Severe psychosis

Contraindication
- Increased ICP
- Cerebral aneurysm
- Cerebral hemorrhage
- Brain tumor
- Acute MI
- Congestive cardiac failure
- Retinal detachment

Methods
- Direct ECT: ECT is given in the absence of muscular relaxation and general anesthesia.
- Modified ECT: (Indirect) ECT is modified by drug-induced muscular relaxation and general anesthesia.

Technique
- Bilateral ECT: This is the standard form of ECT most commonly used. Each electrode is placed 2.5-4 cm above the midpoint, on a line joining the tragus of ear and lateral canthus of eye.
- Unilateral ECT: Electrodes are placed only on onside of head, usually nondominant side. Another one electrodes can place anywhere the head.

Medication
- Thiopentone sodium
- Succinylcholine
- Voltage: 70-120 volt
- Duration: 0.1-1 second

Nursing Care

Before ECT
- Detailed medical psychiatric history, including history of allergies.
- Assessment of patient's and family's knowledge of indication, side effects, therapeutic effects and risk associated with ECT.
- An informed consent should be taken.
- Assess vital signs.
- Patient should be on empty stomach for 6 hrs prior to ECT.

- Withhold night doses of drug which increase seizure threshold like diazepam, barbiturates, etc.
- Withhold oral medication in the morning.
- Any jewellery, prosthesis, metallic objects and tight clothing should be removed from the patient.
- Empty bladder and bowel just before ECT.
- Administer 0.5 mg atropine, muscle relaxant and anesthetic medication as prescribed.

During ECT

- Place the patient comfortably on the ECT table in supine position.
- Assist in administering the anesthetic agent
- Since the muscle relaxant paralyzes, all muscles including respiratory muscles patient airway should be ensured.
- Mouth gag should be inserted to prevent possible tongue bite.
- During seizure monitor vital signs, ECG, oxygen saturation, etc.
- Record positive finding and medication given in patient chart.

After ECT

- Monitor vital signs at least once in 15 minutes and should be able to get in touch with the anesthetist/treating psychiatrist immediately should any problem arises.
- Continue O_2 till spontaneous respiration starts.
- Assess for postical confusion and restlessness.
- Take safety precautions to prevent injury like suctioning to aspirate secretion, etc.
- Reorient the patient after recovery and stay with him until fully oriented.
- Give medication for minor discomfort, such as headache or nausea.
- Document finding as relevant in the patient record.

DISORDERS OF PERCEPTION

- **Illusion:** False perception, e.g. considering a rope as a snake
- **Delusion:** Fixed false belief that no one can change, e.g. A patient admitted in the hospital and complaints to the nurse that his heart has stopped working and my blood become black.
  - *Delusion of grandiosity* (patient consider that he is the supreme power)
  - *Delusion of persecution* (a false belief that he is the object for others harassment)
  - *Somatic delusion* (patient think that he has major illness)
- **Hallucination:** Imaginary perception, e.g. hearing some words (auditory hallucination)

Role of Nurse

- Avoid arguing with the client
- Presenting reality
- Provide psychological support
- Maintain a good relationship with the patient

CLASSIFICATION OF PSYCHIATRIC DISORDERS

There are two important classification in psychiatry.

ICD 10 Classification

- International classification of disease
- In ICD 10 there are A–Z chapters, chapter F deals with mental disorders
- More general terms
- Uses single axial

DSM IV Classification

- Larger number of discrete categories
- Uses a multiaxial system
- Uses term psychotic.

SCHIZOPHRENIA

The word schizophrenia is coined by swiss psychiatrist called as Eugen Bleuler, so it is also called as Bleuler syndrome. Schizophrenia comes from Schizo (splitting) and phrenia (mind), so it is also known as splitting of mind.

Schizophrenia is a chronic mental disorder characterized by disturbance in thinking, emotion and volition (action) with presence of faculties of consciousness.

About 15% of all patients attending OPD are schizophrenia and 50% of all hospital bed is occupied by schizophrenia.

Causes

- Unknown
- Dopamine hypothesis (from the presynaptic area to the post synaptic area there is an excessive transmission of dopamine)
- Enlarged lateral ventricle
- Monozygotic twins
- Stressful situation, over protective parents.

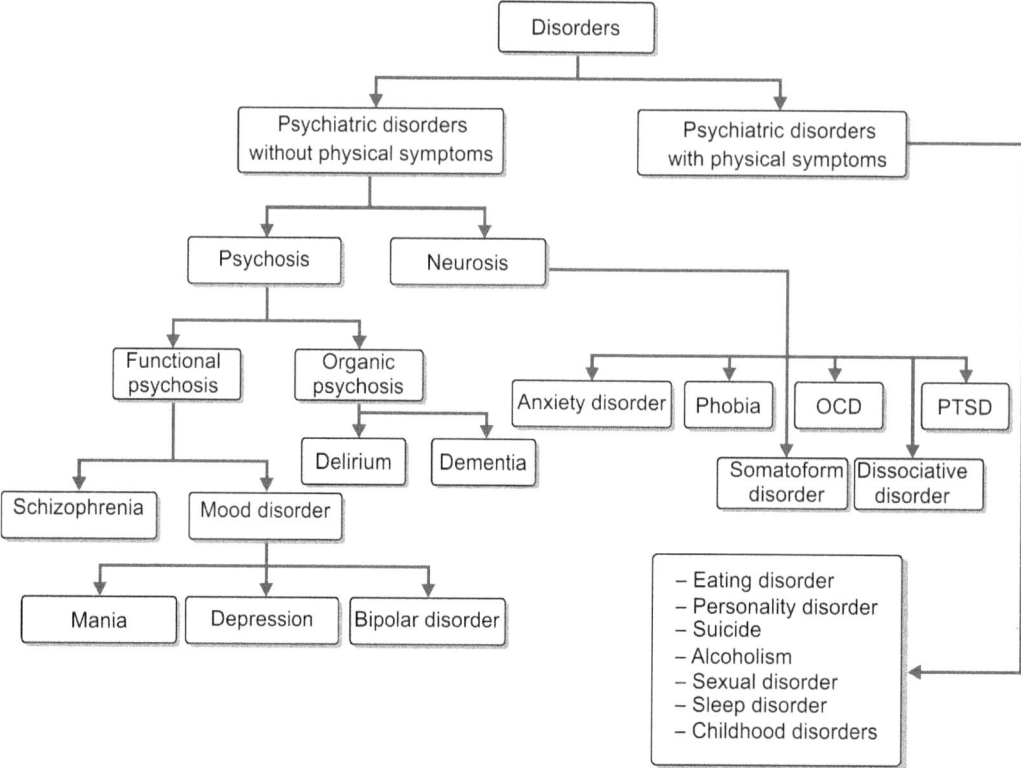

Clinical Manifestation

Bleuler 4As

- A: Affective disturbances
- A: Associative disturbances
- A: Ambivalence
- A: Autistic thinking

Positive symptoms of schizophrenia are delusion, hallucination, speech disturbances, etc.

Negative symptoms of schizophrenia are flat affect, avolition, alogia (lack of speech), anhedonia (inability to experience pleasure).

Types of Schizophrenia

- Paranoid type: Where delusions and hallucinations are present but thought disorder, disorganized behavior, and affective flattening are absent.
- Disorganized type: Also known as hebephrenic schizophrenia in the ICD. Where thought disorder and flat affect are present together.
- Catatonic type: The subject may be almost immobile or exhibit agitated, purposeless movement. Symptoms can include catatonic stupor and waxy flexibility.
- Undifferentiated type: Psychotic symptoms are present but the criteria for paranoid, disorganized, or catatonic types have not been met.
- Residual type: Where positive symptoms are present at a low intensity only.

Management

- Offer self in development of relationship
- Encourage reality orientation
- Remove all harmful objects from the patient side
- Use silence
- Provide psychotherapy
- Administer antipsychotics
- Prepare the patient for ECT

Antipsychotics

The other names of antipsychotics are dopamine blocker or neuroleptics or major tranquilizers. There are two types of antipsychotics.

Typical antipsychotics	Atypical antipsychotics
Treatment of positive symptoms of schizophrenia	Treatment of negative symptoms of schizophrenia
Chlorpromazine (CPZ) 200–600 mg Haloperidol (serenace) 2–10 mg IM Risperidone (risnia) 4–10 mg oral	Olanzapine Clozapine Thiothixene

Antipsychotics are also called as dopamine blockers. It act as a barrier on the post synaptic area thereby prevents the entry of dopamine into the post synaptic area. If the patient is undergoing prolonged antipsychotics, there will be depletion of dopamine in the postsynaptic area and leads to tremor or symptoms of parkinsonism (the side effect of neuroleptics is unintentional tremor).

Side Effect

- CNS (drowsiness, lethargy, mental confusion)
- ANS (dry mouth, blurring of vision, constipation, urinary incontinency)
- Endocrine (infertility)
- Extrapyramidal symptoms
  - Parkinsonism, rigidity, tremor, bradykinesia
  - Acute muscular dystonia, muscle spasm—usually involving linguofacial muscles
  - Tardive dyskinesia (involuntary facial and lip movements)
  - Akathisia (restlessness and feeling of discomfort)
  - Neuroleptic malignant syndrome (occurs rarely with high doses, rigidity, immobility, tremors, and fever)
- Rabbit syndrome
- Ocular side effects (pigmented retinopathy).

Nursing Care

- Monitor for any side effect of the drug
- Administer antiparkinsonism drugs, such as levodopa and carbidopa for a patient with antipsychotics.
- Monitor the intake and output chart
- Monitor for orthostatic hypotension, advice the patient before get down from the bed, allow sitting in the bed and safely moving from bed.

MOOD DISORDERS

A psychological disorder characterized by the elevation or lowering of a person's mood, such as depression or bipolar disorder. It includes:

Mania

It is a mental state characterized by excessive happiness. The onset is before 30 years.

Causes

- Unknown
- Genetic causes
- Serotonin hypothesis (from the presynaptic area to the postsynaptic area, there will be increased transmission of serotonin).

Stages of Mania

Stage I	Euphoria	Mild elevation of mood
Stage II	Elation	Moderate elevation of mood
Stage III	Exaltation	Intense elevation of mood
Stage IV	Ecstasy	Severe elevation of mood or stuporous mania

Clinical Manifestation

- Increased self-esteem or grandiosity
- Heightened energy
- Decreased need for sleep (e.g. one feels rested after only 3 hours of sleep)
- More talkative than usual or pressure to keep talking
- Flight of ideas or subjective experience that thoughts are racing
- Attention is easily drawn to unimportant or irrelevant items
- Increase in goal-directed activity (either socially, at work or school, or sexually) or psychomotor agitation
- Excessive involvement in pleasurable activities that have a high potential for painful consequences.

Management

- Administer antimanic drugs (mood stabilizer)
- Offer finger foods and fluids
- Provide a quiet environment
- Do not argue with the client
- Remove all the harmful objects from the patient
- Set a limit.

Antimanic Drugs (Mood Stabilizers)

Antimanic drugs are agents used to treat bipolar disorders or mania associated with other affective disorders. Mood stabilizers balance certain brain chemicals (neurotransmitters) that control emotional states and behavior, e.g.

- Lithium carbonate
- Carbamazepine
- Valproic acid

Nursing Care

- Lithium is commonly used as an antimanic drug which is metabolized in the kidney. So, monitor serum potassium level and maintain serum sodium level for the patient undergoing lithium therapy.
- Monitor serum lithium level (normal serum lithium level is 0.8–1.2 mEq/L)
- Monitor for any complications of lithium, such as seizures, tremor hypokalemia, etc.

Mild toxicity	1.2–2 mEq/L
Moderate toxicity	2–2.5 mEq/L
Severe toxicity	2.5–3 mEq/L
Fatal	>3 mEq/L

Depression

It is a mental state characterized by excessive sadness.

Causes

- Unknown
- Genetic factors
- Biochemical hypothesis
- Serotonin hypothesis (from the presynaptic area to the postsynaptic area, there is decreased transmission of serotonin).

Clinical Manifestation

- Hopelessness, powerlessness and worthlessness
- Decreased self-esteem
- Decreased ability to perform activities
- Risk for self-injury
- Lack of interest in activities
- Waxy flexibility or stuporous activity

Management

- Administer antidepressants
- Remove harmful objects from the patient side
- Encourage discussion regarding positive and negative aspects of the patient.

Antidepressants

Antidepressants are agents which are used for the treatment of depressive symptoms.

Tricyclic antidepressants (TCA)	Selective serotonin reuptake inhibitors (SSRI)	Monoamine oxidase inhibitors (MAOI)
Imipramine Trimipramine Amitriptyline	Sertraline Citalopram	Phenelzine (Nardil, Nardelzine)

Nursing Care

- Monitor for the complications of tricyclic antidepressants (TCA), the complications are:
  H: Hypotension
  A: Anticholinergic effect like dry mouth
  T: Tachycardia
  S: Sedation
- Instruct the patient to avoid tyramine rich diet if the patient is on MAOI therapy. Tyramine is a chemical which is seen in certain foods, such as wine, hard cheese, vinegar, etc. which react with MAOI and lead to hypertensive crisis. Hypertensive crisis is a severe life-threatening condition. The drug of choice in hypertensive crisis is phentolamine mesylate.
- Be sure that client swallow the medication
- Antidepressant medications are not stopped in between because it may take effect for 2-3 weeks.

OTHER MOOD DISORDERS

- **Bipolar disorders:** It is characterized by mood swings from profound depression to extreme euphoria, with intervening periods of normalcy. During manic episodes, the mood is elevated, expansive, or irritable. Psychotic features may present.
- **Bipolar I disorder:** It is the diagnosis given to an individual who is experiencing, a full syndrome of manic or mixed symptoms. The client may also have experienced episodes of depression.
- **Bipolar II:** At least one hypomanic episode and one or more episodes of major depression.
- **Cyclothymia:** Long-standing pattern of alternating mood episodes that do not meet criteria for major depression or mania, criteria include duration of at least 2 years with recurrent periods of mild depression alternating with hypomania.
- **Seasonal affective disorder (SAD):** Vulnerable to changes in sunlight, especially fall and spring, prevalence rates of 4-6%, found more often in northern latitudes. Many SAD symptoms opposite of those found in major depression—increase in appetite, weight gain, more sleep.
- **Dysthymic disorder:** Characteristics of this mood disturbance are similar to major depressive disorder. Individuals with dysthymic disorder describe their mood as sad or "down in the dumps".

ORGANIC PSYCHOSIS (ORGANIC MENTAL DISORDERS)

Organic mental disorders are behavioral or psychological disorders associated with transient or permanent brain dysfunction which are either primary (primary brain pathology) or secondary (brain dysfunction due to systematic diseases). These are called as amnestic disorders. These disorders can be subcategorized into following categories:

- Delirium
- Dementia
- Organic amnestic syndrome
- Other organic mental disorders

DELIRIUM

It is an organic mental disorder characterized by disturbance in cognition as well as disturbance in consciousness. It is also called as acute brain syndrome or metabolic encephalopathy.

Incidence

- 20-40% of geriatric clients in hospitalization.
- 5-15% of all patients in medical and surgical inpatient units are estimated to develop delirium.
- In postoperative cases, highest incidence was noticed.

Causes

- Delirium due to medical conditions (cancer or major illness)
- Delirium due to substance abuse (alcoholism)
- Delirium due to multiple causes (head injury)

Clinical Manifestation

- Changes in cognition
- Changes in consciousness
- Changes in the sleep wake cycle–insomnia at night, drowsiness at daytime.
- Sun downing syndrome—diurnal variation is marked, usually worsening of symptoms in evening and night.
- Impairment of registration and retention of new memories
- Psychomotor disturbance usually in the form of agitation and occasionally retardation
- Motor symptoms—Asterixis (flapping tremor)

Management

- Identification of causes and its immediate correction
- Symptomatic measures: Benzodiazepines, haloperidol, chlorpromazine
- Supportive medical and nursing care

DEMENTIA

It is an organic mental disorder characterized by disturbance in cognition but there is no disturbance in consciousness. It is also called as senility.

Incidence

- Estimated prevalence of dementia is 1.03% of the population.
- Rises to between 16% and 25% for those over 85 ages, the most common is Alzheimer's disease, which accounts for up to 70% of all cases. Alzheimer's disease is caused by the destruction of certain brain cells leading to the loss of the neurotransmitter acetylcholine.

Causes

- Deposition of beta amyloid in the brain
- Presence of neurofibrillary in the brain
- Deficiency of vitamin B12

Clinical Manifestation

- Memory loss, especially of more recent events
- Difficulty in finding their way around, especially in new or unfamiliar surroundings
- Problems in learning new ideas or skills
- wandering away from home in the late afternoon
- difficulties in meeting activities of daily living

Types

1. Alzheimer's dementia (DAT)
2. Multi Infarct dementia (MID)
3. Hypothyroid dementia
4. AIDS dementia complex
5. Lewy body dementia.

Alzheimer's Disease (Dementia of Alzheimer's Type, DAT)

This is the common cause of dementia, seen in about 70% of all cases of dementia in USA. It is more commonly seen in women—popularly known as "The Disease of Century".

Multi Infarct Dementia (MID)

MID is the second commonest cause of dementia, seen in 10-15% of all cases. It is also one of the important treatable causes of dementia.

Hypothyroidal Dementia

Most important treatable and reversible causes of dementia, hypothyroidism should be suspected in every patient of dementia.

AIDS Dementia Complex

About 50-70% of patients suffering from AIDS exhibit a triad of cognitive, behavioral and motoric deficits of sub cortical dementia type, known as the AIDS-dementia complex.

Lewy Body Dementia

It is now believed to be the second most common cause of degenerative dementias. This is caused by abnormal microscopic deposits of protein, called Lewy bodies, which destroy nerve cells.

NEUROSIS (NEUROTIC DISORDER)

The term neurosis is defined as the presence of a symptom or group of symptoms which cause subjective distress to patient.

In ICD-10, neurotic, stress-related and somatoform disorders are classified into:

- Anxiety disorder
- Phobic anxiety disorder
- OCD
- Post-traumatic stress disorder

- Dissociative disorder
- Somatoform disorder

GENERALIZED ANXIETY DISORDER

Generalized anxiety disorder (GAD) is an anxiety disorder that is characterized by chronic, unrealistic, excessive, uncontrollable and often irrational worry about everyday things that is disproportionate to the actual source of worry. Anxiety is a subjective sense of worry, apprehension, fear and distress.

- **Mild anxiety:** Increase awareness or ability to solve the problem
- **Moderate anxiety:** Moderate increase in tension to solve the problem, have optimal level of learning.
- **Severe anxiety:** Increase vitals, dilated pupils and feeling difficulty in problem-solving.
- **Panic anxiety:** Inability to solve the problem, decrease vitals, increase physical symptoms like chest pain, breathing difficulty, etc.

Nursing Care

- Assess the level of anxiety of the patient.
- Provide outlets by walking and open talks.
- Assist client to recognize own anxiety.
- Promote insight into anxiety and related factors.
- Provide opportunity for learning new adaptive coping responses.
- Involve client and family in educational/support activities.
- Administer antianxiety medications
  - Barbiturates (phenobarbital, secobarbital)
  - Non-barbiturates (chloral hydrate)
  - Benzodiazepines (lorazepam, diazepam, librium).

PHOBIA

A phobia is an unreasonable fear of a specific object, activity or situation.

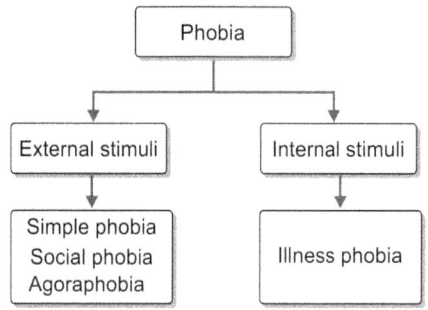

Simple Phobia (Specific Phobia)

Simple phobia is an irrational fear of specific object or stimulus. It is the most common type of phobic disorder in the general population.

Examples

- Acrophobia—fear of heights
- Hematophobia—fear of the sight of blood
- Claustrophobia—fear of closed spaces
- Gamophobia—fear of marriage
- Insectophobia—fear of insects
- AIDS phobia—fear of AIDS

Social Phobia

Social phobia is an irrational fear of performing activities in the presence of other people or interacting with others.

Agoraphobia

It is characterized by an irrational fear of being in places away from the familiar setting of home in crowds or in situations that the patient cannot leave easily.

Internal Stimuli

Illness Phobia (Nosophobia)

It is characterized by an irrational fear of illness. It constitute about 10-20% of phobic patient. It occurs equally in both sexes.

Nursing Care

- Administer antianxiety medications
- Prepare the patient for systematic desensitization
- Teach relaxation therapies

OBSESSIVE-COMPULSIVE DISORDER

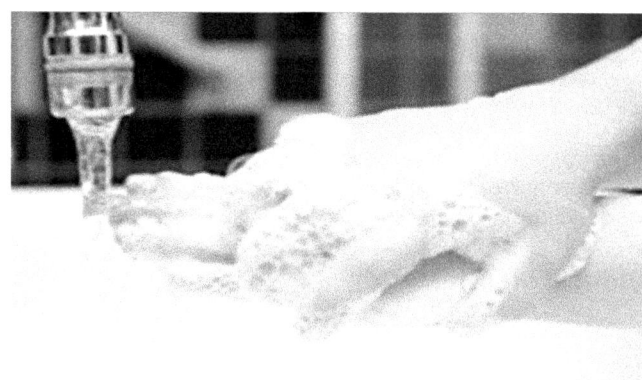

It is an anxiety disorder characterized by obsessional thought and followed by compulsive act. Obsessions are involuntary, seemingly uncontrollable thoughts, images, or impulses that occur over and over again in your mind (feeling of dirt in the hand). Compulsions are behaviors or rituals that you feel driven to act out again and again. (frequent handwashing).

Clinical Manifestation

- Repetitive handwashing
- Extensive hoarding
- Preoccupation with sexual or aggressive impulses, or with particular religious beliefs
- Aversion to odd numbers
- Nervous habits, such as opening a door and closing it a certain number of times before one enters or leaves a room.

Nursing Care

- Allow the impulsive acts, but set some limits
- Encourage the client to perform alternative behavior
- Provide opportunity to perform task that needs perfection.
- Administer antianxiety medications
- Check for the skin integrity as it is a short-term goal and the long-term goal is decrease the number of episodes.
- Prepare the patient for cognitive and behavioral therapy.

POST-TRAUMATIC STRESS DISORDER (PTSD)

An anxiety disorder resulting from exposure to a traumatic event in which an individual has experienced or witnessed to an event that involves actual or threatened death/ serious injury or a threat to the physical integrity of the self or others.

Severe psychological disturbance following a traumatic event characterized by involuntary re-experiencing of elements of the event, with symptoms of hyperarousal, avoidance, and emotional numbing.

Clinical Manifestation

- Re-experiencing the traumatic events
- Nightmares
- Difficulty falling or staying asleep
- Irritability or outbursts of anger
- Difficulty in concentrating
- Hyper vigilance
- Exaggerated startle response

Nursing Care

- Provide safety for client/others.
- Assist client to enhance self-esteem and regain sense of control over feelings/actions.
- Encourage development of assertive, not aggressive, behaviors.
- Promote understanding that the outcome of the present situation can be significantly affected by own actions.
- Assist client/family to learn healthy ways to deal with/ realistically adapt to changes and events that have occurred.

SOMATOFORM DISORDER

Multiple, recurrent somatic complaints of fatigue, backache, nausea, menstrual cramps for many years but there is no organic etiology.

A category of psychiatric disorder characterized by conversion of emotional distress into physical symptoms. It is also called as psychosomatic disorder.

Clinical Manifestation

- History of seeking medical attention from the doctors for prolonged time
- Doctor shopping
- Symptoms range from pain, gastrointestinal, sexual and pseudoneurological
- Will have experienced at least 8 different types of symptoms.

Conversion Disorder

Conversion disorder is an illness of symptoms or deficits that affect voluntary motor or sensory functions which suggest another medical condition. It involves:

- Motor and sensory problems
- May suggest a neurological condition
- Impaired social, occupational and personal ability to function
- Sensory impairment: Tingling, and strong stimulations
- Motor impairment: Arms, legs, vocal chords, tremors and involuntary twitches

Hypochondriasis

It is a condition characterized by:
- Preoccupied with fear of having a serious disease
- Misinterpretation of bodily functions

- Minor abnormalities
- Problems continue without any changes

Body Dysmorphic Disorder

Body dysmorphic disorder is characterized by a preoccupation with an imagined defect in appearance that causes clinically significant distress or impairment in important areas of functioning. The patient believes that there is a problem with appearance.

DISSOCIATIVE DISORDER

A dissociative disorder is the breakdown of one's perception of his/her surroundings, memory, identity, or consciousness. Dissociative disorders is characterized by:
- Severe alterations or detachments
- Affect identity, memory, and/or consciousness
- Severe form of normal perceptual experiences
- Depersonalization: Distortion in perception of reality
- De-realization: Losing a sense of the external world

Clinical Manifestation

- Multiple mannerisms, attitudes and beliefs which are not similar to each other
- Unexplainable headaches and other body pains
- Distortion or loss of subjective time, depersonalization, severe memory loss
- Flashbacks of abuse/trauma
- Sudden anger without a justified cause
- Frequent panic/anxiety attacks
- Unexplainable phobias.

Types

Depersonalization disorder	Frequent episodes where an individual feels detached from his or her mental state or body
Dissociative amnesia	The person loses memory of important personal facts, including personal identity
Dissociative fugue	The person moves away and assumes a new identity, with amnesia for the previous identity
Dissociative identity disorder	Separate, multiple personalities in the same individual
Dissociative trance disorder	Previously known as multiple personality disorder

Nursing Care

- Discuss ways to identify onset of anxiety.
- Discuss ways to intervene to prevent symptoms.
- Teach relaxation techniques.
- Teach assertiveness techniques.
- Administer anxiolytics, antipsychotics, antidepressants.

PERSONALITY DISORDER

Personality refers to all enduring qualities of an individual that are shown in his ways of behaving in a wide variety of circumstances. Personality disorders results when personality traits become abnormal, i.e. inflexible and maladaptive and cause significant social or occupational impairment or significant subjective distress.

A personality disorder is a chronic disturbance in one's relation with self and others and the environment that results in distress or failure to fulfill social roles and obligations.

Causes

- Hereditary factors—chromosomal abnormalities or genetic predisposition can be responsible for a psychopathic personality.
- Relation of personality disorder to mental disorder—psychiatric disorders are associated with the personalities, e.g. schizoid personalities are considered to be partial expressions of schizophrenia. Cluster A personality disorder occurs more frequently in biological relatives of schizophrenia, cluster B among alcohol users and cluster C among anxiety and depression.
- Disturbed parent-child relationship.

Classification of Personality Disorders

According to DSM-IV

The personality disorders are divided into 3 clusters:
1. **Cluster-A (odd and eccentric)**
   - Paranoid personality disorder
   - Schizoid personality disorder
   - Schizotypal personality disorder
2. **Cluster-B (dramatic, emotional and erratic)**
   - Antisocial personality disorder
   - Histrionic personality disorder
   - Narcissistic personality disorder
   - Borderline personality disorder
3. **Cluster-C (anxious and fearful)**
   - Avoidant personality disorder
   - Dependent personality disorder
   - Obsessive-compulsive personality disorder

Paranoid personality disorder	Suspicious, mistrustful, sensitive, argumentative, stubborn, self-important
Schizoid personality disorder	Emotionally cold, aloof, detached humorless, introspective
Schizotypal personality disorder	Inappropriate affect, odd beliefs or magical thinking, social withdrawal
antisocial personality disorder	Failure to sustain relationship, disregard for the feelings of others, impulsive action, tendency to cause violence
Histrionic personality disorder	Dramatic emotionality (emotional blackmail, angry scenes, demonstrative suicide attempts, etc.), attention-seeking behavior
Narcissistic personality disorder	Inflated sense of self-importance, lack of empathy, exploitative behavior
Borderline personality disorder	Unstable relationship, variable moods, lack of control on anger
Avoidant personality disorder	Inferiority complex, unwillingness to become involved with people
Dependent personality disorder	Inability to take decision, feeling uncomfortable or helpless when alone
Obsessive-compulsive personality disorder	Preoccupation with details, rules, lists, order or schedule, perfectionism

Nursing Care

- Convey accepting attitude toward the patient
- Maintain low level of stimuli in the environment
- Help the patient to identify the true object of his hostility and encourage him to gradually verbalize hostile feelings.
- Provide positive feedback for accepting behavior which will encourage repetition of desirable behaviors.
- Help the client to gain insight into his own behavior.

EATING DISORDERS

Eating disorder includes changes in usual eating patterns, regular dieting, skipping meals, and fasting behavior.

ANOREXIA NERVOSA

Anorexia nervosa is a psychiatric disorder characterized by a voluntary refusal to eat. Anorexia nervosa is estimated to occur in about 0.5% to 1% of adolescent girls. It occurs 10–20 times more often in females than males.

Clinical Manifestation

- An intense fear of gaining weight and becoming obese.
- Refuse to eat with their families or in public places.
- Abuse laxatives and even diuretics to lose weight, and ritualistic exercising, extensive cycling, walking, jogging and running are common activities.

BULIMIA NERVOSA

Bulimia is a term that means binge eating, which is defined as eating more food than most persons in similar circumstances and in a similar period of time, accompanied by a strong sense of losing control (excessive eating followed by self-induced vomiting).

Clinical Manifestation

- Persistent sore throat, heartburn
- Tooth staining or discoloration, loss of dental enamel and increased dental carries
- Eating amount of food larger than what most people would eat
- Frequent weight fluctuations, lanugo
- Hypotension and hypothermia
- Abdominal and epigastric pain.

Nursing Care

- Make therapeutic contracts with the client regarding the time, frequency and procedure for weighing the patient.
- Explain the time when meals will be served and the number of meals that are to be eaten each day.
- Provide psychological support.
- Be with the patient for the first 30 minutes after food.
- Monitor for hypotension, lanugo and hypothermia.

SUICIDE

Suicide is one the important psychiatric emergencies which need immediate intervention. It is one of the most common cause of death. It places eight major causes of death.

A murderous attack on an internalized object which has become a source of ambivalence. It is an ultimate act of self destruction.

The attempt of suicide is commonly seen in females but the success is seen in males.

Causes

- Constant failure to the use of normal coping strategies
- Presence of multiple risk factors
- Significant losses
- Perceived abuse
- Biochemical factors
  (When low level of neurotransmitters, e.g. serotonin causes depression)

Types

In 1897, Emile Durkheim classified social categories of suicide. They are:
1. **Egoistic suicide:** One who lost social integration with the social group? It may result from excessive individualism and from the decreasing influence of social norms. It's the response of the individual who feels separated and apart from the main society, e.g. divorce.
2. **Altruistic suicide:** Results from a response to a cultural expectation, or when the degree of social integration is too high, e.g. suicide bomber.
3. **Anomic suicide:** Occurs in response to the changes that occur in an individual's life, e.g. divorce loss of job.
4. **Samsonic suicide or suicide of revenge:** To spite others or experiencing as being unfriendly, e.g. if husband is unfaithful to his wife, she may attempt to commit suicide to take revenge.

Methods of Committing Suicide

There are mainly two classification.
- **Low lethal methods:** Self-poisoning by pill ingestion, wrist cutting
- **High lethal methods:** Gun shooting
  - Hanging and drowning
  - Car crash
  - Fire arms
  - Jumping from height

Recognition of Suicidal Ideas or Facts

- Behavioral clues
- Verbal clues
- Situational clues (life experiences associated with major stress or death of loved ones)
- syndromic clues
- Nonverbal clues (addiction, sleeping too much or too little)
- Emotional and behavior changes associated with suicide.

Assessment of Suicide (SAD PERSONS Scale)

	Factor	Scores
S	Sex	1 if male
A	Age	1 if age 25–44
D	Depression	1 if present
P	Previous attempt	1 if yes
E	Ethanol use	1 if yes
R	Rational thinking loss	1 if yes
S	Social support lack	1 if yes
O	Organized plan	1 if yes
N	No spouse	1 if yes
S	Sickness	1 if any major illness

Points

- Send home if score 0–2
- Close follow-up 3–4
- Strongly consider hospitalization 5–6
- Strict hospitalization 7–10.

Levels of Intervention

Nursing interventions for suicide takes place in three levels.
- Primary intervention: It include activities that provide support, information and education to prevent suicide.
- Secondary intervention: It is the treatment of actual suicidal crisis.
- Tertiary intervention: It refers to the intervention with the family and friends of a person who committed suicide to reduce the traumatic after effects.

ALCOHOLISM

Alcoholism refers to the use of alcoholic beverages to the point of causing damage to individual, society or both. It is a CNS depressant.

A concentration of 80 to 100 mg of alcohol per 100 mL of blood is considered intoxication. A person with 200 mg to 250 mg will be toxic, sleepy, confused and thought process will be altered. If the blood level is 300 mg/100 mL of blood the person may lose consciousness. A concentration of 500 mg/100 mL is fatal.

Complications

- Gastritis, peptic ulcer, reflux esophagitis, carcinoma of stomach and esophagus.
- Fatty liver, cirrhosis of liver, hepatitis, liver cell carcinoma.
- Acute and chronic pancreatitis
- Alcoholic cardiomyopathy
- High risk for myocardial infarction
- Peripheral neuropathy
- Epilepsy
- Head injury
- Cerebral degeneration
- Protein malnutrition
- Vitamin deficiency disorder
- Peripheral muscle weakness
- Sexual dysfunction in males, failure of ovulation in females
- Damage to the fetus.

Clinical Manifestation

Psychiatric disorders due to alcohol dependence:
1. Acute intoxication
2. Withdrawal syndrome
3. Alcohol-induced amnestic disorders
4. Alcohol-induced psychiatric disorders

Acute Intoxication

Acute intoxication develops during or shortly after alcohol ingestion. It is characterized by clinically significant maladaptive behavior or psychological changes, e.g. inappropriate sexual or aggressive behavior, mood lability, impaired judgment, slurred speech, incoordination, unsteady gait, impaired attention and memory finally resulting in stupor or coma.

Withdrawal Syndrome

- **Simple withdrawal syndrome:** The common withdrawal syndrome is hangover on the next morning. Mild tremors, nausea, vomiting, weakness, irritability, insomnia and anxiety are also common withdrawal symptoms.
- **Delirium tremens:** It occurs usually within 2–4 days of complete or significant abstinence from heavy alcohol drinking. It is characterized by:
  - Clouding of consciousness with disorientation in time and place.
  - Poor attention span and distractibility.
  - Visual hallucinations and illusions.
  - Marked autonomic disturbance with tachycardia, fever, sweating, hypertension and papillary dilation, insomnia, with a reversal of sleep-wake pattern.
  - Dehydration with electrolyte imbalance.

Alcohol-induced Amnestic Disorders

Chronic alcohol abuse associated with thiamine (vitamin B) deficiency is the most frequent cause of amnestic disorders. This condition is divided into:

- **Wernicke's syndrome:** This is characterized by prominent cerebellar ataxia, palsy of the 6th cranial nerve, peripheral neuropathy and mental confusion.
- **Korsakoff's syndrome:** The prominent symptom in Korsakoff's syndrome is gross memory disturbance. Other symptoms include disorientation, confusion, confabulation, poor attention span and distractibility, impairement of insight.

Alcohol-induced Psychiatric Disorders

- Alcohol-induced dementia
- Alcohol-induced mood disorders
- Suicidal behavior
- Alcohol-induced anxiety disorder
- Alcoholic seizures (rum fits)
- Alcoholic hallucinosis

Agencies concerned with Alcohol-related Problems

- Alcoholic anonymous (AA): This is a self-help organization founded in the USA by two alcoholic men, Dr Bob Smith and Bill Wilson on 1935.
- Al-Anon family groups: It is a group started by Mrs Anne, wife of Dr Bob to support the spouses of alcoholics.
- Alateen: Provide support to their teenage children.
- Hostels: These are intended mainly for those rendered homeless due to alcohol-related problems. They provide rehabilitation and counseling.

Management

- Administer antianxiety medications (diazepam)
- The priority management of a patient with alcohol withdrawal is administer diazepam.
- Administer vitamin B
- Alcohol deterrent therapy (administer disulfiram or monosulfiram to produce an unpleasant taste).
- Provide psychotherapy

SUBSTANCE ABUSE DISORDER

The word drug addiction and drug addict were dropped from scientific use due to their derogatory connotation. Instead 'drug abuse', 'drug dependence', and 'psychoactive substance use disorders' are the terms used in the current nomenclature. A psychoactive drug is one that is capable of altering the mental functioning.

There are four important patterns of drug use disorders, which may overlap with each other.
- Acute intoxication
- Withdrawal state
- Dependency state and
- Harmful use

Acute Intoxication

According to ICD-10, acute intoxication is a transient condition following the administration of alcohol or other psychoactive substance, resulting in disturbances in level of consciousness, cognition, perception, affect or behavior, or other psychophysiological functions and responses. This is usually associated with high blood level of the drug.

Withdrawal State

This is characterized by a cluster of symptoms, often specific to the drug used, which develop on total or partial withdrawal of a drug, usually after repeated and/or high dose use. This, too, is a short lasting syndrome with usual duration of few hours to few days. Typically, the patients reports that withdrawal symptoms are relieved by further substance use.

The withdrawal state is further classified as:
- Uncomplicated
- With convulsions
- With delirium

Dependence Syndrome

According to the ICD-10, the dependence syndrome is a cluster of physiological behavioral and cognitive phenomena in which the use of a substance or a class of substances takes on a much higher priority for a given individual than other behaviors that once had greater value.

Harmful use

Harmful use is characterized by:
- Continued drug use despite awareness of harmful medical and/or social effect of the drug being used.
- A pattern of physically hazardous use of drug (e.g. driving during intoxication).
- The diagnosis requires that actual damage should have been caused to the mental or physical health of the user.

Psychoactive Substances

The major dependence producing drugs are:
1. Alcohol
2. Opioids
3. Cannabinoids, e.g. Cannabis
4. Cocaine
5. Amphetamine and other sympathomimetics
6. Hallucinogens, e.g. LSD, phencyclidine
7. Sedatives and hypnotics, e.g. barbiturates
8. Inhalants
9. Nicotine
10. Other stimulants (e.g. caffeine)

Opioid Use Disorders

Dried exudates obtained from unripe seed capsules of papaver somniferum has been used and abused for centuries. The most important dependence producing derivatives are morphine and heroine. They both like majority of dependency producing opioids.

This is characterized by apathy, bradycardia, hypotension, respiratory depression subnormal core body temperature and pinpoint pupils. In severe intoxication, mydriasis may occur due to hypoxia.

Management

- Administer opioid antagonist (Naloxone)
- Administer methadone for detoxification

Cannabis Use Disorders

Cannabis is derived from the hemp plant, cannabis sativa, which has several varieties named after the region in which it is found. Cannabis produces a very mild physical dependence, with a relatively mild withdrawal syndrome characterized by fine tremors, irritability, restlessness, nervousness, insomnia, decreased appetite and craving. The syndrome begins within few hours of stopping cannabis use and lasts for 4–5 days.

Mild cannabis intoxication is characterized by mild impairment of consciousness and orientation, light-headedness, tachycardia, a sense of floating in the air, a euphoric dream-like state, alternation in psychomotor activities and tremors in addition to photophobia, lacrimation, tachycardia, reddening of conjunctiva, dry mouth and increased appetite.

Cocaine Use Disorders

Cocaine is an alkaloid derived from the coca bush, Erythroxylum coca, found in Bolivia and Peru. Cocaine is a central stimulant which inhibits the reuptake of dopamine along with that of nor epinephrine and serotonin.

Acute cocaine intoxication is characterized by pupillary dilatation, tachycardia, hypertension, sweating, and nausea or vomiting. Later judgment is impaired and there is impairment of social and occupational functioning.

Management

- Monitor for anxiety level and seizure episodes
- Administer oxygen
- Administer IV diazepam or thiopentone
- Administer bromocriptine (dopaminergic agonist) and amantadine.

Amphetamine Use Disorders

Amphetamine refers to a unique chemical which is precisely phenylisopropylamine. It is a powerful CNS stimulant, with peripheral sympathomimetic effects. The signs and symptoms of acute amphetamine intoxication are primarily cardiovascular (tachycardia, hypertension, hemorrhage, cardiac failure and cardiovascular shock) and central (seizures, hyperpyrexia, tremors, ataxia, euphoria, pupillary dilatation and coma). The neuropsychiatric manifestations include anxiety, panic, insomnia, restlessness, irritability and hostility.

LSD Use Disorders

Lysergic acid diethylamide, first synthesized by Albert Hoffman in 1938 and popularly known as 'acid', is a powerful hallucinogen. LSD presumably produces its effects by an action on the 5-HT levels in brain.

Although tolerance and psychological dependence occur with LSD use, no physical dependence or withdrawal syndrome is reported.

The characteristic features of acute LSD intoxication are perceptual changes occurring in clear consciousness and autonomic hyperactivity. These changes are usually associated with marked anxiety or depression, thought euphoria is more common in small doses. Sometimes, acute LSD intoxication presents with an acute panic reaction, known as a bad trip, in which an individual experiences a loss of control over his self. The recovery usually occurs within 8–12 hours of the last dose.

Barbiturate Use Disorders

Barbiturate use disorders are now subsumed under the sedative, hypnotic and anxiolytic use disorders. The commonly abused barbiturates are secobarbital, pentobarbital and amobarbital. Barbiturates produce marked physical and psychological dependence. Tolerance (both central and metabolic) develops rapidly and is usually marked. There is also a cross tolerance with alcohol.

Acute intoxication, typically occurring as an episodic phenomenon, is characterized by irritability, increased productivity of speech, incoordination, attention and memory impairment, and ataxia. Intravenous use can lead to skin abscesses, cellulites, embolism and hypersensitivity reaction.

Nursing Management for Substance Use Disorders

- Recognition of alcohol abuse: The CAGE questionnaire may be adopted for this purpose.
    - C: Have you ever felt you ought to CUT down on your drinking?
    - A: Have people ANNOYED you by criticizing your drinking.
    - G: Have you ever felt GUILTY about your drinking.
    - E: Have you ever had a drink first thing in the morning (an EYE-OPENER) to steady your nerves or get rid of a hangover?
- Be suspicious about 'at-risk' factors: problems in the marriage and family, at work, with finances or with the law; at risk occupations; withdrawal symptoms after admission; alcohol-related physical disorders; repeated accidents.
- If at risk factors raise suspicion, the next step is to ask tactful but persistent questions to confirm the diagnosis.
- Monitor the behavioral changes, such as absence from school or work, negligence of appearance, minor criminal offences and adoption of new friends in a drug culture.
- Prepare the patient for laboratory tests:
    - Raised gamma-glutamyl transpeptidase.
    - Raised mean corpuscular volume.
    - Blood alcohol concentration.
    - Most drugs can be detected in urine, the notable exception being LSD.

SLEEP DISORDERS

Sleep is generally characterized by a reduction in voluntary body movement, temporary blindness, and decreased reaction to external stimuli, loss of consciousness, a reduction in audio receptivity, an increased rate of anabolism and a decreased rate of catabolism.

Normal Sleep Requirements and Patterns

Sleep duration and quality vary among persons of all age groups:
- Infants: 16 hours/day
- Toddlers: 12 hours/day
- Preschoolers: 11 hours/day
- Schoolers: 9–10 hours/day
- Adolescents: 8–9 hours/day
- Adults: 6–8 hours/day

Normal Sleep Cycle

Normal sleep cycle requires, a restorative sleeping pattern has two distinct stages of sleep:
1. Nonrapid eye movement (NREM)
2. Rapid eye movement (REM)

During the NREM sleep cycle, an individual initially enters the first of 4 stages of sleep, repeating them in a cycle fashion throughout the sleep episode. The individual first enters to stage 1 NREM sleep upon closing his or her eyes and drifting into light sleep state. The EEG of an individual who is in stage 1 NREM shows many alpha waves. The person is able to be aroused in this stage of sleep cycle. If not awakened during this stage 1 NREM sleep, the person will enters to stage 2 NREM sleeps, where he or she will be less easily aroused. The predominant EEG recording during this stage reflects high K complexes and spindle like tracings at frequencies of 12–14 Hz. Soon thereafter the person will enters to stage 3 NREM sleep where theta and delta wave activity will appear on the EEG recordings. During this stage of NREM sleep the vital recordings usually reflects a decline from baseline values, and the individual is in a deeper sleep state when compared to the previous 2 NREM stages. Progressively, an individual will enters to stage 4 NREM sleep, where arousal is difficult. Vital recordings are usually at their lowest level from base line recordings, the muscles are very relaxed and the EEG brain wave activity reflects a predominance of delta wave, or slow wave activity.

After moving from wakefulness through stages 1 through 4 NREM sleep, the person goes back from stage 4 to stage 2 NREM sleep. Then the individual enters the active sleep stage known as REM sleep. The first REM period of sleep episode takes place approximately 90 min after the individual first falls asleep, with subsequent REM periods occurring four to five times, at 90 minutes interval, throughout the sleep episode. The duration of each REM period usually lasts from 5–30 minutes, depending on the individual. For example, if the individual is extremely tired, REM sleep is shorter or does not occur at all during the sleep episode. However, once the individual become less fatigued, the REM periods typically increases in frequency and duration throughout the sleep cycle.

Sleep pattern disturbance is a nursing diagnosis that is defined as a disruption of sleep time that causes discomfort or interferes with a desired life cycle.

Causes of Sleep Disorders

- Due to any medical conditions, such as cardiac, respiratory, endocrine, etc.
- Due to any psychiatric conditions, such as depression, PTSD, anxiety, etc.
- Due to any environmental problems, such as stressful job, shifts.

Clinical Manifestation

- Difficulty falling asleep
- Waking up frequently during the night
- Difficulty returning to sleep
- Waking up too early in the morning
- Unrefreshing sleep
- Daytime sleepiness
- Difficulty concentrating
- Irritability

Classification of Sleep Disorders

The sleep disorders are mainly classified in to two, they are:
- **Dyssomnias:** Characterized by abnormalities in amount, quality or timing of sleep.
- **Parasomnias:** Characterized by abnormal behavior or physiologic events occurring in association with sleep or sleep-wake transitions.

Dyssomnias

The disorders include:
- **Insomnia:** It is defined as persistent difficulty in initiating or maintaining sleep. The individual complains of difficulty in falling asleep, difficulty in maintaining sleep. The sleep disturbance occurs at least 3 times a week for at least 1 month.
  - Primary insomnia begins in early to middle adulthood and increases with age
  - More common in women than in men.
- **Hypersomnias:** Hypersomnia or somnolence can be defined as excessive sleepiness or seeking excessive amount of sleep. It refers to a condition where the affected individual obtains sufficient sleep at night but still cannot stay awake during the day.
  - It begins in late adolescence or early adulthood
  - It is more common in men than in women
- **Narcolepsy:** Narcolepsy is one of the disorders characterized by excessive daytime sleepiness. The client also experiences disturbed nocturnal sleep and repeated episodes of almost irresistible daytime drowsiness followed by brief periods of sleep, especially when engaged in monotonous activities.
  - Onset of narcolepsy occurs most frequently in the adolescence or early adulthood.
  - This disorder is equally common in men and women.
- **Breathing-related sleep disorder:** Breathing-related sleep disorder is characterized by sleep disruption leading to excessive sleepiness or insomnia caused by a sleep-related breathing disturbance. Two disorders of the respiratory system that can produce hypersomnia are sleep apnea and central alveolar hypoventilation.
- **Circadian rhythms sleep disorder** (sleep-wake schedule disorder): Circadian rhythm sleep disorders are a group of sleep pattern disturbances with a persistent or recurrent pattern of sleep disruption that results from difference in an imposed sleep-wake cycle and the individuals own circadian sleep-wake pattern requirements.

  Circadian rhythm sleep disorders result from:
  - Jet lag type
  - Shift work type
  - The delayed sleep phase
  - Unspecified type
    - **Jet lag type:** This type of sleep disorder has periods of sleepiness and alertness that occur at an inappropriate time of day, relative to local time. These patterns of sleep and wakefulness occur after repeated travel across more than one time zone.
    - **Shift work type:** It is usually the result of night shift work or frequently rotating shift work. It also takes place in individuals with irregular sleeping schedules. The individual with this type of sleep pattern disturbance typically experience insomnia during the major sleep period or excessive sleepiness during the major awake period. These symptoms are usually most pronounced right after the individual changes schedule, but, in some cases, the symptoms do not improve with the passage of time.
    - **The delayed sleep phase:** This occurs when the individual has persistent pattern of late sleep onset and late awakening times and is unable to fall asleep and wake up at the desired earlier times. Once sleep can be maintained, however, it may be uninterrupted until the normal awakening period.

Parasomnias

This includes:
- **Nightmare disorder:** Nightmare disorder is one type of parasomnia, that usually takes place during the REM period late in the sleep cycle. Individuals with this disorder frequently experience fragmented sleep as a result of waking up during the night with frightening dreams that threaten their survival, security, or self-esteem.
- **Sleep-terror disorders:** An individual with this disorder experiences arousal during non-REM sleep. This individual will typically awaken during the early part of the night. This awakening is usually caused by manifestations of extreme anxiety and panic. It is not unusual for the person to scream, or cry and appear disoriented during a sleep terror episode. As with sleep walking, the individual with sleep terror disorder is usually not able to recall the event.
- **Sleep-walking disorder:** This disorder is also called as somnambulism. Individuals with a sleep-walking disorder typically will repeatedly engage in such complex behaviors, such as walking, dressing, toileting, and driving while they are in a deep non-REM stage of sleep. While sleep-walking, the individual appears to be in a trance, and arousal is difficult.

Management

- Encourage activities that prepare one for sleep; soft music, relaxation exercises, warm bath, etc.
- Discourage strenuous activities within 1 hour of bedtime
- Provide a high carbohydrate snack before bedtime
- Instruct the client not to use alcoholic beverages to relax
- Discourage smoking and use of other tobacco products near sleep time
- Discourage daytime napping. Increase program of activities to keep the person busy
- Individuals with chronic insomnia should use sleeping medications judiciously.

SEXUAL DISORDERS

Sexuality is the constitution and life of an individual relative to characteristics regarding intimacy. It reflects the totality of the person and does not relate exclusively to the sex organ or sexual behavior. The common sexual disorders are:
- **Paraphilias:** Culturally inappropriate or dangerous patterns of sexual arousal.
- **Sexual dysfunctions:** Involves either a disturbance of sexual arousal or of performance.
- **Gender identity disorders:** Dissatisfaction with one's biological gender and a desire to become a member of the opposite gender.

Paraphilias

The term paraphilia is used to identify repetitive or preferred sexual fantasies or behaviors. Paraphilias are sometimes referred to as sexual deviations or perversions. Paraphilias include fantasies, behaviors, or sexual urges focusing on unusual objects, activities, or situations. The common types are:
- **Exhibitionism:** Exhibitionism is a tendency to sexually expose oneself to others. For example, a man's behavior is exhibitionistic when he exposes a part of his naked body, usually his genitals.
- **Fetishism:** People with a fetish experience sexual urges and behavior which are associated with non-living objects. For example, the object of the fetish could be an article of female clothing, like female underwear. Usually, the fetish begins in adolescence and tends to be quite chronic into adult life.
- **Frotteurism:** Men have a paraphilia called frotteurism when the focus of their sexual urges are related to the touching or rubbing of their body against a non-consenting, unfamiliar woman. Usually, the male rubs his genital area against the female.
- **Pedophilia:** A pedophile is a person, most frequently a man, who focuses his sexual fantasies and behavior toward children. People who enjoy child pornography or "kiddie porn" are pedophiles.
- **Masochism:** Masochism is the getting of pleasure, often sexual, from being hurt or humiliated. Sometimes the masochistic acts are limited to verbal humiliation or blindfolding. However, masochistic behavior might include being bound or beaten.
- **Sadism:** Sadism is deriving pleasure, often sexual, from mistreating others. Like other paraphilias, some people have fantasies which are sadistic, but they never act upon them. Also, some people have sexual urges of a sadistic nature, and they find a willing partner who agrees to participate in the sadistic activity.
- **Transvestism:** Cross-dressing by heterosexual males is called transvestic fetishism or transvestism. The male with this fetish usually has a variety of female clothes that he uses to cross-dress. While some males will wear only one special piece of female apparel, others fully dress as a female and use full facial make-up to achieve a total female appearance.
- **Voyeurism:** Voyeurism is seeking sexual pleasure by secretly observing another. Another name for the behavior is "peeping" or "peeping Tom". The activity brings on sexual excitement and may conclude with

masturbation by the voyeur. Voyeurism usually starts in adolescence and tends to persist into adulthood.

CHILDHOOD DISORDERS

Child psychiatry is a specialized branch of psychiatry which deals with the diagnosis, treatment and prevention of disorders which are affecting the children. The common childhood disorders are:
- Mental retardation
- Autism
- ADHD
- TIC disorder
- Tourette disorders
- Conduct disorders

MENTAL RETARDATION

Mental retardation is a developmental disorder characterized by the IQ (intelligence quotient) is less than 70. Normal IQ of an individual is 80-120.

IQ = Mental Age/Chronological Age × 100.

Causes

- Chromosomal abnormalities or fetal exposure to drugs or toxins
- Maternal rubella infection
- Environmental deprivation
- Problems of pregnancy and the perinatal period
- Hereditary abnormalities, such as inborn errors of metabolism or chromosomal aberrations.
- Medical conditions of infancy or childhood.

Types

Mild MR	Moderate MR	Severe MR	Profound MR
80–85% of cases	10% of cases	4–5% of cases	1% of cases
IQ: 50–70	IQ: 35–50	IQ: 20–35	IQ: < 20
Educable	Trainable	Nontrainable	Nontrainable

Management

- Provide psychotherapy
- Teach rehabilitation techniques
- Provide genetic counseling

AUTISM

Autistic disorder/autism spectrum disorder (ASD) is a range of complex neurodevelopment disorders, characterized by social impairments, communication difficulties, and restricted, repetitive, and stereotyped patterns of behavior.

Clinical Manifestation

- Marked impairment in the use of nonverbal behaviors
- Failure to develop peer relationships appropriate to developmental level
- A lack of spontaneous seeking to share enjoyment, interests, or achievements
- Lack of social or emotional reciprocity
- Marked impairment in the ability to initiate or sustain a conversation with others in individuals that can speak
- Stereotyped mannerisms
- Persistent preoccupation with parts of objects.

ATTENTION DEFICIT HYPERACTIVITY DISORDER (ADHD)

Attention deficit hyperactivity disorder is one of the most common childhood disorders and can continue through adolescence and adulthood. The classical manifestations of ADHD are hyperactivity, inattention and impulsivity.

Incidence

- Occurs in 4–12% of children who are 6 to 12 years of age
- Symptoms are usually present around age 3 or 4
- 68% of children with ADHD have problems as adults.

Clinical Manifestation

- Hyperactivity (talk nonstop)
- Running away from the home
- Violating the rules and regulations
- Not seem to listen when spoken to
- Daydream, become easily confused, and move slowly
- Have difficulty processing information as quickly and accurately as others
- Struggle to follow instructions
- Detachment from social relationship

CONDUCT DISORDER

Conduct disorder is defined as marked by repetitive, persistent, aggressive conduct in which basic rights are violated. It is commonly seen in older children and adolescents. The disorder is more common among boys than girls. Conduct disorder occurs with greater frequency in the children of parents with antisocial personality disorder and alcohol dependence than in the general population.

Clinical Manifestation

- Often bullies, threatens, or intimidates others
- Often initiates physical fights
- Has used a weapon that can cause serious physical harm to others (e.g. a bat, brick, broken bottle, knife, gun)
- Has been physically cruel to people
- Has been physically cruel to animals
- Has stolen while confronting a victim (e.g. mugging, purse snatching, extortion, armed robbery)
- Has forced someone into sexual activity
- Destruction of property
- Deceitfulness or theft
- Serious violations of rules

Management

- Individual therapy
- Family therapy
- Group therapy
- Behavior therapy

TIC DISORDER

It is a sudden, abnormal, involuntary, rapid, repetitive and purposeless contraction of a small group of muscles involving face, throat and shoulder.

Clinical Manifestation

- Grunts
- Barks
- Sniffs
- Echolalia
- Coprolalia (the spontaneous utterance of socially objectionable or taboo words or phrases)
- Learning difficulties
- Neurological signs—hyperactivity

Management

- Administer medications, such as haloperidol or baclofen groups
- Provide support and empathetic environment.
- Improve social relationship, enhance situational support.
- Client education and counseling.
- Promote self-esteem, self-confidence of the client by implementing positive behavior modification techniques and comprehensive nursing process.

TOURETTE SYNDROME

Tourette is defined as part of a spectrum of tic disorders, which includes transient and chronic tics. Tourette's disorder is an inherited neuropsychiatric disorder with onset in childhood, characterized by multiple physical (motor) tics and at least one vocal (phonic) tic.

Chapter 17

Maternity Nursing

Chapter Objectives

- Keynotes in maternity nursing
- Anatomy of female reproductive system
- Antepartum disorders
- Intrapartum period
- Postpartum changes

KEY TERMS

Placenta   APH
GDM   Lochia
PPH   Cystitis

KEYNOTES

- The pH of vaginal fluid is 4.5–5.5, i.e. it is acidic in nature.
- The pH of seminal fluid is 7–7.5, i.e. it is alkaline in nature.
- Bacterial vaginosis is a condition characterized by abnormal vaginal discharge.
- The classical manifestation of placenta previa is painless vaginal bleeding.
- The classical manifestation of abruptio placentae is painful vaginal bleeding.
- The priority nursing care of a pregnant woman admitted in the hospital with increased BP is monitor for urine protein in order to rule out pre-eclapmsia.
- The priority nursing care of a pregnant woman admitted in the labor room is monitor the FHS.
- If there is any variability in the FHS change the position of the mother because variability is due to cord compression.
- Lochia rubra is seen in first three days after delivery.
- Progestin only pills are safe during lactation (for contraception).
- Demerol or meperidine is contraindicated in pregnancy.
- An antenatal mother admitted in the antenatal clinic with complaints of frequent muscle cramps, the priority nursing care is instruct the mother to take one glass of milk everyday (muscle cramps are due to hypocalcemia. Milk is a good source of calcium).
- The best time to perform breast self examination is 7–10 days after menstruation.
- The drug of choice for breast cancer is tamoxifen citrate.
- The main cause of thrombophlebitis in pregnant women is increased intra-abdominal pressure.
- The hormone that causes vomiting in pregnancy is human chorionic gonadotropin (HCG).
- Classical symptoms of pre-eclampsia are edema, weight gain and proteinuria.
- Complications of pre-eclampsia are hemolysis, elevated liver enzyme, lowered platelet (HELLP).
- The life of ovum is 12–24 hours.
- The life of sperm is up to 7 days in female body.
- Administer indomethacin in polyhydramnios to prevent preterm delivery.

FEMALE REPRODUCTIVE SYSTEM

Anatomy

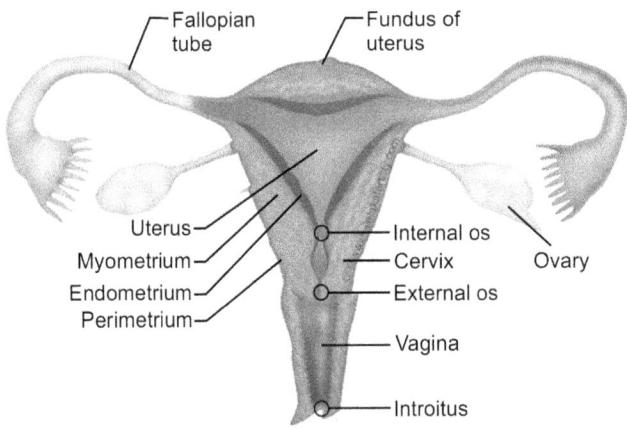

The female reproductive system is designed to carry out several functions. It produces the female egg cells necessary for reproduction, called the ova or oocytes. The system is designed to transport the ova to the site of fertilization. Conception, the fertilization of an egg by a sperm, normally occurs in the fallopian tubes. The next step for the fertilized egg is to implant into the walls of the uterus, beginning the initial stages of pregnancy. If fertilization and/or implantation does not take place, the system is designed to menstruate (the monthly shedding of the uterine lining).

FEMALE REPRODUCTIVE STRUCTURES

External Structures

- **Labia majora:** The labia majora enclose and protect the other external reproductive organs. Literally translated as "large lips," the labia majora are relatively large and fleshy, and are comparable to the scrotum in males. The labia majora contain sweat and oil-secreting glands. After puberty, the labia majora are covered with hair.
- **Labia minora:** Literally translated as "small lips," the labia minora can be very small or up to 2 inches wide. They lie just inside the labia majora, and surround the openings to the vagina and urethra.
- **Bartholin's glands:** These glands are located beside the vaginal opening and produce a fluid (mucus) secretion.
- **Clitoris:** The two labia minora meet at the clitoris, a small, sensitive protrusion that is comparable to the penis in males. The clitoris is covered by a fold of skin, called the prepuce, which is similar to the foreskin at the end of the penis. Like the penis, the clitoris is very sensitive to stimulation and can become erect.

Internal Structures

- **Vagina:** The vagina is a canal that joins the cervix (the lower part of uterus) to the outside of the body. It also is known as the birth canal.
- **Uterus (womb):** The uterus is a hollow, pear-shaped organ that is the home to a developing fetus. The uterus is divided into two parts: the cervix, which is the lower part that opens into the vagina, and the main body of the uterus, called the corpus. The corpus can easily expand to hold a developing baby. A channel through the cervix allows sperm to enter and menstrual blood to exit.
- **Ovaries:** The ovaries are small, oval-shaped glands that are located on either side of the uterus. The ovaries produce eggs and hormones.
- **Fallopian tubes:** These are narrow tubes that are attached to the upper part of the uterus and serve as tunnels for the ova (egg cells) to travel from the ovaries to the uterus. Conception, the fertilization of an egg by a sperm, normally occurs in the fallopian tubes. The fertilized egg then moves to the uterus, where it implants into the lining of the uterine wall.

At birth, there are approximately 1 million to 2 million eggs; by the time of puberty, only about 300,000 remain. Of these, only about 500 will be ovulated during a woman's reproductive lifetime. Any remaining eggs gradually die out at menopause.

PELVIS

A large bony frame near the base of the spine to which the hind limbs or legs are attached in humans and many other vertebrates in which the child passes during birth.

Pelvis is subdivided into:
- **True pelvis** or the lesser pelvis, below the pelvic brim, consist of the pelvic inlet, pelvic cavity and pelvic outlet.
- **False pelvis** or the greater pelvis, above the pelvic brim. A shallow upper basin of the pelvis supports the enlarging uterus.
- **Android pelvis:** Narrow heart-shaped male pelvis
- **Anthropoid pelvis:** Narrow oval-shaped with greater anteroposterior diameter.
- **Gynecoid pelvis:** Classic female pelvis with wide and well rounded in all directions.
- **Platypelloid pelvis:** Wide but flat and may still allow vaginal delivery.

BREAST

A pair of mammary glands which are located on the anterior chest wall between the second and sixth rib. It is responsible for the ejection of milk after delivery. Both in males and females breast originate from the same embryonic tissue. Estrogen and progesterone in female enhance the development of breast in female and testosterone suppresses the growth in male, so it is enlarged in females.

MENSTRUAL CYCLE

Stage I: Menstruation

First days of the cycle when endometrium is shed, when the fertilization does not occur endometrial shedding occurs.

Stage II: Proliferative Phase or Follicular Phase

Major hormone involved is estrogen which influences build up of endometrium.

Stage III: Ovulation Phase

Release of the ovum usually in the 14 days (plus or minus 2).

Stage IV : Secretory Phase or Luteal Phase

Major hormone is progesterone which influences myometrium.

HUMAN SEXUAL RESPONSE CYCLE

1. **Desire stage**: Lasts for minutes to hours sexual fantasies and the desire for sexual intimacy.
2. **Excitement stage:** Foreplay, in male's penile erection and in female's vaginal lubrication, nipple erection and vasocongestion of the external genitalia. In late phase (seconds to minutes), male—drops of fluid at head of penis and in female—tightening of outer 1/3 of the vagina and, breast engorgement.
3. **Orgasmic stage:** 5-15 seconds
   In males—ejaculation and involuntary muscular contractions of pelvis obligatory refractory period.
   In females—contractions of the outer 1/3 of the vagina and involuntary pelvic thrusting multiple orgasms.
4. **Resolution stage:** Detumescence feelings of relaxation and well-being.

FERTILIZATION OR IMPLANTATION

The fusion of male gamete (sperm) and female gamete (ovum) results in a fertilized ovum. It is also called as zygote. Each gamete consists of 23 chromosomes (X and Y), so a total of 46 chromosomes. XX denotes the female and XY denotes the male. It occurs in the outer third of the fallopian tube (ampulla). From the ampulla, it enters to the uterus and attach to the top of uterus know as nidation or implantation. After 7-10 days of fertilization, the zygote develops into a trophoblastic stage. The chorionic villi appear on the trophoblast secrete human chorionic gonadotropin (HCG) which acts as the basis of pregnancy test. This inhibits further ovulation.

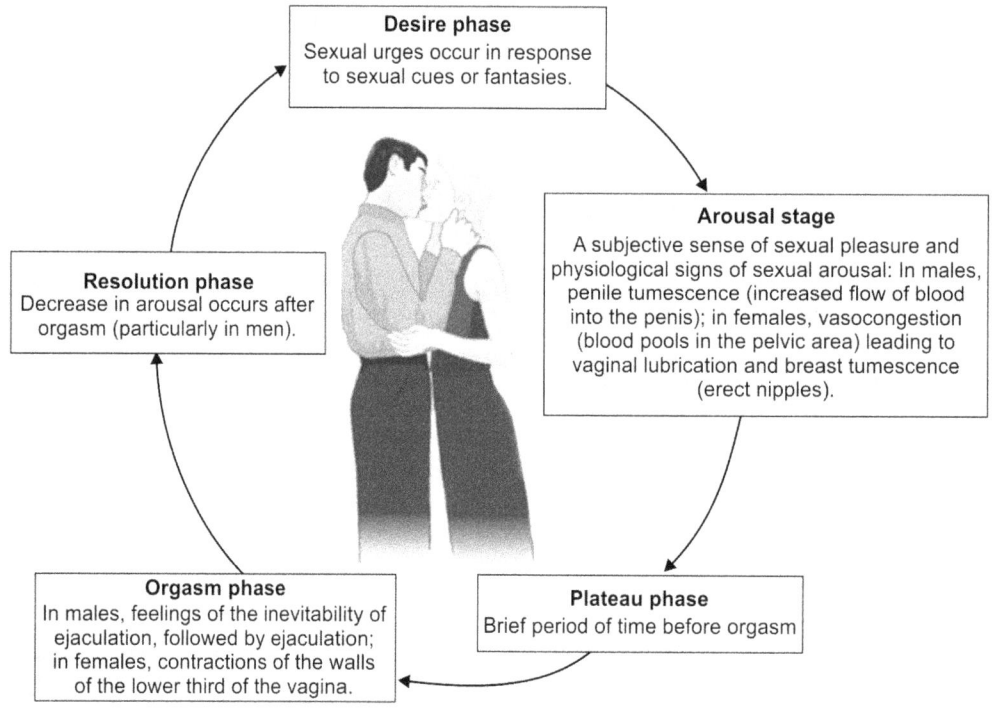

Amniotic Fluid

- Amniotic fluid or liquor amnii is a clear yellowish fluid surrounding the developing fetus. It protects the growing fetus.
- Normal amount of amniotic fluid is 800-1000 mL
- pH of amniotic fluid is 7.0-7.5
- Green or brown amniotic fluid indicates meconium stained
- Dark color indicated intrauterine fetal death
- Red color indicates bleeding
- Alkaline pH indicates the rupture of membrane
- Amniotic fluid index (AFI) is the estimate of amniotic fluid
- Normal AFI is 5-15 cm
- In oligohydramnios, the amniotic fluid is less than 400 mL (AFI less than 5 cm)
- In polyhydramnios, the amniotic fluid is greater than 1900 mL (AFI greater than 24 cm)

Umbilical Cord

- Connecting link between mother and fetus
- Carry oxygen and nutrients to the fetus
- Length of umbilical cord is 50 cm (20 inches)
- Contains two arteries and one vein
- Wharton's jelly is substance seen on the umbilical cord which prevents kinking and knotting
- There is no pain receptors in the umbilical cord
- Clamp the umbilical cord about 3-4 cm (1½-2 inches) from your baby's belly button with a plastic clip

Placenta

- The placenta is an organ that develops in your uterus during pregnancy. This structure provides oxygen and nutrients to your growing baby and removes waste products.
- It has fetal and maternal part
- Length of placenta 22 cm
- Weight of placenta 500 gm
- It is dark red or crimson color
- Produce hormones to maintain pregnancy (estrogen, progesterone and HPL)

Fetal Heart Rate

A normal fetal heart rate (FHR) usually ranges from 120 to 160 beats per minute (bpm) in the in utero period. It is measurable sonographically from around 6 weeks and the normal range varies during gestation, increasing to around 170 bpm at 10 weeks and decreasing from then to around 130 bpm at term.

- FHR less than 120 bpm is fetal bradycardia
- FHR greater than 180 bpm is fetal tachycardia
- Notify the physician in case of fetal bradycardia or tachycardia and administer oxygen.

Fetal Circulation

The umbilical arteries carry impure blood and umbilical vein carries pure (oxygenated blood). The placenta accepts the bluest blood (blood without oxygen) from the fetus through blood vessels that leave the fetus through the umbilical cord (umbilical arteries, there are two of them). When blood goes through the placenta it picks up oxygen and becomes red. The red blood then returns to the fetus via the third vessel in the umbilical cord (umbilical vein). The red blood that enters the fetus passes through the fetal liver and enters the right side of the heart.

Gestation

- Time from the fertilization of the ovum until the estimated date of confinement or estimated date of delivery.
- About 280 days or 9 calendar months or 3 trimester or 40 plus or minus 2 weeks
- To calculate estimated date of delivery (EDC) by Naegele's rule
- First day of the last menstrual period (LMP) + add seven days + 9 months
- EDC = LMP + 7 days + 9 months
- For example, LMP of pregnant women is September 12, 2011
- EDC = June 19, 2012

Gravidity or Parity

- Gravida refers to pregnant women
- Gravidity refers to number of pregnancies
- Nullipara—never pregnant
- Primi—first time pregnant
- Multi—more than one time
- To calculate the gestational age use GTPAL
  - Where G is the gravidity
  - T is term birth (greater than 37 weeks)
  - P is preterm birth (before 37 weeks)
  - A is abortion or miscarriage
  - L is current living children

FETAL DEVELOPMENT

Week 1	Blastocyst is free floating
Weeks 2–4	Blood circulation begins, lung buds appear. Heart begins to beat
Week 5	Double heart chambers are visible. Limb buds form
Week 8	Eyelids begin to fuse, circulatory system through the cord is well established, every organ systems present
Week 12	Face is well-formed, limbs are long, kidney begins to form urine, sex is usually recognizable, heart beat detected by Doppler between 10 and 12 weeks
Week 16	Active movements present, lanugo hairs begin to develop, skeletal ossification occurs
Week 20	Heart beat detected by regular fetoscope, quickening developed, lanugo covers entire body, length 16–18.5 cm and weight 300 gm
Week 24	Hair on head developed, vernix caseosa covers the entire body, length 23 and weight 600 gm
Week 28	Limbs are well flexed, brain developing rapidly, provide gas exchange, length 27 cm and weight 1100 gm
Week 32	Fully developed bone, subcutaneous fat developed, skin smooth and pink, Lecithin-sphingomyelin ratio (L/S) developed
Week 36	Length 35 cm and weight 2200–2900 gm, lanugo disappear and body is rounded
Week 40	Length 40 cm and weight 3200 gm, baby is active, skin is pinkish. In males, testis will descend to scrotum and in females labia majora developed

PHYSIOLOGICAL CHANGES IN PREGNANCY

Common Signs of Pregnancy

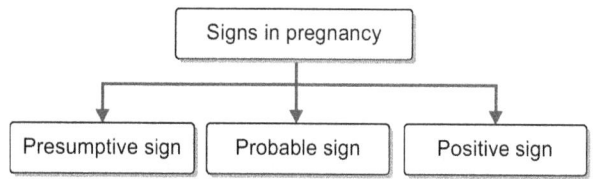

Presumptive Signs

- Amenorrhea (absence of menstruation)
- Nausea and vomiting
- Enlarged nipple
- Discoloration of vaginal mucosa
- Fatigue
- Increased size and feeling of fullness in the breast
- Increased urinary frequency
- Quickening (first perception of fetal movement by the mother in 16-20 weeks of gestation)

Probable Signs

- Uterine enlargement
- Hegar's sign (softening of the lower uterine segment occurs about 6 weeks)
- Goodell's sign (softening of the cervix that occurs at the beginning of 2nd month)
- Chadwick's sign (violet discoloration of the mucous membrane of the cervix, vagina, vulva that occurs at about 4 weeks)
- Ballottement (rebounding of the fetus head against the examiner's fingers on palpation)
- Braxton hicks contraction (irregular painless contractions that may occur intermittently throughout the pregnancy)
- Positive pregnancy test for determination of HCG

Positive Signs

- FHR detected by electronic devices (doppler) at 10-12 weeks and by nonelectronic device (fetoscope) at 20 weeks of gestation.
- Active fetal movement palpated by the examiner
- Outline of fetus by radiography or ultrasonography

Physiological Changes

System	Changes
Cardiovascular system	Heart rate increases by 15–20 bpm Cardiac output increases by 30–50% Increase blood volume Increase cardiac palpitation
Respiratory system	Increased tidal volume Increased oxygen consumption Elevated diaphragm, epistaxis
Gastrointestinal system	Nausea and vomiting (due to HCG) Hemorrhoids and constipation, anorexia Pregnancy gingivitis and gum bleeding (estrogen) Excessive secretion of saliva
Renal system	Increased GFR and urinary frequency Decreased bladder tone and renal threshold for sugar Decreased BUN, creatine and uric acid
Endocrine system	Increased enlargement and activity of thyroid gland Increased basal metabolic rate Pituitary gland enlarges
Musculoskeletal system	Increased lumbosacral curve (lordosis) Altered center of gravity Duck waddling gait

Contd...

Contd...

System	Changes
Integumentary system	Increased skin pigmentation Facial mark, acne vulgaris, dermatitis Vascular spider nevi Linea nigra (streaks on abdomen) and striae
Uterus	Increased size and weight Braxton hicks contraction and cervical softening Increased fibrous connective tissue
Breast	Increased breast size and heaviness Tingling and fullness Darkening of nipple and thin watery secretion
Vagina	Hypertrophy and hyperplasia of the lining Increased thick white secretion
Nutrition	Normal weight gain is 20–30 lbs Increased need for water Increased caloric intake by 300 cal per day Increased folic acid and iron requirement

Measurement of Fundal Height

- It is measured to evaluate the gestational age
- At 12th week, measure at the level of symphysis pubis
- At 16th week, half way between umbilicus and pubis
- At 20th week, at the level of umbilicus
- At 36 week, at the level of xyphoid process
- In the second and third trimesters, fundal height is equal to the gestational age plus or minus 2
- Assess for any supine hypotension syndrome while monitoring fundal height because the gravid uterus may compress inferior vena cava and results in decreased cardiac output, so provide left lateral position with a pillow.

DIAGNOSTIC MEASURES

Ultrasound

An ultrasound scan is a diagnostic technique which uses high-frequency sound waves to create an image of the internal organs. A screening ultrasound is sometimes done during the course of a pregnancy to check normal fetal growth and verify the due date. Ultrasounds may be performed at various times throughout pregnancy for different reasons:
- To establish the dates of a pregnancy
- To diagnose an ectopic pregnancy or miscarriage
- In some cases to detect fetal abnormalities
- To examine the fetal anatomy for presence of abnormalities
- To check the amount of amniotic fluid
- To examine blood flow patterns
- To determine the position of a fetus
- To assess the placenta

Genetic Screening

Many genetic abnormalities can be diagnosed before birth. Examples of genetic disorders that can be diagnosed before birth include the following:
- Cystic fibrosis
- Duchenne muscular dystrophy
- Hemophilia A
- Thalassemia
- Sickle cell anemia
- Polycystic kidney disease
- Tay-Sachs disease

Glucose Tolerance Test

A glucose tolerance test, usually conducted in the 24 to 28 weeks of pregnancy, measures levels of sugar (glucose) in the mother's blood. Abnormal glucose levels may indicate gestational diabetes.
- An initial fasting sample of blood is drawn from a vein.
- You will be given a special glucose solution to drink.
- Blood will be drawn several times over the course of several hours to measure the glucose levels in your body.

Chorionic Villus Sampling

Chorionic villus sampling (CVS) is a prenatal test that involves taking a sample of some of the placental tissue. This tissue contains the same genetic material as the fetus and can be tested for chromosomal abnormalities and some other genetic problems. Testing is available for other genetic defects and disorders depending on the family history and availability of laboratory testing at the time of the procedure.

Amniocentesis

An amniocentesis is a procedure used to obtain a small sample of the amniotic fluid that surrounds the fetus to diagnose chromosomal disorders and open neural tube defects (ONTDs), such as spina bifida. Testing is available for other genetic defects and disorders depending on the family history and availability of laboratory testing at the time of the procedure. An amniocentesis is generally offered to women between the 15th and 20th weeks of pregnancy who are at increased risk for chromosome abnormalities, such as women who are over age 35 years of age at delivery, or those who have had an abnormal maternal serum screening test, indicating an increased risk for a chromosomal abnormality or neural tube defect.

Alpha-fetoprotein Screening (AFP)

This blood test measures the level of alpha-fetoprotein in the mothers' blood during pregnancy. AFP is a protein normally produced by the fetal liver and is present in the fluid surrounding the fetus (amniotic fluid), and crosses the placenta into the mother's blood. The AFP test is also known as MSAFP (maternal serum AFP). It is used to rule out:
- Open neural tube defects, such as spina bifida
- Down syndrome and other chromosomal abnormalities
- Defects in the abdominal wall of the fetus.

ANTEPARTUM DISORDERS

Hyperemesis Gravidarum

Excessive vomiting in the early pregnancy leads to dehydration and metabolic acidosis. It is due to the increase in HCG levels.

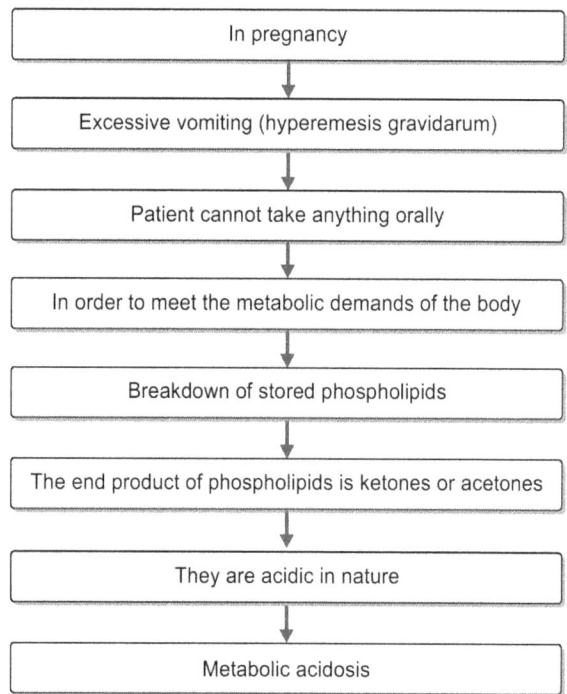

Nursing Care

- Monitor urine acetone to rule out metabolic acidosis
- Administer more fluids to prevent dehydration
- Monitor the electrolyte levels
- Monitor for weight loss
- Assist the patient for parenteral nutrition

ABORTION

Pregnancy that ends before 20 weeks of gestation, may be spontaneous or elective.

Types

- Spontaneous: Abortion that occurs due to natural cause
- Induced: Termination of pregnancy due to any therapeutic or elective reason
- Threatened abortion: Spotting and cramping occurs, cervix begins to dilate and efface
- Inevitable abortion: Loss of some products of conception
- Complete abortion: Loss of all products of conception
- Missed abortion: Products of conception retained in the uterus after fetal death
- Habitual abortion: Spontaneous abortion occurs in three or more successful pregnancies

Signs and Symptoms

- Spontaneous vaginal bleeding
- Uterine cramping and contraction
- Hemorrhage and shock-like symptoms

Nursing Care

- Monitor the vitals
- Provide proper bed rest
- Count the perineal pads to detect the amount of blood loss
- Maintain IV fluids
- Prepare the patient for D&C (Dilation and curettage)

ANEMIA

Iron deficiency anemia is a common type of anemia seen in pregnancy due to the inadequate amount of iron in the blood.

Signs and Symptoms

- Fatigue
- Tachycardia and palpitation
- Hb less than 10 gm/dL
- Hct less than 30 gm/dL
- Pallor and cyanosis

Nursing Care

- Monitor Hb and Hct level every two weeks
- Administer iron preparations: In case of oral iron preparations, administer along with Vitamin C to increase the absorption
- Avoid administering iron preparations along with tea, coffee, milk, egg, etc. Administer along with citrus juice, such as orange juice

- Administer folic acid supplements
- In severe anemia, administer parenteral iron preparation.

ECTOPIC PREGNANCY

Implantation of the fertilized ovum outside the uterine cavity.

Signs and Symptoms

- Missed menstrual period
- Abdominal pain
- Vaginal spotting or bleeding (dark red or brown color).

Nursing Care

- Monitor the vital signs
- Monitor for bleeding
- Administer methotrexate preparation to inhibit cell division
- Administer immunoglobulin.

GESTATIONAL DIABETES MELLITUS (GDM)

GDM is a newly detected diabetes mellitus at the time of gestation. It is common between 20 and 28 weeks of gestation. The management of GDM is insulin therapy. Educate the women that the GDM will subside soon after the delivery of placenta.

- From the mother to the fetus nutrients are transferred through the placenta
- During the transmission, a number of hormones are developed in the placenta
- Among that hormones, HPL (human placental lactogen) is a hormone having an anti-insulin effect
- So, there is increase in the blood glucose level

Signs and Symptoms

- Polyuria
- Polyphagia
- Polydipsia
- Increased blood glucose level

Nursing Care

- Prepare the patient for oral glucose tolerance test
- Administer insulin as prescribed

PREGNANCY-INDUCED HYPERTENSION (PIH)

Development of new arterial hypertension (BP greater than 140/90 mm Hg) in a pregnant women after 20 weeks of gestation without the presence of protein in the urine.

Causes

- Family history of pre-eclampsia
- Women greater than 40 years or less than 19 years
- History of renal disease
- Rh incompatibility

Pre-eclampsia

It is the gestational hypertension with BP greater than 140/90 mm Hg and proteinuria (urine protein 3+).

Signs and Symptoms

- Urine protein 3+
- Headache and vomiting
- Edema and weight gain
- Increased BP

Eclampsia

It is tonic-clonic seizures appear in a pregnant with high BP and proteinuria.

Signs and symptoms

- Increased BP
- Convulsions
- Coma

Nursing Care

- Administer antihypertensive as prescribed (drug of choice is methyldopa)
- Monitor for urine protein
- In case of eclampsia, provide a dark room and limit the number of visitors
- Use side rails for the patient to prevent falls associated with seizure episodes
- Monitor for HELLP syndrome
  - H: Hemolytic anemia
  - EL: Elevated liver enzymes
  - LP: Low platelet count

HYDATIDIFORM MOLE (GESTATIONAL TROPHOBLASTIC DISORDER)

It is manifested as edematous grape-like clusters that may be nonmalignant or may develop into choriocarcinoma.

Signs and Symptoms

- Elevated HCG
- Fetal heart rate not detectable
- Vaginal bleeding after 12 weeks (dark red to brownish)
- Elevated BP
- Snow storm pattern on USG

Nursing Care

- Prepare the patient for uterine evacuation
- Administer oxytocin for uterine contraction
- HCG should be monitored for every one to two weeks until normal pregnancy obtained and then check every 1-2 months for 1 year

ANTEPARTUM HEMORRHAGE (APH)

Placenta Previa

Placenta is improperly implanted in the lower uterine segment. It may be:
1. **Partial placenta previa:** The lower border of placenta is within 3 cm from the internal OS.
2. **Marginal placenta previa:** Placenta reaches the margin of internal OS but does not cover it.
3. **Complete or total placenta previa:** Internal OS covered entirely.

Signs and Symptoms

- Painless vaginal bleeding
- Soft and nontender uterus

Nursing Care

- Administer IV fluids
- Monitor for fetal heart rate
- Provide bed rest in side lying position in case of heavy bleeding

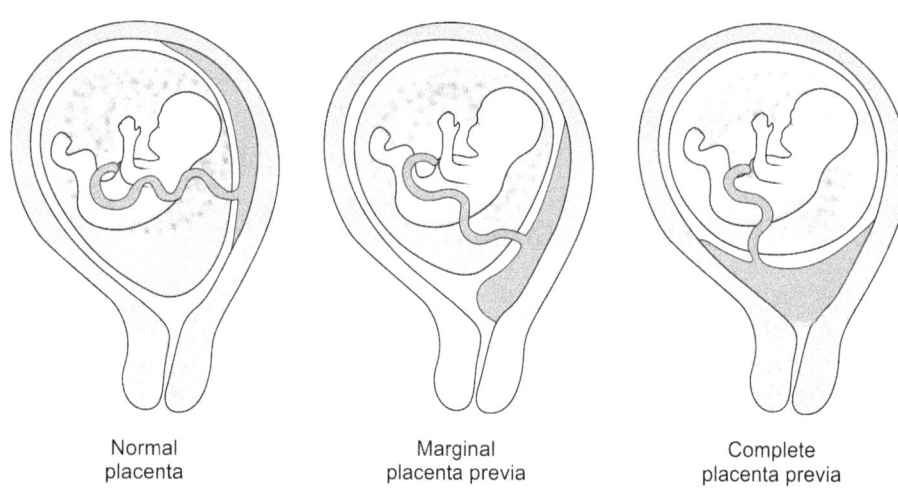

Normal placenta   Marginal placenta previa   Complete placenta previa

- Monitor for the amount of blood loss
- Avoid vaginal examination as it stimulates uterine activity

Abruptio Placentae

Premature separation of placenta after 20 weeks of gestation before delivery of fetus.

Signs and Symptoms

- Painful vaginal bleeding
- Severe abdominal pain rigid and tender uterus.

Nursing Care

- Assess for excessive bleeding
- Place the client in a trendelenburg position to decrease the pressure of the fetus on placenta
- Monitor for any coagulation problem
- Prepare for emergency surgery as indicated

SUPINE HYPOTENSIVE SYNDROME

It is the sudden fall in blood pressure due to diminished venous return caused by compression of the vena cava by the gravid uterus when the pregnant woman rests flat on her back. The low venous return also results in decreased placental perfusion and potentially in fetal hypoxia.

Clinical Manifestation

- Pallor
- Tachycardia (early sign)
- Bradycardia (very late sign)
- Sweating
- Nausea
- Hypotension and dizziness
- Edema of the lower extremities
- Signs of fetal hypoxia or distress
- Decreased femoral pulse

Management

- Place patient in left lateral recumbent position or elevate right hip and support the gravid uterus.
- If suspected trauma or spinal injury secure to backboard, tilt backboard to left.
- High flow oxygen via non-rebreather.

UTERINE FIBROIDS

Uterine fibroids are noncancerous growths of the uterus that often appear during childbearing years. It is also called leiomyomas or myomas; they aren't associated with an increased risk of uterine cancer. Uterine fibroids develop from the smooth muscular tissue of the uterus (myometrium) and it is associated with imbalance in estrogens and progesterone.

Clinical Manifestation

- Heavy menstrual bleeding
- Prolonged menstrual periods—seven days or more of menstrual bleeding
- Pelvic pressure or pain
- Frequent urination
- Difficulty emptying your bladder
- Constipation
- Backache or leg pains

Management

Administer gonadotropin-releasing hormone (GnRH) agonists, such as leuprolide (Lupron), will cause your estrogen and progesterone levels to drop.

BACTERIAL VAGINOSIS

Normal bacterial flora is replaced by anaerobic bacteria. It is common in 18–45 years.

Administer metronidazole for bacterial vaginosis, instruct the patient to avoid alcohol along with metronidazole as it cause disulfuiram-like reaction when ingested along with alcohol.

INTRAPARTUM PERIOD (LABOR)

It starts from the onset of labor to the end of stage 3 or up to immediate postpartum period. Labor is the culmination of pregnancy or it is the fruitful outcome of pregnancy.

4Ps of Labor

1. P: Power of the mother to expel the fetus
2. P: Passenger, the fetus
3. P: Passage way, the birth canal
4. P: Psychic energy or mental energy of the mother to expel the fetus.

Leopold maneuvers is a method of abdominal palpation to know the position of fetus inside the uterus. It is very difficult to perform in obese and women with polyhydramnios.

Tokophobia is the fear of childbirth.

Baby blues, a least severe form of postpartum depression in which the women experiences sadness and changes in emotion soon after the delivery. It is also known as postpartum blues.

Lie of Fetus

1. Longitudinal lie: Fetal spine parallel to maternal spine
2. Transverse lie: Fetal spine perpendicular to maternal spine

Labor

1. True labor: Contraction increases in duration and intensity. The cervical dilation occurs and effacement is progressive
2. False labor: Contractions are irregular and do not produce any dilation and effacement.

Position

1. LOA (left occiput anterior): Fetal occiput is on maternal left side and toward front. Face is down and it is a favorable position for delivery.
2. ROA (right occiput anterior): Fetal occiput is on maternal right side and toward the front. Face is down and it is favorable for delivery.
3. LOP (left occiput posterior): Fetal occiput is on maternal left side and towards back. Face is up and presents problem with delivery.
4. ROP (right occiput posterior): Fetal occiput is on maternal right side and towards back. Face is up and presents problem with delivery.

Mechanism of Labor

1. Engagement—fetal presenting part as its widest diameter reaches the level of the ischial spine of the pelvis.
2. Descent—movement of the biparietal diameter of the fetal head downward until it reaches the pelvic inlet.
3. Flexion—fetal head reaches the pelvic floor; head bends forward onto chest, presenting the smallest anteroposterior diameter.
4. Internal rotation—fetus enters pelvic inlet to the maternal pelvis, allows longest fetal head to match the longest maternal pelvic diameter.
5. Extension—internal rotation is complete, fetal head passes beneath the symphysis pubis while in flexion.
6. External rotation (restitution)—allow the shoulders to rotate internally to fit the pelvis.
7. Expulsion—occurs first as the anterior, then the posterior shoulder passes under the symphysis pubis.

Bishop's Score (Prelabor Score or Cervical Score)

The Bishop's score is a set of scores, ranging from 0–13, given before a woman is in labor to assess her likelihood of success with labor induction.

Parameter	0	1	2	3
Position	Posterior	Middle	Anterior	-
Consistency	Firm	Medium	Soft	-
Effacement	0–30%	40–50%	60–70%	>80%
Dilation	Closed	1–2 cm	3–4 cm	5+ cm
Fetal station	–3	–2	– 1, 0	+1, +2

- Score 5 or less—labor less likely to start
- Score 9 or more—labor most likely to start
- Total score is 15.

Dilation of cervix: It is the opening of cervix, entrance of the uterus for the childbirth. It occurs in the first stage of labor. It is measured in centimeters. Complete cervical dilation is 10 cm.

Effacement: It is also called as thinning of the cervix which occurs in pregnant women as labor and delivery get closer. It is measured in percentage.

Fetal station: It describes the position of the fetus head in relation to the distance from the ischial spines. Negative numbers indicate that the head is further inside than the ischial spines and positive numbers show that the head is below the level of the ischial spines.

STAGES OF LABOR

There are four stages of labor.

Stage I: Onset of labor

It is the beginning of labor. It commences with the onset of true pain and uterine contractions, which bring about gradual opening up of the cervix. The opening of cervix is assessed in terms of "centimeters". When the cervix is fully opened or dilated as it is medically referred to, it is approximately 10 cm in diameter. The duration is 6-24 hours. In primigravida, it is longer than multigravida.

The first stage of labor is divided into three phases:

1. **Latent phase:** This first phase of the first stage of labor is called the latent phase, but can also be referred to as early labor, or just simply the first stage of labor. During this phase the cervix will start dilating and you will be having contractions, and they are normally not painful and you are able to move around, talk, laugh and function through them as normal. The length of cervical dilation is 0-4 cm.
2. **Active phase:** This second phase of the first stage of labor results in your cervix dilating from 4-8 centimeters, and during this phase, your contractions will normally come between 2 and 5 minutes apart, and last up to a minute in duration. The active phase can last an average of 3-4 hours, but can go on longer, or end sooner, depending on your body and your labor.
3. **Transition phase:** The third and last phase of the first stage of labor results in your cervix dilating between 8 and 10 centimeters, and is the phase where your pain will be at its worst. During this time, your contractions will seem to be coming one right on top of the other, and may last up to two minutes each in duration. During this stage, the contractions are pushing your baby further down through the cervix, allowing his head to enter the vagina to prepare for birth. This stage normally lasts between 10 minutes and an hour.

Stage II: Expulsion of Fetus

Once the cervix is fully dilated (10 cm diameter), the baby can now pass out of the uterus, through the vagina and be delivered. This part of labor from full dilation of the cervix to delivery of the baby is called the second stage of labor. During this stage, the contractions are extremely strong and come every 2-3 minutes.

Stage III : Placental Stage

Once the baby is delivered, the uterus contracts and shrinks in size. Due to this, the placenta separates from the inner surface of the uterus and is expelled out. The period after delivery of the baby to the delivery of the placenta is called as placental stage or third stage of labor. This usually last for more than 30 minutes.

Stage IV: Immediate Postpartum Period

This is the period 1-4 hours after delivery or immediate postpartum period.

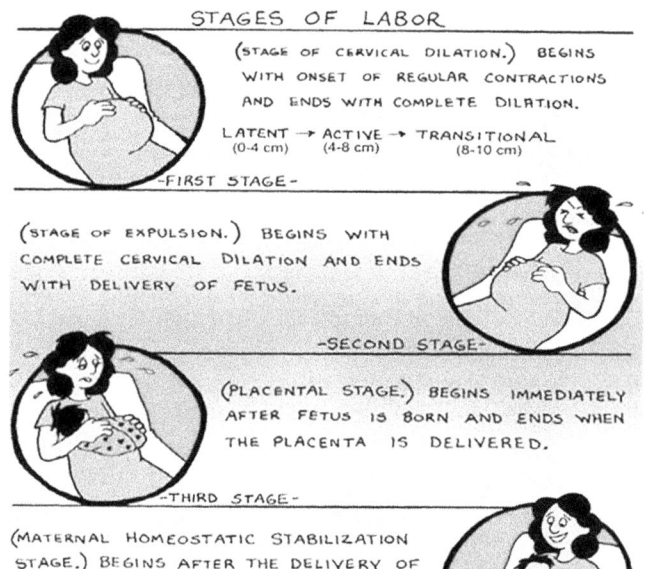

Episiotomy

An incision made in the perineum to enlarge the vaginal opening.

Nursing Care

- Care of the episiotomy wound begins immediately after delivery
- Provide local wound care and pain management.
- During the first 12 hours after delivery, an ice pack may be helpful in preventing both pain and swelling of the site of the episiotomy.
- The incision should be kept clean and dry to avoid infection.
- Frequent sitz baths (soaking the area of the wound in a small amount of warm water for about 20 minutes several times a day) can help keep the area clean.
- The episiotomy site should also be cleaned after a bowel movement or after urination; this can be accomplished with use of a spray bottle and warm water. A spray bottle may also be used during urination to decrease the pain that occurs when urine comes in contact with the wound. After the site has been sprayed or soaked, the area should be dried by gently blotting with tissue paper.

Forceps Delivery

In a forceps delivery, the obstetrician applies forceps, an instrument-shaped like a pair of large spoons or salad tongs to the baby's head to help guide the baby out of the birth canal. This is typically done during a contraction while the mother pushes.

Nursing Care

- After a forceps delivery, thorough examination of both the mother and the newborn is advisable. Maternal cervical, vaginal, and perineal lacerations must be excluded. In addition, maternal vulvar edema may be significant.
- Most operators institute measures, such as perineal ice to ameliorate edema and pain.
- Administer pain medications as ordered.
- Monitor for bleeding, these patients are at increased risk for hemorrhage, and a postoperative hemogram should be obtained and the condition corrected as needed.
- Before discharge, pelvic and rectal examinations may help to confirm the integrity of pelvic organs and may exclude such entities as pelvic hematoma, rectal tears, and misplaced sutures.
- The newborn must be examined for lacerations, bruising, and other injuries. The pediatric service should be made aware of the circumstances of delivery.

Cesarean Section

Cesarean delivery is defined as the delivery of a fetus through surgical incisions made through the abdominal wall (laparotomy) and the uterine wall (hysterotomy).

Indications

- Repeat cesarean delivery
- Obstructive lesions in the lower genital tract, including malignancies
- Pelvic abnormalities that preclude engagement or interfere with descent of the fetal presentation in labor
- Situations in which neonatal morbidity and mortality could be decreased by the prevention of trauma
- Malpresentations (e.g. preterm breech presentations, non-frank breech term fetuses)
- Certain congenital malformations or skeletal disorders
- Infection and prolonged acidemia.

Preoperative Nursing Care

- NPO from mid night (at least 2 hours from clear liquids, 6 hours from a light meal, and 8 hours from a regular meal)
- Administer IV fluids
- Place a Foley's catheter and check the urine output
- Placement of an external fetal monitor and monitors for the patient's blood pressure, pulse, and oxygen saturation
- Administer antibiotics as ordered
- Check routine investigations.

Postoperative Nursing Care

- Monitor vitals
- Palpate and measure the fundal height
- Administer pain medications
- Ambulation on postoperative day 1; advance as tolerated
- If patient plans to breastfeed, initiate within a few hours after delivery; if patient plans to bottlefeed, she may use a tight bra or breast binder in the postoperative period.
- Discharge on postoperative day 3 or 4, if no complications.
- Teach about contraception as well as refraining from intercourse for 4-6 weeks postpartum.

DISORDERS IN INTRAPARTUM PERIOD

Preterm Delivery

Labor that occurs before 37 weeks of gestation.

Causes

- Pregnancy-induced hypertension
- Material injury

- Infections
- Placental abnormalities
- Cervical incompetence
- Polyhydramnios

Management

- Monitor fetal heart rate continuously
- Provide side lying position in case of severe fetal distress
- Administer indomethacin to prevent preterm delivery
- Administer betamethasone (betnesol) to improve lung maturity
- Administer medications to decrease uterine contraction, such as terbutaline, magnesium sulfate, duvadilan or Isoxsuprine.

POST-TERM DELIVERY

Labor that occurs after 42 weeks of gestation.

Causes

- Previous post-term pregnancies
- Maternal obesity
- Sulfatase deficiency in the placenta
- Central nervous system abnormalities
- Anencephaly (loss of major portion of brain tissue)

Management

- Prepare the patient for labor induction
- Monitor for complications, such as meconium aspiration, fetal macrosomia
- Perform continuous monitoring of fetal and maternal vitals.

FETAL DISTRESS

Fetal distress is an uncommon complication of labor. It typically occurs when the fetus has not been receiving enough oxygen. Fetal distress may occur when the pregnancy lasts too long (postmaturity) or when complications of pregnancy or labor occur.

Causes

- Cord compression
- Placental abnormalities

Clinical Manifestations

- Decelerations in the FHR
- Meconium-stained amniotic fluid

Management

- Check the fetal heart rate
- Change the position of the mother to relieve compression
- Provide left side
- Administer oxygen

DYSTOCIA

Dystocia is also known as obstructed labor, is a condition in which, even though the uterus is contracting normally, the baby does not exit the pelvis during childbirth due to being physically blocked. It is associated with cephalopelvic disproportion.

Management

- Prepare oxytocin infusion
- Monitor the mother and fetus continuously
- Prepare for cesarean delivery

PRECIPITOUS LABOR

Precipitous labor is defined as expulsion of the fetus within less than 3 hours of commencement of regular contractions. It is an emergency delivery without client's physician or midwife.

Causes

- An efficient uterus that contracts with unusual strength
- An above-average "pelvic outlet"
- A well-aligned pelvis, pubic bone and birth canal
- An unusually small baby
- A baby positioned extremely well to come out
- Having a female relative who also experienced fast labors

Management

- Administer medications to decrease the force of contraction
- Monitor the client's desire to push the baby
- Observe for any perineal bulging or bleeding
- Monitor for any complications for the mother and baby
- In some cases, prepare the patient for cesarean section.

AMNIOTIC FLUID EMBOLISM

Escape of amniotic fluid into the maternal circulation and act as an emboli resulting in fatal conditions.

Clinical Manifestation

- Bleeding
- Cyanosis
- Pulmonary edema
- Shortness of breath
- Signs of shock (hypotension)

Management

- Administer oxygen
- Administer medications to control bleeding
- Prepare for emergency delivery.

POSTPARTUM PERIOD

A postpartum period or postnatal period is the period beginning immediately after the birth of a child and extending for about six weeks.

Changes in Postpartum Period

Involution of Uterus

Rapid decrease in the size of the uterus. The weight of uterus decreases from approximately 2 lbs to 2 oz within 6 weeks. Uterus is palpated after delivery below the umbilicus, the uterus regresses approximately 1 finger breadth (1 cm) per day and by the end of second week it cannot be palpated abdominally.

Lochia

Lochia is a discharge consists of blood and blood vessels. Foul smelling lochia indicates infection.

1. **Lochia rubra:** Dark red in color, first 3 days after delivery
2. **Lochia serosa:** Pinkish brown in color, 4–10 days after delivery
3. **Lochia alba:** Yellowish in color, 11–14 days after delivery

Cardiovascular Changes

Cardiovascular changes in the puerperium are dramatic. Blood volume increases by about 50% at the time of delivery. There is an average 500 mL blood loss at vaginal delivery, and a gradual replacement of this with an "autotransfusion" of 500–750 mL as the uterus contracts. Most of the hemodynamic recovery occurs in the first 2 weeks postpartum, with more gradual shifts continuing over the next 4 or 5 months.

Renal Changes

Renal anatomic changes of pregnancy (particularly dilated ureters) persist for at least 5 days postpartum, and in some patients may persist much longer. Renal function (plasma flow and glomerular filtration rate) are at prepregnant levels by 6 weeks postpartum.

Breast Changes

Changes in the breast begin well before delivery but become most dramatic in postpartum. Several hormones interact to allow smooth production and excretion of milk, including the withdrawal of estrogen and progesterone, along with prolactin, glucocorticoid, insulin, and thyroid hormone activity. For approximately 3 days postpartum, the breast secretes colostrum, distinct from milk in having higher amounts of immunoglobulins and white blood cells and lower amounts of fat and lactose. Over 2 weeks, the milk assumes its typical nutritional properties.

In lactating mothers, high level of prolactin immediately after delivery, initial secretion is colostrum and true breast milk appearing between 48 and 96 hours.

In nonlactating mothers, prolactin levels fall rapidly, may still secrete colostrum for 2-3 days, breast engorgement occurs due to the temporary congestion of veins and lymphatic circulation.

Menstruation (Reappearance)

Resumption of menses after delivery is highly variable. For most non-breastfeeding mothers, the first postpartum menses occur at approximately 55 to 60 days (range 20–120) post delivery. Breastfeeding may delay in return of menses by several months, especially if the child is getting no other supplemental source of nutrition. Although the first several cycles may be anovulatory, ovulation has been demonstrated in 52% of women whose menses resumed less than 60 days following delivery.

POSTPARTUM DISORDERS

Postpartum Hemorrhage

Bleeding of 500 mL or more after delivery resulting in decreased BP and increased pulse.

Types

1. **Primary postpartum hemorrhage:** Bleeding before 24 hours after delivery
2. **Secondary postpartum hemorrhage:** Bleeding after 24 hours of delivery

Causes

- Atonic uterus
- Trauma
- Any hematoma formation
- Hb level less than 10 gm/dl in the antepartum period

Nursing Care

- Massage the fundus
- Monitor restlessness and hemorrhage
- Maintain Hb level
- Count the perineal pad for checking the amount of blood loss.

POSTPARTUM INFECTION

Any infection in the reproductive tract associated with delivery, usually occurs within 10 days.

Causes

- Cesarean delivery
- Trauma
- Maternal anemia

Nursing Care

- Monitor the temperature (temperature of 100 degree Fahrenheit or 38.9 degree Celsius or more for 2 consecutive days)
- Monitor the vaginal discharge for any foul smell
- Monitor the WBC count
- Administer more fluids
- Administer medications as ordered
- Encourage high calorie high protein diet to promote wound healing
- Provide semi to high Fowler's position.

MASTITIS

Inflammation of the breast caused by cracked nipples in the nursing mothers.

It occurs in 5% of breastfeeding women and is associated with fevers that can be quite high, erythema of a portion of a breast, induration, exquisite tenderness, and systemic findings, such as chills and malaise.

Causative organism is *Staphylococcus aureus*. The organism is commonly transferred from the infant's mouth during breastfeeding.

Management

- Treatment includes thorough and frequent expression of milk (there is no risk to the infant of continuing to breastfeed, if the patient's pain threshold will allow it; otherwise she should be instructed to manually express her breasts at frequent intervals) to prevent stasis.
- Administer analgesics, such as aspirin or acetaminophen.
- Provide local comfort measures, such as a well-supporting bra and local heat, and a semisynthetic penicillin (erythromycin or cephalosporins are acceptable alternatives).

POSTPARTUM PSYCHOSIS

Postpartum psychosis (or puerperal psychosis) is a term that covers a group of mental illnesses with the sudden onset of psychotic symptoms following childbirth. A typical example is for a woman to become irritable, have extreme mood swings and hallucinations, and possibly need psychiatric hospitalization.

Most women experience some period of transient depressed mood within the 1st week of delivery, referred to as *postpartum blues*. This may represent a combination of physical exhaustion, an overwhelming sense of the responsibilities of parenthood, and massive hormonal and metabolic shifts. This period is brief (days to a week) and manageable. Some patients, however, continue down the slope to feelings of despair, gross inadequacy, isolation, and depersonalization. In some cases, this can become a psychotic condition, leading to suicide or homicide.

SUBINVOLUTION OF UTERUS

The failure of the uterus to revert to prepregnant state during postpartum period is called as subinvolution of uterus.

Causes

- Infections
- Retained products of placenta
- Uterine fibroid

Clinical Manifestation

- Uterus remains enlarged
- Fundus higher in abdomen
- Heavy bleeding

Management

- Administer medications, such as ergonovine
- Monitor for bleeding

SHEEHAN'S SYNDROME

Sheehan syndrome, also known as Simmonds syndrome, postpartum hypopituitarism or postpartum pituitary gland necrosis, may occur following profound hemorrhage or eclampsia. The mechanism of injury is thought to be hypoxic because the anterior pituitary is the area of the brain most sensitive to hypoperfusion.

Causes

- Ischemic necrosis
- Hypovolemic shock due to bleeding

Clinical Manifestation

- Absence of lactation, amenorrhea
- Loss of axillary and pubic hair
- Genital and breast atrophy
- Super involution of the uterus
- Infertility
- Hypothyroidism (fatigue, cold intolerance, edema)
- Adrenocortical insufficiency (fatigue, anorexia, weight loss, decreased skin pigmentation, abnormal stress response).

CONTRACEPTIVES

- These are hormonal preparations used for birth control
- These are preparations of estrogen and progesterone
- Progestin only pills are safe in lactating mothers
- Contraceptives suppress ovulation
- Medications containing progestin are less effective
- Contraceptives are contraindicated in hypertension, thromboembolic diseases, CAD, pregnancy, etc.
- Contraceptives interfere with activities of bromocriptine, anticoagulants, antidepressants and antibiotics.

Nursing Care

- Monitor the blood glucose in diabetes patients
- Instruct the client that contraceptives will take 1 week to 10 days for full contraceptive activity.
- Instruct the client to perform breast self-examination (BSE) monthly
- If a woman is using contraceptive for the past 6 months and now she wants to conceive a child, then instruct the woman to use an alternative method like condoms for 1 month period to ensure the complete removal of hormonal agent.
- Teach the client regarding the harmful effect of taking prolonged contraceptives, it may sometime suppress ovulation and resulting in infertility.
- Educate the women regarding various fertility hormones (Menotropins, folitropins, HCG, etc.).

Previous Questions and Answers

Part 1

1. A client is taking phenelzine (nardil) 15 mg PO, three times a day. The nurse is about to administer the 1 pm dose when the client complaints of a throbbing headache. Which of the following would the nurse do next?
   a. Give the client an analgesic ordered PRN
   b. Call the physician to report the symptom
   c. Administer the client's next dose of phenelzine
   d. Obtain the client's vital signs

2. When assessing a client for suicidal risk, which of the following methods of suicide would the nurse identify as the most lethal?
   a. Aspirin overdose
   b. Use of a gun
   c. Head hanging
   d. Wrist-cutting

3. A client who overdosed on barbiturates is being transferred to the inpatient psychiatric unit from the intensive care unit. The nurse receiving the client would anticipate which of the follow as a priority?
   a. Nutrition
   b. Sleep
   c. Safety
   d. Hygiene

4. The nurse assesses the child with chronic renal failure who is receiving peritoneal dialysis for edema. Which of the following would the nurse expect to find?
   a. Absence of pulmonary crackles
   b. Decreased dialysate outflow
   c. Normal blood pressure
   d. Pallor

5. Which of the following diet plan would be appropriate for the nurse to discuss with the family of a child with acute renal failure?
   a. High carbohydrate and protein
   b. High fat and carbohydrate
   c. Low fat and protein
   d. Low in carbohydrate and fat.

6. A child with nephritis is placed on prednisone. The dose is 2 mg/kg/day to be administered twice a day. The child weight is 25 pounds. How many milligrams will the child receive each dose?

7. The toddler with nephrotic syndrome responds to treatment and is ready to go home. When helping the family plan for home care, which of the following instructions would the nurse include in the teaching?
   a. Administer pain medication is needed
   b. Keep the child away from others with an infection
   c. Notify the physician if there is an increase in the child's urine output.
   d. Administer acetaminophen daily

8. Commercial formula contains 20 calories for the 1 day old infant weight this morning was 8 pounds and was fed 45 cc at 2.00 am, 5.30 am, 8.00 am, 11.00 am, 2.00 pm, 4.30 pm, 8.00 pm and 10.30 pm. What is the total amount of calories the infant received today?

9. Approximately, 90 minutes after birth, the nurse encourages the mother of a term neonate to do which of the following:
   a. Feed the neonate
   b. Allow the neonate to sleep
   c. Get to know the neonate
   d. Change the neonate's diaper

10. While making a home visit to a primigravida client and her 3 days old son, the nurse observes the mother changing the baby's disposable diapers. Before putting the clean diaper, the mother begins to apply baby powder to the neonate's buttocks. Which of the following statements about baby powder would the nurse relate to the mother?
    a. It may cause pneumonia to develop
    b. It helps to prevent diaper rash
    c. It keeps the diaper from adhering the skin
    d. It can result in allergies in later life

11. A client has undergone surgery for retinal detachment. A priority nursing goal would be:
    a. To control pain
    b. Prevent increase in intraocular pressure
    c. Promote a low sodium diet
    d. Maintain darkened environment

12. A client with burns is admitted, the nurse should anticipate that the drug to be administered as soon as possible after admission is:
    a. Tetanus toxoid
    b. Gamma globulin
    c. Isoproterenol (Isopures)
    d. Phytonadione (Aquamephyton)
13. When caring for a client with a cervical laminectomy, the nurse:
    a. Should maintain the client head in a flexed position
    b. Has the responsibility of removing oral secretions
    c. Must keep the client's head at 45° angle from the spine
    d. Should provide ROM exercise early during POP period
14. When assessing a client with cancer of the tongue in the specific manifestation, the nurse should expect to find is:
    a. Halitosis
    b. Leukoplakia
    c. Bleeding gums
    d. Substernal pain
15. After incision and drainage of an oral abscess, the client should be instructed to notify the physician if there is:
    a. Foul odor to the breath
    b. Pain and swelling after 1 week
    c. Pain associated with swallowing
    d. Tenderness to the mouth when chewing
16. The nurse is caring for a 48 years old woman whose blood pressure over the past two months has range between 140/88 and 148/94—the nurse explain to her that her pressure is considered elevated because the current upper limit for normal systolic:
    a. 110 mm Hg
    b. 120 mm Hg
    c. 140 mm Hg
    d. 160 mm Hg
17. The nurse is having difficulty in assessing peripheral pulses. The most appropriate action for the nurse to take is to:
    a. Ask him to lie on his stomach
    b. Have him do 20 jumping jacks
    c. Ask him to flex and extend his foot
    d. Ask him to elevate his leg
18. The nurse is caring for a woman who had a lumbar laminectomy with a spinal fusion immediately after surgery which of the following should the nurse expect the client to manifest?
    a. Absence of lower extremity movement
    b. Response to pin prick sensation
    c. Severe muscle spasm
    d. Weak pedal pulses
19. The patient has suffered a chemical burn. The best initial action is to:
    a. Roll the patient in a blanket
    b. Secure lead lined gloves and move the patient away from the chemical
    c. Flush the area with copious amount of water or normal saline
    d. If the chemical is an acid neutralize with a base
20. Mrs. Smith has a ventricular demand pacemaker that is set at 72 beats per minute the nurse knows that her pacemaker is functioning correctly if which of the following appears on the ECG?
    a. Pacemaker spikes instead of QRS complex
    b. Pacemaker spikes followed by QRS complex
    c. Pacemaker spikes appearing only if the heart rate is over 72
    d. Pacemaker lead
21. A client with diverticulosis is admitted to the hospital, the nurse can expect that this client with be placed on:
    a. A bland low residue client
    b. A low protein high carbohydrate diet
    c. A soft, but high fiber diet
    d. Saline cathartics to increase intestinal peristalsis
22. The nurse is assessing a client who was raped a month ago. The client cannot describe any feelings related her rape. She focuses on the need for better law enforcement and rape prevention programs. The client is using which defense:
    a. Denial
    b. Conversion
    c. Introjections
    d. Isolation
23. A client with an acute exacerbation of rheumatoid arthritis is admitted to the hospital for treatment. Which drug is used to treat client with rheumatoid and has both an anti-inflammatory and immune suppressive effect:
    a. Gold sodium thiomalate (myochrysine)
    b. Azathioprine (imuran)
    c. Prednisone (wysolone)
    d. Naproxen (naprosyn)
24. Mrs. Freddy is pregnant for the first time calls the clinic to say she is bleeding, to obtain important information the nurse should next ask:
    a. When did you last feed the baby one?
    b. How long have you been pregnant?

c. When was your pregnancy test done?
d. Are you having any uterine cramping?

25. **An adult is newly diagnosed with graves' disease asks the nurse why do I need to take propranolol (inderal) based on the nurses understanding of the medication and graves' disease the best response would be:**
    a. The medication will limit thyroid hormone secretion
    b. The medication will inhibit synthesis of thyroid hormones
    c. The medication will relieve the symptoms of craves disease
    d. The medication will increase the symptoms of thyroid hormone

26. **The plan of care for a client with acute myocardial infarction (MI) contains the nursing diagnosis risk for activity intolerance related to fatigue. The nurse plans to:**
    a. Provide positive reinforcement and encouragement during physical activity.
    b. Provide adequate fluid intake before and after physical activity.
    c. Provide assistants with self care needs and provide frequent rest periods
    d. Administer oxygen as needed.

27. **A clinic nurse is reviewing the record of a client with a suspected diagnosis of Meniere's disease. Which finding documented in the client's record is unrelated to this disorder?**
    a. Tinnitus
    b. Sensorineural hearing loss on the involved side
    c. Conductive hearing loss on the involved side
    d. Vertigo accompanied by nausea and vomiting

28. **In planning nutrition for the client with hypoparathyroidism, which diet would be appropriate?**
    a. High in calcium and low in phosphorus
    b. Low in vitamins A, D, E and K
    c. High in sodium with no fluid restriction
    d. Low in water and insoluble fiber.

29. **A nurse is planning care for a client with a diagnosis of thyrotoxicosis (thyroid storm) which of the following would the nurse include in the plan of care of the client?**
    a. Use of hypothermic (cooling) blanket
    b. Restriction of fluid intake
    c. Administration of levothyroxine (synthroid)
    d. Administration of enemas and stool softeners as needs

30. **A client with Guillain-Barrè syndrome asks the nurse what caused the disorder. In formulating a response, the nurse incorporates the understanding that the theory of causation:**
    a. Is unknown
    b. Relates to a previous central nervous system injury
    c. Is a fungal infection
    d. Relates to previous musculoskeletal injury

31. **An oral powder form of nelfinavir (Viracept) is prescribed for a client with HIV, the nurse provides instructions regarding the preparation of the medication, and tells the client to mix the powder with:**
    a. Milk
    b. Orange juice
    c. Apple juice
    d. Grapefruit juice

32. **The nurse is caring for a pregnant client who is receiving an intravenous (IV) infusion of magnesium sulfate. To provide a safe environment, the nurse ensures that which priority item is at the bed side?**
    a. Tongue blade
    b. Percussion hammer
    c. Potassium chloride injection
    d. Calcium gluconate injection

33. **The nurse is assisting the client with hepatic encephalopathy to fill out the dietary menu. The nurse advices the client to avoid which of the following entre items that could aggravate the client's condition:**
    a. Tomato soup
    b. Fresh fruit plate
    c. Vegetable Lasagna
    d. Ground beef patty

34. **A client with bipolar disorder is beginning medication therapy with lithium carbonate (intalith). The nurse plans to teach the client the importance of having blood levels drawn how often until therapeutic medication level is reached?**
    a. Daily
    b. Weekly
    c. Monthly
    d. Every 3 months

35. **A client has been diagnosed with acute pyelonephritis. The nurse assess the client for which manifestation of this disorder?**
    a. Low-grade fever
    b. Flank pain on the unaffected side
    c. Chills and nausea
    d. Pale, dilute urine

36. A client has just been diagnosed with acute renal failure (ARF) the laboratory telephones to report a serum potassium level of 6.1 mg/dl for the client the nurse take which important action?
    a. Call the physician
    b. Check the sodium level
    c. Encourage the client to drink an extra 500 ml of fluid
    d. Asks the dietary department to deliver additional vegetables on the client's diet tray

37. The nurse is preparing to care for a client who has undergone (esophagogastroduodenoscopy (OGD) after checking the vital signs what should be the nurse's next priority.
    a. Monitor for sharp epigastric pain
    b. Give ware gargles for sore throat
    c. Check for a return of the gag reflex
    d. Monitor for the complaints heart burn

38. A client with trigeminal neuralgia undergoes surgery for pain relief. In the postoperative period which nursing intervention will prevent an episode of facial pain?
    a. Instruct the client to brush the teeth thoroughly following meals
    b. Bring the client room temperature water for washing
    c. Peach the client to chew on the affected
    d. Offer the client ice chips between meals

39. The client is scheduled to have an arterial blood gas drawn from the radial artery. The nurse plans to determine which if the following before the sample is drawn:
    a. Patency of brachial artery
    b. Whether the client is allergic to Beparine sodium (heparin sodium)
    c. Whether the client has weakness in the extremity in which the blood will be drawn
    d. Perform Allen test

40. An adult has been reported in a motor vehicle accident. She has a 4 inch laceration on her forehead that is bleeding profusely. Her left ankle has an obvious deformity and is splinted. Her vital signs are BP 100/60. P. 110 R. 16. What is the first action the nurse should take:
    a. Start an IV line
    b. Place a Foley's catheter
    c. Get an ECG
    d. Check her neurologic status

41. Which assessment is most important for the nurse to make when monitoring a client with a pituitary tumor that secretes ACTH?
    a. Height
    b. Blood pressure
    c. Pulse rate
    d. Output

42. The pregnant woman asks the nurse if there are any special problems that she might encounter during labor and delivery because she has diabetics. The nurse responds that during labor and delivery, diabetic mothers may develop:
    a. Hypoglycemia
    b. Hyperglycemia
    c. Hyperosmolar nonketotic coma
    d. Hypokalemia

43. An adult presents with severe rectal bleeding and 16 diarrheal stools a day. Severe abdominal pain tenesmus and dehydration. Because of these symptoms, the nurse should be alert for complication associated which of these diseases
    a. Crohn's disease
    b. Ulcerative colitis
    c. Diverticulitis
    d. Peritonitis

44. A nurse is caring for a client with a fractured tibia and fibula few hours after a long leg cast is applied; the client reports a significant increase in pain level even after administration of the prescribed dose of opioid analgesic. The appropriate initial nursing action is to:
    a. Contact the physician
    b. Administer another dose of pain medication
    c. Elevate the casted leg
    d. Check the neurovascular status of the toes on the casted leg

45. A nurse is reviewing the record of a client who has just been told that a pregnancy test is positive. The physician has documented the presence of Goodell's sign. The nurse determines that this sign indicates:
    a. A softening of the cervix
    b. The presence of fetal movement
    c. The presence of HCG in the urine
    d. A soft blowing sound that corresponds to the maternal pulse during auscultation of the uterus.

46. The nurse is developing a plan of care for a client with pulmonary edema. The nurse establishes a goal to have the client participate in activities that reduce cardiac workload. The nurse identifies which client action as contributing to this goal?
    a. Elevating the legs when in bed
    b. Sleeping in the supine position
    c. Using seasonings to improve the taste of food
    d. Using a bedside commode

47. A client with a first degree heart block has an electrocardiogram (ECG) during an episode of chest pain. The nurse knows that which ECG finding indicates first degree heart block?
    a. Prolonged PR interval
    b. Widened QRS complex
    c. Tall, peaked T waves
    d. Presence of Q waves

48. A nurse is conducting an initial assessment on a client in crisis. When assessing the client's perception of the precipitating event that led to the crisis, the appropriate question to ask is:
    a. With whom do you live?
    b. Who is available to help you?
    c. What leads you to seek help now?
    d. What do you usually do to feel better?

49. A client with suspected primary hyperparathyroidism is undergoes diagnostic testing. The nurse would assess for which of the following as a sign of this disorder?
    a. Polyphagia
    b. Weight gain
    c. Diarrhea
    d. Polyuria

50. A pediatric client with ventricular septal defect repair is placed on a maintenance dosage of digoxin (Lanoxin) elixir. The dosage is 0.07 mg/kg/day, and the client's weight is 7.2 kg. The physician prescribes the digoxin to be given twice daily. A nurse prepares how much digoxin to administer to the client at each dose?
    a. 0.5 mg
    b. 2.5 mg
    c. 0.25 mg
    d. 0.37 mg

51. A client is to undergone pleural biopsy at the bedside. Knowing the potential complications of the procedure, the nurse plans to have which of the following items available at the bedside?
    a. Chest tube and drainage system
    b. Intubation tray
    c. Portable chest X-ray machine
    d. Morphine sulfate injection

52. An immobile client is at risk for tissue osteoporosis. The nurse understands that which of the following substances plays an important role in the bone remodeling process?
    a. Vitamin C
    b. Vitamin A
    c. Calcitonin
    d. Thyroid hormone

53. A nurse is assessing an electrocardiogram (ECG) rhythm strip for a client. The P waves and QRS complexes are regular. The PR interval is 0.14 sec, and the QRS complexes measure 0.08 sec. The overall heart rate is 82 beats/min. The nurse interprets the cardiac rhythm to be:
    a. Sinus bradycardia
    b. Sick Sinus syndrome
    c. Normal Sinus rhythm
    d. 1st degree heart block

54. A patient who has left frontal lobe tumor has undergone craniotomy. Four hours after surgery, the following data are obtained by the nurse. Which of the following data would be most indicative of increasing intracranial pressure?
    a. A patient's blood pressure is 160/94 mm Hg, up from 140/90 mm Hg
    b. The patient is difficult to arouse
    c. The patients Babinski's reflex is negative
    d. The patient is incontinent of urine

55. To which of the following nursing measures should a nurse give priority in the care of a patient who is receiving vincristine sulfate (oncovin)?
    a. Limiting environmental stimuli
    b. Observing for gum hyperplasia
    c. Monitoring for cardiac dysrhythmias
    d. Increasing dietary fiber content

56. When caring for an adolescent who is diagnosed with idiopathic scoliosis a nurse should recognize that the priority concern for the adolescent is related to:
    a. Body image
    b. Activity limitations
    c. Financial burden
    d. Imposed dependence

57. The patient's blood test results reveal that hematocrit level of 66 mm/dl. To which of the following nursing diagnosis would a nurse give priority?
    a. Ineffective breathing pattern
    b. Activity intolerance
    c. Hyperthermia
    d. Dysreflexia

58. A patient who had surgery on his right eye (occipital dysplasia, OD) for glaucoma complains of pain and nausea postoperatively. The nurse initially should carry out which of the following measures:
    a. Remove the dressing and assess for bleeding
    b. Administer acetylsalicylic acid (aspirin) for pain
    c. Position the patient on his/her right side
    d. Notify the physician

59. A patient taking the drug glipizide (Glucotrol) should be assessed by the nurse for which of the following side effects:
    a. Agranulocytosis
    b. Vitamin B1 deficiency
    c. Hyperlipidemia
    d. Hypernatremia
60. The physician evaluates the most recent set of arterial blood gas of a patient with ARDS and orders an increase in the Positive End Expiratory Pressure from 5 cm of H_2O to 10 cm of H_2O. Based on this change in therapy, the nurse should anticipate which of the following ABG findings:
    a. Decreased PaO_2
    b. Increased PaO_2
    c. Decreased HCO_3
    d. Increased $PaCO_2$
61. An 82 years old patient is experiencing confusion and forgetfulness. He is diagnosed with vascular dementia. The family asks the nurse for the information about the cause of this disorder. Which of the following statements made by the nurse is correct?
    a. The cause of this type of dementia is unknown
    b. Vascular dementia is the result of many small strokes damaging areas of the brain
    c. Vascular dementia is caused by a viral infection
    d. The dementia symptoms are caused by the medications he is taking
62. An 86 yrs old male is admitted to the hospital for renal insufficiency, the first night he becomes extremely disoriented, confused after being given a low dose tricyclic antidepressant. The nurse should be aware that such behavior is indicative of:
    a. Dementia
    b. Delirium
    c. Psychosis
    d. Depression
63. A psychiatric patient continues to disrupt the unit items by pacing up and down the hall. The nurse responds by placing the patient in the seclusion room. As a result of her actions, the nurse may be held responsible for which of the following legal implications?
    a. False imprisonment
    b. Battery
    c. Invasion of privacy
    d. Defamation of character
64. When allotting a new nurse to the psychiatric unit, an experienced nurse should provide which of the following explanations regarding the use of patient restraints?
    a. PRN order for restraints is unacceptable
    b. Documentation must be done every eight hours while a patient is restrained.
    c. A restraint order, once written, is in effect for the entire hospitalization.
    d. The vest restraint is the safest type of restraint to use.
65. At 16 weeks gestation, no fetal heart rate was detected during assessment of a pregnant patient. An ultrasound confirmed a hydatidiform molar pregnancy. Which of the following actions should the nurse tell the patient to expect during her one-year following up?
    a. Multiple serum chorionic gonadotropin levels will be drawn
    b. An intrauterine device will be used to decrease vaginal bleeding
    c. Pregnancy will be restricted for another year
    d. Oral contraceptives will not be prescribed because they will increase the risk of cancer
66. A patient admitted with a diagnosis of bipolar disorder, mania. Which of the following nursing diagnoses would be a priority?
    a. Decisional conflict related to making health care choices.
    b. Self-care deficit, bathing/hygiene, related to take of attention
    c. Hopelessness related to impending depression
    d. Fatigue related to hyperactivity
67. A client with cirrhosis vomits bright red blood and the physician suspects bleeding esophageal varices. The physician decides to insert a Sengstaken—Blakemore tube. The nurse should explain to the client that the tube acts by:
    a. Providing a large diameter for effective gastric lavage
    b. Applying direct pressure to gastric bleeding sites.
    c. Blocking blood flow to the stomach and esophagus.
    d. Applying direct pressure to the esophagus.
68. The client's wife asks the nurse whether the intravenous infusion is meeting her husband's nutritional needs because he has vomited several times. The nurses response should be based on the knowledge that 1 liter of 5% dextrose in normal saline delivers:
    a. 170 calories
    b. 250 calories
    c. 340 calories
    d. 500 calories

69. Attempts to stops a client's preterm labor are unsuccessful and her baby is weighing 4 pounds 2 ounces which of the following observations of this newborn suggest a gestational age of less than 40 weeks?
    a. Small amounts of lanugos and vernix, testes descended, and palmar and plantar creases.
    b. Parchment like skin, no lango, and full areolas in breasts
    c. Upper pinna of ear well curved with instant recoil, small amount of lanugos and pink in color.
    d. Dark red skin, testes undescended with few rugations, and abundant lanugos.

70. To prevent complications of bed rest imposed on a client with gangrene, which nursing action would be contraindicated?
    a. Inspect the client's feet
    b. Teach about appropriate foot care
    c. Restricted fluid intake
    d. Exercise joints and muscle

71. Which of the following snacks would be the best choice for a child with nephrosis?
    a. I ounce processed cheese spread, celery sticks and Kool-Aid.
    b. ½ cup Vanilla pudding and grape juice.
    c. ½ peanut butter sandwich, apple slice and ½ cup hot cocoa
    d. ½ cup corn flakes, milk, raisins.

72. The wife of a client with bipolar disorder, manic phase states to the nurse, "He is acting so crazy. What did he do to get this way?" The nurse bases the response to the client's wife on the understanding of which of the following about this disorder?
    a. It is caused by underlying psychological difficulties
    b. It is caused by disturbed family dynamics in the client's early life.
    c. It is the result of an imbalance of chemicals in the brain
    d. It is the result of a genetic inheritance from someone in the family.

73. The parent of a child who is taking an antibiotic for bilateral otitis media tells the nurse that he has stopped the medicine since his child is better sawing the rest of the medications to use the next time the child gets sick which of the following would be the nurse's best response?
    a. It is important to give the medicines as ordered.
    b. How do you know your child's cares are cured?
    c. Your child needs all of the medicine so that the infection clears.
    d. Stopping the medicine is not what's best for your child.

74. What is the purpose of I.V. replacement therapy for a client with nasogastric (NG) tube?
    a. Maintain bladder function
    b. Facilitate osmotic dieresis
    c. Equalize water intake and output
    d. Maintain fluid and electrolyte balance

75. There is discussion about how to treat a third degree burn is the nursing room. Which is the most preferable method?
    a. Peel off burned dead skin
    b. Using antiseptic creams
    c. Pierce the opened blisters
    d. Administering morphine

76. How to manage a client having deep vein thrombosis in her right leg?
    a. Encourage the client to ambulate twice a shift
    b. Have the client do active leg exercises hourly with both legs
    c. Keep the right leg elevated above heart level
    d. Assess the edema of the right leg every 4 hrs.

77. A lady call the health center and tell about her problems that is her husband physically abused her. She requested the registered nurse to give any remedies for this. In which option should opted by the nurse in such situation?
    a. Give the telephone number of safe shelter and advice her use this if necessary.
    b. Advise her to react against her husband
    c. Advise her to make a request to the neighbors.
    d. Advise her to leave the house

78. Pick the suitable reason for pediculosis in a child?
    a. Child got this from the pet animals
    b. If happened from person to person by direct relation
    c. He got it from new climate
    d. Child got this from junk foods

79. What are the side effects of gentamycin I.V. application for an infection case?
    a. Hepatomegaly
    b. Dementia
    c. Ototoxicity
    d. Cardiac arrhythmias

80. Which of the following is normal breath sound?
    a. Vesicular
    b. Bronchotracheal
    c. Bronchovesicular
    d. Adventitious

81. Which of the following option indicates promotion of urinary continence in the patient?
    a. Increased fluid intake
    b. Better bladder control
    c. Timed voiding
    d. Obedience with drinking schedule and voiding

82. Which type of room has been appropriate for an infant who got diarrhea?
    a. Not a room, preferable for ward
    b. A two-bed room with same disease infants
    c. A two-bed room with no other patients
    d. There is no cause of admission

83. Which of the following meal choice is suitable for a 6 months old infant?
    a. Egg white, formula and orange juice
    b. Apple juice, Carrots, whole milk
    c. Rice cereal, apple juice, formula
    d. Melba toast, egg yolk, whole milk

84. The client scheduled for electroconvulsive therapy tells the nurse, "I'm so afraid. What will happen to me during the treatment?" which of the following statements is most therapeutic for the nurse to make?
    a. You can expect to be supply and confused for a time after the treatment
    b. You will be given medicine to relax you during the treatment
    c. The treatment might produce nausea and headache
    d. The treatment will produce a controlled "grand mal seizure"

85. A 6 years old with cystic fibrosis has an order for creon. The nurse knows that the medication will be given?
    a. Daily in the morning
    b. With meals and snacks
    c. At bedtime
    d. Twice daily

86. A teen hospitalized with anorexia nervosa is now permitted to leave her room and eat in the dining room. Which of the following nursing interventions should be included in the client's plan of care?
    a. Placing high protein foods in the canter of the clients plate
    b. Weighing the client after she eats
    c. Providing the client with child size utensils
    d. Having a staff member remain with her for 1 hrs after she eats.

87. A client taking Dilantin (Phenytoin) for grand mal seizures is preparing for discharge. Which information should be included in the client's discharge care plan?
    a. The clients will need to avoid a high carbohydrate diet
    b. The medication can cause dental staining.
    c. The client will need a regularly scheduled CBC
    d. The medication can cause problems with drowsiness.

88. The nurse is conducting nutritional counseling for a patient with cholecystits. which of the following information is important to communicate?
    a. The patient should limit sweets and sugary drinks
    b. The patient should limit fatty foods
    c. The patient must maintain a high protein/low carbohydrate diet
    d. The patient must maintain a low calorie diet.

89. A patient with history of DM is in the second postoperative day following cholecystectomy. She has complained of nausea and isn't able to eat solid foods. The nurse enters the room to find the patient confused and shaky. Which of the following is the most likely explanation for the patient's symptoms?
    a. Hyperglycemia
    b. Hypoglycemia
    c. Anesthesia reaction
    d. Diabetic ketoacidosis

90. A client with DKA who is receiving intravenous fluid and insulin complaints of tingling, shortness of breath, numbness of fingers and toe and ECG shows appearance of U wave that nurse should recognize that these symptoms indicate:
    a. Hypercalcemia
    b. Hyponatremia
    c. Hypoglycemia
    d. Hypokalemia

91. When assessing for hemorrhage after a client has a total hip replacement, the most important nursing action should be:
    a. Check vital signs every 4 hours
    b. Examine the bleeding under the client
    c. Observe for ecchymosis at the operative site
    d. Measure the girth of the thigh

92. The nurse is preparing postoperative discharge instruction for a client who had one adrenal gland removed. The nurse should include which of the following:
    a. The reason for maintaining a diabetic diet
    b. Teaching proper application of an ostomy pouch

c. Instructing about early signs of a wound infection
d. The need for lifelong replacement of adrenal hormones

93. A client is admitted to the emergency department after a burn injury sustained in a house fire. The skin on its back is waxy white color. The nurse interpret that this clients burn should be documented as:
    a. Partial thickness
    b. Moderate partial thickness
    c. Full thickness
    d. Deep full thickness

94. A patient is admitted in the hospital with diagnosis of hypoparathyroidism the nurse recovered the laboratory results of the client. Which diet the nurse can administer for this patient?
    a. Low in vit A, D, E, K
    b. High in calcium and low in phosphorus
    c. High in sodium
    d. High protein and low calcium diet

95. The client is admitted with a pH of 7.10 $PaCO_2$ 50 and HCO_3 of 30. The nurse should assess the finding as which of the following:
    a. Metabolic acidosis
    b. Metabolic alkalosis
    c. Respiratory alkalosis
    d. Respiratory acidosis

96. A pregnant client with DM arrives at the health care clinic for a follow-up visit. What priority assessment should the nurse monitor?
    a. Urine for specific gravity
    b. For the presence of edema
    c. Urine for glucose and ketones
    d. Blood pressure, pulse and respirations

97. A nurse assists a client who is at 38 weeks of gestation to lie down on the examining table in the obstetricians' office. The client suddenly become dizzy and light-headed and skins become cool. The nurse should take which of the following measure:
    a. Place a cool wash cloth on the client's forehead
    b. Explain the reason for these symptoms
    c. Measure blood pressure, pulse and respirations
    d. Position the client on her side

98. The nursing assessment in a client exhibiting symptoms of myxedema should reveal:
    a. Increased pulse rate
    b. Decreased temperature
    c. Fine tremors
    d. Increased radioactive iodine uptake level

99. A client admitted with atrial fibrillation. What medication protocol would be most important to implement?
    a. Inderal
    b. Isuprel
    c. Lidocaine
    d. Verapamil

100. A client is experiencing ARDS, which of the following would be the most effective nursing intervention?
    a. Maintain low flow oxygen via nasal cannula
    b. Encourage oral intake of at least 3000 ml fluids per day
    c. Ask open-ended questions to promote expression of anxiety
    d. Position the client in semi high Fowler's position with support to back

Answers (Part 1)

1. **Ans. is (d) Obtain the client's vital signs**

   The nurse would first take the client's vital signs, because the client could be experiencing a hypertensive crisis, which requires prompt intervention.

2. **Ans. is (b) Use of a gun**

   A crucial factor in determining the lethality of a method is the amount of time that occurs between initiating the method and the delivery of the lethal impact of the method.

3. **Ans. is (c) Safety**

   Client safety is the priority to prevent further self harm. Nutrition, sleep, hygiene are important concerns, but they are secondary to safety.

4. **Ans. is (d) Pallor**

   With edema, pallor can occur following to hemodilution as intestinal fluid moves to vascular space. The child would exhibit pulmonary crackles secondary to pulmonary congestion and edema.

Dialysate outflow would decrease, not increases as the body attempts to conserve fluid. The child's blood pressure would be increased because of excessive fluid volume.

5. **Ans. is (b) High fat and carbohydrate**

   The child with acute renal failure needs extra calories to reduce tissue metabolism, metabolic acidosis and uremia. Using high fat and carbohydrate diet helps to supply the necessary extra calories. If the child is able to tolerate oral foods, concentrated food sources that are high in carbohydrate and fat but low in protein, potassium and sodium may be provided.

6. **Ans. is 22.72 mg,** 25 pounds = 11.3 kg

   11.3 kg × 2 mg = 22.7 mg/day

7. **Ans. is (b) Keep the child away from others with an infection**

   A child recovering from nephrotic syndrome should be protected from infection. Therefore, the nurse would teach the parents to keep the child away from others with an infection. Because pain is not associated with this disorder, pain medication typically is not needed. The physician should be notified if urine output decreases, in children recovering from nephrotic syndrome, there is no reason to administer acetaminophen daily.

8. 240, 45 cc = 1.5 oz, 1.50 z × 8 feedings = 12

   12 × 20 calorie = 240 calories

9. **Ans. is (b) Allow the neonate to sleep**

   As part of the neonate's physiological adaptation to birth. At 90 mts after birth, the neonate typically is in the rest or sleep phase. During this time, the heart and respiratory rate slow and the neonate sleeps, unresponsive to stimuli at this time, the mother shown rest and allow the neonate to sleep

10. **Ans. is (a) It may cause pneumonia to develop**

    The nurse should inform the mother that baby powder can enter the neonate's lungs and result in pneumonia secondary to aspiration of the particles.

11. **Ans. is (b) Prevent increase in intraocular pressure**

12. **Ans. is (a) Tetanus toxoid**

    Clostridium tetani can develop in partial and full thickness burns that contain dead tissue

13. **Ans. is (b) Has the responsibility of removing oral secretions**

    Removing the oral secretions

14. **Ans. is (b) Leukoplakia**

    Leukoplakia are white thickened patches that tend to tissue become malignant ulceration of the mouth or the tongue may indicate cancer.

15. **Ans. is (b) Pain and swelling after 1 week**

    Pain and swelling should subside before 1 week postoperatively. Continued pain may indicate infection the breath may have an odor because of dried blood in the oral cavity; this is to be expected during in the postoperative period.

16. **Ans. is (c) 140 mm Hg**

    140 mm Hg, the normal range for blood pressure is between 95 and 140 mm Hg systolic pressure and between 60 and 90 mm Hg diastolic.

17. **Ans. is (a) Ask him to lie on his stomach**

    Asking the client to lie in the prone position will provides greater exposure to the popliteal space and thereby make assessment easier.

18. **Ans. is (b) Response to pin-prick sensation**

19. **Ans. is (c) Flush the area with copious amount of water or normal saline**

    Water will neutralize most chemicals while decreasing the heart rate.

20. **Ans. is (b) Pacemaker spikes followed by QRS complex**

    The ventricular pacemaker stimulate the ventricle if no atrial impulse is transmittal through the AV node. the appearance of the QRS complex shows that the ventricle has resonated to the stimulus.

21. **Ans. is (c) A soft, but high fiber diet**

    A soft but high fiber elicit to increase the bulk of the stool, there by promoting defecation. Fluid intake of 22 day is recommended unless otherwise contraindicated. Seeds are not allowed.

22. **Ans. is (d) Isolation**

    Isolation is separating unacceptable feelings from one's thoughts.

23. **Ans. is (c) Prednisone (wysolone)**

    Prednisone is used to treat person with acute exacerbations of rheumatoid arthritis. This medication is give for its anti-inflammatory and immunesuppressive effects.

24. **Ans. is (b) How long have you been pregnant?**

25. **Ans. is (c) The medication will relieve the symptoms of Graves' disease**

    Propranolol is a beta-adrenergic blocker that wills relieves the symptoms of Graves' disease caused by increased circulating thyroid hormone.

26. **Ans. is (c) Provide assistants with self care needs and provide frequent rest periods**

    Progressive gradual increases in activity should be done after MI. Gradual increases in activity prevent or minimize overload of the heart and fatigue. The nurse's role is to monitor and adjust the client's activity level according to individual tolerance. Providing positive reinforcement and encouragement during physical activity and providing adequate fluid intake will not prevent or minimize activity tolerance. Administer oxygen is not the best intervention in terms of the subject activity intolerance and fatigue.

27. **Ans. is (c) Conductive hearing loss on the involved side**

    The three characteristic symptoms of Meniere's disease are tinnitus, sensorineural hearing loss on the involved side and severe vertigo accompanied by nausea and vomiting.

28. **Ans. is (a) High in calcium and low in phosphorus**

    Hypocalcemia is the result of hypoparathyroidism because of either a lack of parathyroid hormone (PTH) secretion or ineffective PTH influence on tissue. Calcium is the major controlling factor of PTH secretion. Because of this diet need to be high in calcium but low in phosphorus because these two electrolytes must exist in inverse proportions in the body. Other options are not dietary interventions hypoparathyroidism.

29. **Ans. is (a) Use of hypothermic (Cooling) blanket**

    Use a hypothermic blanks, thyroid storm is a potentially fatal acute episode of thyroid over activity characterized by high fever, severe tachycardia, delirium, dehydration and extreme irritability. Because it is an emergency, thyroid storm requires heroic interventions for control. The high fever is treated with hypothermic blanket and dehydration is reversed with intravenous fluids.

30. **Ans. is (a) Is unknown**

    Guillain-Barre syndrome is an inflammatory disease of unknown origin that involves degeneration of the myelin sheath of peripheral nerves.

31. **Ans. is (a) Milk**

    Nelfinavir is an antiviral medication used in the treatment of HIV infection. It is available in both tablet and powder form. The powder form is prepared by mixing the dose with a small amount of water, milk, soy milk or dietary supplements. The powder is not mixed with acidic foods or juices.

32. **Ans. is (d) Calcium gluconate injection**

    Toxic effects of magnesium sulfate may cause loss of deep tendon reflexes, heart block, respiratory paralysis, and cardiac arrest. The antidote for magnesium sulfate is calcium gluconate and should be available at the client's bedside.

33. **Ans. is (d) Ground beef patty**

    Clients with hepatic encephalopathy have impaired ability to convert ammonia to urea and must limit intake of protein and ammonia containing foods in the diet. The client should avoid foods, such as chicken, beef, cheese, buttermilk, onions, peanut butter, etc.

34. **Ans. is (b) Weekly**

    Blood levels are usually drawn weekly when a client beginning with lithium therapy. The literature varies somewhat and states that blood levels may be drawn initially from 3 times a week to biweekly during this phase. After therapeutic levels are achieved, blood level draws may be reduced to monthly. If levels are stable after 6–12 months, the frequency may be further reduced to every 3 months.

35. **Ans. is (c) Chills and nausea**

    Typical manifestations of acute pyelonephritis include high fever, chills, nausea and vomiting, flank pain on the affected side.

36. **Ans. is (a) Call the physician**

    The client with hyperkalemia is at risk of developing cardiac dysrhythmias and result cardiac arrest, because of this, the physician must be notified at once that the client may receive definitive treatment.

37. **Ans. is (c) Check for a return of the gag reflex**

    The nurse place highest priority on assessing for the return of the gag reflex, which is part of maintaining the client's airway.

38. **Ans. is (b) Bring the client room temperature water for washing**

    Temperature and touch or pressure are important factors to consider when caring for this postoperative client.

39. **Ans. is (b) Whether the client is allergic beparine sodium (heparin sodium)**

    Patency of ulnar artery, before drawing an arterial sample from the radial artery performs the Allen test. This involves compression of the radial and ulnar artery and then releasing either of them to determine patency of that vessel.

40. **Ans. is (a) Start an IV line**

    Vital signs indicate that she is probably going into shock. Fluids are the first action to do after assessing ABCS.

41. **Ans. is (b) Blood pressure**

    ACTH secreting tumors can cause Cushing's syndrome which can elevate the blood pressure to dangerously high levels.

42. **Ans. is (a) Hypoglycemia**

43. **Ans. is (b) Ulcerative colitis**

44. **Ans. is (d) Check the neurovascular status of the toes on the casted leg**

    An increase in pain level in an extremity is at risk for neurovascular compromise (Compartment syndrome) often is the first sign of increasing pressure within a tissue compartment.

45. **Ans. is (a) A softening of the cervix**

    Goodell's sign is an indication of pregnancy. It is a significant softening of the vaginal portion of the cervix from increased vascularization. This vascularization is a result of hypertrophy and engorgement of the vessels below the growing uterus. Others are not correct for Goodell's sign.

46. **Ans. is (d) Using a bed side commode**

    Using a bedside commode decreases the work of getting to the bathroom or struggling to use the bedpan. Elevating the client's legs increases venous return to the heart, increasing cardiac workload. The supine position increases respiratory effort and decreases oxygenation. This increases cardiac workload.

47. **Ans. is (a) Prolonged PR interval**

    A prolonged PR interval indicates first degree heart block. A widened QRS complex indicates a delay in interventricular conduction, such as bundle branch block. Tall, peaked T waves may indicate hyperkalemia. The development Q wave indicates myocardial necrosis.

48. **Ans. is (c) What leads you to seek help now?**

    A nurse's initial tasks when assessing a client in crisis is to assess the individual or family and the problem. The more clearly the problem can be defined better the chance a solution can be found. Option 'C' would assist in determinate data related to the precipitating event that led to the crisis.

49. **Ans. is (d) Polyuria**

    Hypercalcemia classically occurs with hyperparathyroidism. Elevated serum calcium levels produce osmotic dieresis.

50. **Ans. is (c) 0.25 mg**

    Calculate the dosage by weight first. The physician prescribes digoxin twice daily; two doses in 24 hrs will be administered.

51. **Ans. is: (a) Chest tube and drainage system**

    Complications following pleural biopsy include hemothorax, preumothorax and temporary pain from intercostals nerve injury. The nurse has a chest tube and drainage system available at the bedside for use if hemothorax and pneumothorax develops.

52. **Ans. is (c) Calcitonin**

    Bone remodeling is the result of osteoblastic and osteoclastic activities, which are influenced by the degree of stress that is placed on the bone to three substances which play an important role in this process are parathyroid hormone (which regulates calcium levels and bone reabsorption), vitamin D (which is active in bone formation and calcium reabsorption from bone) and calcitonin (which antagonizes parathyroid hormone and inhibits bone reabsorption).

53. **Ans. is (a) Sinus bradycardia**

    Normal sinus rhythm. Normal sinus rhythm is defined as a regular rhythm with an overall rate of 60 to 100 beats/min. The PR and QS measurements are normal, measuring 0.12 to 0.20 second and 0.04 to 0.10 sec respectively.

54. **Ans. is (a) A patient's blood pressure is 160/94 mm Hg, up from 140/90 mm Hg**

    As intracranial pressure increases, the patient becomes less alert and more difficult to rouse. This change in consciousness is one of the earliest sign of increased ICP.

55. **Ans. is (d) Increasing dietary fiber content**

    Oncovin can cause severe constipation and paralytic ileus. A prophylactic regimen, such as increasing dietary fiber, should be started against these complications at the beginning of treatment.

56. **Ans. is (d) Imposed dependence**

    It is difficult for a child to be restricted at any phase of development but the teenagers need continual positive reinforcement encouragement and as much independence as can be safely assumed during this time. Adolescents appreciate guidance and assistance regarding participation in social activities. Socialization with peers should be encouraged and every effort made to help the adolescent feel worthwhile.

57. **Ans. is (b) Activity intolerance**

    Hematocrit is an effective indicator of body fluid volume. Increased hematocrit levels can indicate shock due to a large fluid loss and hemoconcentration. Activity Intolerance would be the priority nursing diagnosis for this patient.

58. **Ans. is (d) Notify the physician**

    Discomfort postcataract surgery should be minimal to moderate and may be relieved by use of acetaminophen. Severe pain and nausea are not characteristic in the patient who has had cataract surgery. The physician should be notified immediately to prevent damage to the eye.

59. **Ans. is (a) Agranulocytosis**

    Glipizide is a second-generation sulfonylurea agent used to treat type 2 diabetes mellitus in patients with some pancreatic beta-cell function remaining. While hypoglycemia is the most common side effect, this drug can also cause hematologic reactions, such as agranulocytosis.

60. **Ans. is (b) Increased PaO_2**

    Based on the change in therapy, the nurse should anticipate an increased PaO_2. PEEP causes a constant increase in the pressure in the airways and alveoli, helping them to stay open. PEEP is usually needed to maintain adequate blood oxygen levels in acute respiratory distress syndrome (ARDS).

61. **Ans. is (b) Vascular dementia is the result of many small strokes damaging areas of the brain**

    Vascular (or multi infarct) dementia is second only to Alzheimer's disease in incidence. Multiple small cerebral infarctions, or small strokes, result in multi-infarct dementia. Cerebral damage occurs because of disruption of blood supply to the brain.

62. **Ans. is (b) Delirium**

    Delirium has an abrupt onset and usually manifests in impaired orientation, recent and immediate memory impairment and variable psychomotor behaviors. In delirium, the cause lie outside the nervous system. The severity of delirium is related to the physiologic disturbance and degree of cerebral oedema. Both can occur with renal insufficiency. Symptoms often are worse at night.

63. **Ans. is (a) False imprisonment**

    There is no indication for the use of seclusion with this patient. The use of seclusion or restraint that is not defensible as being necessary and is the clients best interest may result in false imprisonment of the client and liability for the nurse.

64. **Ans. is (a) PRN order for restraints is unacceptable**

    Physical restraints, usually leather strips, are used to immobilize a person who is clearly dangerous to self or others. In almost all cases, a specific physicians order is required for each episode, as is clearly documented evidence that the restraints were needed. A standing PRN order in not legally sufficient.

65. **Ans. is (a) Multiple serum chorionic gonadotropin levels will be drawn**

    Frequent serum chorionic gonadotropin levels will be needed until the level falls below normal and stays there for three weeks monthly levels will be drawn for six months, and then bimonthly levels are drawn for the remainder of the year.

66. **Ans. is (d) Fatigue related to hyperactivity**

    A patient with a bipolar disorder displays excessive and constant motor activity and is unable to sleep or eat for several days. Fatigue related to hyperactivity is a priority concern for this patient, and nursing care must be directed toward preventing exhaustion and cardiac collapse.

67. **Ans. is (d) Applying direct pressure to the esophagus**

    The Sengstaken-Blakemore tube has a small gastric balloon that anchors the tube and applies pressure to the area of the cardiac sphincter. The large esophageal balloon applies direct pressure on the bleeding sites in the esophagus. A tube passing through the balloons allows for aspiration and irrigation.

68. **Ans. is (a) 170 calories**

    Each liter of 5% dextrose in normal saline solution contains 170 calories. The nurse should consult with the physician and dietician when a client is on intravenous therapy or in NPO for any extended period, because further electrolyte supplementation or alimentation therapy may be needed.

69. **Ans. is (d) Dark-red skin, testes undescended with few rugations, and abundant lanugos**

    These signs are all indicative of a gestational age of less than 40 weeks. Lanugos and vernix are shed in utero as the foetus matures. Palmar and plantar creases increase with age. Development in the ears, breast tissue, and scrotum occurs with age. Testes begin descent at approximately 36 weeks of gestation. Dark-red skin in the premature infant is reflective of lack of subcutaneous fat. Parchment like skin is typical of the position infant.

70. **Ans. is (c) Restricted fluid intake**

    When bed rest is prescribed for a client, fluids are increased, not decreased in order to prevent urinary stasis.

71. **Ans. is (c) ½ peanut butter sandwich, apple slice and ½ cup hot cocoa**

    Children with nephrosis need low sodium, high protein diet to combat edema. This snack in highest in potassium and protein and low in sodium.

72. **Ans. is (c) It is the result of an imbalance of chemicals in the brain**

    Bipolar disorder is a biochemical disorder caused by an imbalance of neurotransmitter in the brain. Manic episodes seem to be related to excessive levels of norepinephrine, serotonin, and dopamine. Bipolar disorder could be genetic or inherited from someone in the family. But, it is best for the client and family to understand the disease concept related to neurotransmitter imbalance.

73. **Ans. is (c) Your child needs all of the medicine so that the infection clears**

    Frequently when a child appears better, the parents stop the medication. Unfortunately the infection remains. Therefore the nurse needs to explain that all of the medication is needed to clear up the infection.

74. **Ans. is (d) Maintain fluid and electrolyte balance**

    The importance of the fluid therapy of a client is to maintain fluid and electrolyte balance. I.V. fluids are required to replace the fluid and electrolyte loss.

75. **Ans. is (d) Administering morphine**

    The third degree burns are the most dangerous type of burns.

76. **Ans. is (c) Keep the right leg elevated above heart level**

    The extremity should be kept elevated, and apply some heat for treat the inflammation and pain, this gets decrease chances of dislodging a thrombus.

77. **Ans. is (a) Give the telephone number of safe shelter and advice her use this if necessary**

    Give the telephone numbers of safe shelter and advice her use this if necessary. It is the most appropriate step that the nurse should provide the information about safe shelters to the lady.

78. **Ans. is (b) If happened from person to person by direct relation**

    Pediculosis (body louse infestation) is not happened from animals and it only got from the direct contacts among the people.

79. **Ans. is (c) Ototoxicity**

    Ototoxicity is a serious side effect of gentamycin. Tinnitus and dizziness are common.

80. **Ans. is (a) Vesicular**

    Vesicular breath sounds are normal breath sounds, which is heard over all healthy lung field, except the main bronchi.

81. **Ans. is (a) Increased fluid intake**

    Promotion of urinary continence is the main target and tried to increase fluid intake and timed voiding.

82. **Ans. is (c) A two-bed room with no other patients**

    Diarrhea makes high risk of infection and it is important to prevent it. The best thing is place the diarrhea patient in a private room.

83. **Ans. is (c) Rice cereal, apple juice, formula**

    Rice, cereal, apple juice, and formula are suitable foods for the 6 months old infant whole milk, orange juice and eggs are not suitable for the young infant.

84. **Ans. is (b) You will be given medicine to relax you during the treatment**

    The client will receive medication that relaxes skeletal muscles and produces mild sedation.

85. **Ans. is (b) With meals and snacks**

    Pancreatic enzyme replacement is given with each meal and each snack.

86. **Ans. is (b) Weighing the client after she eats**

    Having a staff member remain with the client for 1 hrs after meals will help to prevent self-induced vomiting.

87. **Ans. is (c) The client will need a regularly scheduled CBC**

    Adverse effect or side effect of dilantin includes agranulocytosis and aplastic anemia. Therefore, the client will need frequent CBCs.

88. **Ans. is (b) The patient should limit fatty foods**

    Cholecystitis is the inflammation of the gall bladder, is most commonly caused by the presence of gall stones which may block bile from entering the intestine. Patient should decrease dietary fat by, imiting foods like fatty meats, fried foods, etc.

89. **Ans. is (b) Hypoglycemia**

    A postoperative patient with DM who is unable to eat is likely to be suffering from hypoglycemia; confusion and shakiness are common symptoms. Anesthesia reaction would not occur on the second postoperative day.

90. **Ans. is (d) Hypokalemia**

91. **Ans. is (b) Examine the bleeding under the client**

92. **Ans. is (c) Instructing about early signs of wound infection.**

93. **Ans. is (c) Full thickness**

94. **Ans. is (b) High in calcium and low in phosphorus**

95. **Ans. is (d) Respiratory acidosis**

96. **Ans. is (c) Urine for glucose and ketones**

97. **Ans. is (d) Position the client on her side**

98. **Ans. is (b) Decreased temperature**

99. **Ans. is (d) Verapamil**

100. **Ans. is (d) Position the client in semi high Fowler's position with support to back**

     ARDS produce severe dyspnea and life-threatening abnormalities of blood gases; therefore, positioning the client in upright position will promote gas exchange and help to relieve dyspnea. The client with ARDS requires high oxygen usually by mask or ventilator.

Part 2

1. **What is the first priority to do in a patient with burn?**
   a. Check pulse
   b. Check breathing
   c. Open the airway
   d. Intravenous fluids
   e. Coverage of the patient

2. **What is not true about placenta previa?**
   a. Do vaginal examination to evaluate the presenting part
   b. Painless vaginal bleeding
   c. Administer betamethasone
   d. CBR is required

3. **Which of the following discharge teachings to include in patient with cataract to prevent increase of IOP?**
   a. Avoid ambulation, with comfort room privileges
   b. Work with lifting up to 7 kg
   c. Daily exercise
   d. Drug instructions

4. **A nurse is putting together an educational seminar on advance directives. What information would be included in the materials?**
   a. A patient may change a treatment decision in an advance directive if the patient's health care agent approves the change.
   b. When admitted to the hospital, a patient must appoint a Durable Power of Attorney for health care decisions.
   c. A health care facility must provide a patient informational material advising them of their rights to declare their desires concerning treatment decisions.
   d. A health care facility is required to provide a patient an attorney when the patient is signing a living will.

5. A nurse provides dietary instruction to the parents of a child with a diagnosis of cystic fibrosis. The nurse tells the parents that the diet should be:
   a. Fat free
   b. Low in protein
   c. Low in sodium
   d. High in calories
6. Which of the following factors should be the primary focus of nursing management in a patient with acute pancreatitis?
   a. Nutritional management
   b. Fluid and electrolyte balance
   c. Management of hypoglycemia
   d. Pain control
7. Patient is prone of having bed sores, what would be the best nursing intervention you could do?
   a. Massage the bony prominences
   b. Use moisturizing lotion on dry skin
   c. Move the patient on sliding motion
   d. Wash the skin with warm water and soap
8. A nurse in the newborn nursery is planning for the admission of a large for gestational age (LGA) infant. In preparing to care for this infant, the nurse obtains equipment to perform. Which diagnostic test?
   a. Serum insulin level
   b. Heel stick blood glucose
   c. Rh and ABO blood typing
   d. Indirect and direct bilirubin levels
9. The nurse is admitting a client with a diagnosis of hypothyroidism to the hospital. The nurse performs which of the following that will pro-vide data related to this diagnosis?
   a. Inspects facial features
   b. Auscultates lung sounds
   c. Percusses the thyroid gland
   d. Assesses the client's ability to ambulate
10. While a client is being prepared for discharge, the nasogastric (NG) feeding tube becomes clogged. Teach the client's family how to deal with it at home, what should the nurse do?
    a. Irrigate the tube with cola
    b. Advance the tube into the intestine
    c. Apply intermittent suction to the tube
    d. Withdraw the obstruction with a 30 ml syringe
11. A client is ordered to start receiving digoxin 0.25 mg P.O. Which parameter should be checked first before administering digoxin?
    a. Apical pulse
    b. Blood pressure
    c. Radial pulse
    d. Respiratory rate
12. In what position should the nurse place the head of the bed to obtain the most accurate reading of jugular vein distention?
    a. High Fowler's
    b. Raised 10 degree
    c. Raised 30 degree
    d. Supine
13. When assessing for a patient on chemotherapy, for CA esophagus what can we expect?
    a. Alopecia
    b. Hyper salivation
    c. Gingivitis
    d. Peptic ulcer
14. Macewen's sign is a manifestation of which disease?
    a. Hydrocephalus
    b. Meningitis
    c. Appendicitis
    d. cerebral palsy
15. A nurse is advising a patient with chronic fatigue syndrome on infection control procedures. Which of the following statements by the patient indicates that the patient understands the advice?
    a. I'm going to a basketball game tonight.
    b. I should avoid anyone with cold symptoms.
    c. I should have a blood test.
    d. I'm not going to attend functions with large crowds.
16. The nurse is caring for a client with a spinal cord injury who has spinal shock. The nurse performs an assessment on the client, knowing that which assessment will provide the best information about recovery from spinal shock?
    a. Reflexes
    b. Pulse rate
    c. Temperature
    d. Blood pressure
17. Why is there a need for licensure exam for the nurse?
    a. To ensure minimum knowledge
    b. To ensure excellent knowledge in specialized area
    c. To assess if the nurse fit to practice
    d. To assess continuing
18. Which of the following medications is not given to the patient with pulmonary embolism?
    a. Heparin
    b. Warfarin

c. Streptokinase
d. Digoxin

19. What is the first nursing intervention for the MI patients?
    a. Morphine and Aspirin
    b. Morphine
    c. Morphine and Oxygen
    d. Aspirin

20. Which of the following neurologic changes indicates that the client is in the progressive stage of shock?
    a. Restlessness
    b. Confusion
    c. Incoherent speech
    d. Unconsciousness

21. The nurse is caring for a male client with a diagnosis of chronic gastritis. The nurse monitors the client knowing that this client is at risk for which vitamin deficiency?
    a. Vitamin A
    b. Vitamin B12
    c. Vitamin C
    d. Vitamin E

22. Patient arrived in emergency room with severe burn and on shock. What would be the best fluids you could give?
    a. 0.9 sodium chloride with 70% albumin solution
    b. D25 solution
    c. 0.45% sodium chloride injection
    d. D5 water

23. The client sustains a contusion of the eyeball following a traumatic injury with a blunt object. Which intervention is initiated immediately?
    a. Notify the physician
    b. Irrigate the eye with cold water
    c. Apply ice to the affected eye
    d. Accompany the client to the emergency room

24. In which of the following ways can the nurse promote the sense of taste for an older adult?
    a. Mix foods together on the dinner tray
    b. Avoid cologne, air freshners, or room deodorizers
    c. Encourage the client to chew food thoroughly
    d. Discourage the use of salt or seasonings with prepared food

25. Physiological integrity to enhance the percutaneous absorption of nitroglycerine ointment, it would be MOST important for the nurse to select a site that is:
    a. Muscular
    b. Near the heart
    c. Nonhairy
    d. In legs

26. Which of the following clients is at highest risk for colorectal cancer?
    a. The client who smokes
    b. The client who has been treated for Crohn's disease for 20 years
    c. The client who has a family history of lung cancer
    d. The client who eats a vegetarian diet

27. The registered nurse will be assisting in admitting Ms. McNamara for observation and post procedure care after undergone esophagogastroduodenoscopy (EGD). The nurse would plan to do which of the following first once Ms. McNamara arrives?
    a. Measure Ms. McNamara's temperature
    b. Monitor Ms. McNamara's nasoesophageal pH level
    c. Monitor Ms. McNamara for the return of the gag reflex
    d. Give Ms. McNamara warm water

28. Which of these steps in the administration of eye drops to a client is correct?
    a. Warming the medication to body temperature
    b. Having the client look downward as the head is tilted forward before administration
    c. Placing the number of prescribed drops directly on the cornea.
    d. Applying gentle finger pressure to the client's inner canthus for one or two minutes after administration.

29. Mr. Mathew has orders for a physical therapy consult. The nurse contacts the appropriate department but 12 hours later, no one has come to see the client. Which is the most appropriate action of the nurse?
    a. Call the supervisor and file a complaint against the physical therapy department
    b. Contact the physician to notify him that the orders were not carried out
    c. Assess the client's activity level by assisting with ambulation using a gait belt
    d. Contact the physical therapy department again and repeat the order

30. Which of the following nursing interventions is appropriate for a client who is suffering from a fever?
    a. Avoid giving the client food
    b. Increase the client's fluid volume

c. Provide oxygen
d. All of the above
e. Both b and c

31. **A nurse is assessing an African American client for risks of a pressure ulcer. Which of the following best describes what the nurse might find with an early pressure ulcer in this client?**
    a. Skin has a purple/bluish color
    b. Capillary refill is 1 second
    c. Skin appears blanched at the pressure site
    d. Tenting appears when checking skin turgor

32. **Clients with type I diabetes may require which of the following changes to their daily routine during periods of infection?**
    a. No changes
    b. Less insulin
    c. More insulin
    d. Oral ant diabetic agents

33. **Calcitonin should be administered for patient with hypercalcemia, which route nurse use:**
    a. Intradermal
    b. Subcutaneous
    c. Intramuscular
    d. Oral

34. **Which of the following is classified as a prerenal condition that affects urinary elimination?**
    a. Nephrotoxic medications
    b. Pericardial tamponade
    c. Neurogenic bladder
    d. Polycystic kidney disease

35. **A client has been diagnosed with a form of terminal cancer and has started receiving hospice care. The nurse notes that both the client and his family avoid talking about the diagnosis. All attempts at discussion result in changing the subject. The nurse recognizes that this family is exhibiting:**
    a. Closed awareness
    b. Mutual pretense
    c. Open awareness
    d. Powerless assessment

36. **An RN at night duty what to make to net feel sleepy?**
    a. Wash her face frequently
    b. Wear cloth not make her warm
    c. Make frequent round for patients
    d. All of the above

37. **Overweight nurse is planning to reduce weight, how much calories should reduce daily, to lose 1lb/week**
    a. 500 calories
    b. 1000 calories
    c. 3000 calories
    d. 5000 calories

38. **A nurse caring for a child with congestive heart failure who will be discharged to home provides instructions to the parents regarding the administration of digoxin (Lanoxin).Which statement by the mother indicates a need for further instructions?**
    a. I will mix the medication with food.
    b. I will check my child's pulse before giving the medication.
    c. If my child vomits after I give the medication, I will not repeat the dose.
    d. I will check the dose of medication with my husband before I give the medication.

39. **When feeding a patient with gastrostomy tube, which of the following intervention should be the nurse's priority:**
    a. Elevate HOB at least 30
    b. Initially flush the ostomy with 30 ml water
    c. Check patency by auscultation
    d. Heat formula in room temperature

40. **Which is the test for long standing hyperglycemia**
    a. Random blood sugar
    b. Fasting blood sugar
    c. Oral glucose tolerance
    d. HbA1c

41. **Which ensures the effectiveness of atropine administration to a preoperative patient you should check:**
    a. Pulse rate
    b. Dryness of the mouth
    c. Blood pressure
    d. Pupil constriction

42. **The best position for a patient having burn in his head and neck is :**
    a. High Fowler
    b. Prone
    c. Semi Fowler
    d. Supine

43. **The doctor ordered 2000 ml of a solution to be given in 24 hrs. How should the nurse give the solution?**
    a. Give 1000 cc regulate at 83 cc/hr then replace after 12 hrs
    b. Give 1000 cc, regulate at 42 cc/hr then replace after 12 hrs
    c. Give 500 cc, regulate at 83 cc/hr then replace after 12 hrs
    d. Give 500 cc, regulate at 42cc/hr then replace after 12 hrs

44. The following clients present to a walk-in clinic at the same time. Which should the nurse schedule to be seen first?
    a. 25 years old with high fever, vomiting and diarrhea
    b. 38 years old with sore throat, fever, and swollen lymph glands
    c. 40 years old with severe headache, vomiting and stiff neck
    d. 44 year old limping on a very swollen bruised ankle

45. Test results indicate that your patient is HIV positive. The patient has stated that her choice of infant feeding is breast milk. Your postpartum plan of care should be based on the knowledge that:
    a. Breastfeeding should be encouraged for all new mothers to foster maternal child bonding.
    b. Formula feeding should be encouraged because the mother is not likely to live long enough to successfully breastfeed the infant
    c. The mother's HIV status should not influence her decision on how to feed her infant.
    d. Breastfeeding is contraindicated for HIV positive mothers

46. A nursing assistant tells the charge nurse that another nursing assistant never cleans up the utility room at the end of the shift. The most effective approach to resolving the conflict would be to:
    a. Acknowledge that the nursing assistant who is supposed to clean the utility room may feel overworked.
    b. Tell the nursing assistant who never helps clean that she needs to help
    c. Bring both parties together to discuss underlying issues of conflict
    d. Develop a schedule for rotating responsibility for the department's utility room

47. A patient is admitted to the unit with a tentative diagnosis of Hodgkin's disease. Which of the following findings are most significant in supporting this diagnosis?
    a. Change in mental status
    b. Dependent edema
    c. Distended abdomen
    d. Enlarged lymph nodes

48. Which of the following statements, if made by a 44 yrs old female, would support a nursing diagnosis of knowledge deficit: early detection of breast cancer?
    a. I should not examine my breast or have mammogram during my menstrual period
    b. I include the underarm area when I examine my breasts
    c. Women who practice regular breast examination find breast lumps earlier than women who do not
    d. Breast self-examination is not necessary if I get regular mammograms

49. ABCD in cancer EXCEPT?
    a. Asymmetry in shape
    b. Border irregularities
    c. Color is not uniform
    d. Diameter >6 mm

50. A transparent film dressing used for what kind of wound?
    a. Minor burn
    b. Draining wound
    c. Pressure ulcer
    d. Full thickness burn

51. Pain behind eyes
    a. Migraine
    b. Cluster headache
    c. Tension headache
    d. Headache

52. The nurse is caring for a client who is scheduled to have a hysterectomy. The nurse understands that the more common conditions requiring a hysterectomy are:
    a. Polyps
    b. Fibroids
    c. Vaginal prolapsed
    d. Prolonged bleeding

53. 12 weeks pregnant rush to emergency hospital with vaginal bleeding. The nurse should know?
    a. d and c
    b. Use gram HCG to monitor her
    c. Spontaneous abortion
    d. Instruct bed rest to reduce further vaginal bleeding

54. When feeding a patient with gastrostomy tube, which of the following intervention should be the nurse's priority?
    a. Elevate HOB at least 30
    b. Initially flush the ostomy with 30 ml water
    c. Check patency by auscultation
    d. Heat formula in room temperature

55. In dealing with a severely depressed client what is essential with regards to therapeutic communication
    a. The process is focused on the patient
    b. Nurse-patient process recording

c. Show sympathy
d. Divulge nurse's personal info to gain the client's trust

56. Mother who is O-, she should receive rhogam if she delivers:
   a. A+ baby
   b. Baby
   c. O+ baby
   d. O- Baby

57. Which of the following vaccine when administered may tamper the result of a tuberculin test?
   a. Diphtheria
   b. Tetanus
   c. Varicella
   d. MMR

58. A school age child has been hospitalized to roll out congenial heart disease. What room you should place the child?
   a. Multi bed room with another child
   b. Two beds with 1 adult
   c. Private room
   d. Respiratory isolation

59. Corticosteroids are potent suppressors of the body's inflammatory response. Which of the following conditions or actions do they suppress?
   a. Cushing syndrome
   b. Pain receptors
   c. Immune response
   d. Neural transmission

60. After starting hemodialysis, your patient starts complaining of abdominal pain, you should:
   a. Stop – discontinue – dialysis
   b. Continue dialysis
   c. Put patient on supine position
   d. Give patient diuretics and continue dialysis

61. Position for asthma in adult and child?
   a. Sitting position (upright position)
   b. Prone position
   c. Standing position
   d. Supine positions

62. Patient had sunstroke, what hemodynamic results may result:
   a. Respiratory acidosis
   b. Respiratory alkalosis
   c. Metabolic acidosis
   d. Metabolic alkalosis

63. A patient is agitated, lethargy and dry mouth was rush to emergency unit with potassium level of 5.8 meq/L and sodium of 135 meq/L. What would be the anticipated solution to be use to correct the problem?
   a. Dextrose 5% water
   b. Lactated ringers solution
   c. 1/2 normal saline with 4 meq Kcl
   d. Normal saline solution

64. The most common cause of Melena is?
   a. Colorectal cancer
   b. Anal fissure
   c. Hemorrhoid
   d. Peptic ulcer disease

65. The person responsible for collaborating the care of patients in a surgical team is?
   a. Circulating nurse
   b. First assistant
   c. Scrub nurse
   d. Surgeon

66. What solution to administer to cause fluid shift into cell
   a. Hypotonic
   b. Hypertonic
   c. Isotonic
   d. Colloid

67. You are caring for a client who is newly diagnosed with renal failure and has recently started on peritoneal dialysis. During the infusion of the dialysate, the client begins to complain of abdominal pain. Which action by the nurse is appropriate?
   a. Slow the infusion
   b. Explain that the pain will subside after the first few exchanges.
   c. Decrease the amount to be infused.
   d. Stop the dialysis

68. A nurse caring for a client with hypocalcemia would expect to note which of the following changes on the electrocardiogram?
   a. Widened T wave
   b. Prominent U wave
   c. Prolonged QT interval
   d. Shortened ST segment

69. The most common and serious complication of burns that often lead to death is:
   a. Hypovolemic shock
   b. Hypothermia
   c. Sepsis.
   d. Infection

70. The type of burn in which all the dermis and epidermis, is destroyed and there is involvement of underlying structures is called:
   a. Superficial or first degree burn
   b. Partial thickness or second degree burn

c. Full-thickness or third degree burn
d. Fourth degree burn

71. Which situation should have standard precaution other than using gloves?
    a. Barium enema administration
    b. Interstitial radiation on oral cancer
    c. Renal arteriogram
    d. Vomiting patient on brachytherapy

72. The nurse admits a client who is in sickle cell crisis to the hospital. Which does the nurse prepare as the priority in the management of the client?
    a. Pain management
    b. Fluid administration
    c. Oxygen administration
    d. Red blood cell transfusion

73. During breastfeeding, mother complaints of breast pains. The nurse tells the mother that after pains are more painful due to secretion of?
    a. Oxytocin
    b. Prolactin
    c. Estrogen
    d. Progesterone

74. What solution makes fluid to go into the cell?
    a. Isotonic
    b. Isometric
    c. Hypertonic
    d. Hypotonic

75. What type of anemia needs frequent checking of feet?
    a. Sickle cell
    b. Polycythemia vera
    c. Pernicious
    d. Thalassemia

76. When administering mannitol for raised ICP, which one of the following lab tests is the priority?
    a. Serum arginine vasopressin (AVP)
    b. Urine specific gravity
    c. Serum creatinine
    d. Serum osmolality

77. A patient is prescribed with drug bleomycin. Which of the following test will be prescribed for the client?
    a. Liver function test
    b. Glucose tolerance test
    c. Pulmonary function test
    d. Creatinine clearance test

78. The nurse is teaching a mother whose daughter has iron deficiency anemia. The nurse determines the parent understood the dietary modifications, if she selects?
    a. Bread and coffee
    b. Fish and Pork meat
    c. Cookies and milk
    d. Oranges and green leafy vegetables

79. Which of the following is the most common clinical manifestation of G6PD following ingestion of aspirin?
    a. Kidney failure
    b. Acute hemolytic anemia
    c. Hemophilia A
    d. Thalassemia

80. The nurse assesses a client with an ileostomy for possible development of which of the following acid-base imbalances?
    a. Respiratory acidosis
    b. Metabolic acidosis
    c. Metabolic alkalosis
    d. Respiratory alkalosis

81. The nurse anticipates which of the following response in a client who develops metabolic acidosis.
    a. Heart rate of 105 beats/min
    b. Urinary output of 15 ml
    c. Respiratory rate of 30 beats/min
    d. Temperature of 39 degree Celsius

82. A client has a phosphorus level of 5.0 mg/dL. The nurse closely monitors the client for?
    a. Signs of tetany
    b. Elevated blood glucose
    c. Cardiac dysrhythmias
    d. Hypoglycemia

83. A nurse is caring for a child with pyloric stenosis. The nurse would watch out for symptoms of?
    a. Vomiting large amounts
    b. Watery stool
    c. Projectile vomiting
    d. Dark-colored stool

84. The nurse responder finds a patient unresponsive in his house. Arrange steps for adult CPR.
    a. Assess consciousness
    b. Give 2 breaths
    c. Perform chest compression
    d. Check for serious bleeding and shock
    e. Open patient's airway
    f. Check breathing

85. Which of the following is mostly likely to occur, when there is continuous bubbling in the water seal chamber of the closed chest drainage system?
    a. The connection has been taped too tightly
    b. The connection tubes are kinked

c. Lung expansion
   d. Air leak in the system
86. Which of the following young adolescent and adult male clients are at most risks for testicular cancer?
   a. Basketball player who wears supportive gear during basketball games
   b. Teenager who swims on a varsity swim team
   c. 20-year-old with undescended testis
   d. Patient with a family history of colon cancer
87. The nurse plans to frequently assess a post-thyroidectomy patient for?
   a. Polyuria
   b. Hypoactive deep tendon reflex
   c. Hypertension
   d. Laryngospasm
88. An 18-month-old baby appears to have a rounded belly, bowlegs and slightly large head. The nurse concludes?
   a. The child appears to be a normal toddler
   b. The child is developmentally delayed
   c. The child is malnourished
   d. The child's large head may have neurological problems.
89. Several patients from a reported condominium fire incident were rushed to the emergency room. Which should the nurse attend first?
   a. A 15-year-old girl, with burns on the face and chest, reports hoarseness of the voice
   b. A 28-year-old man with burns on all extremities
   c. A 4-year-old child who is crying inconsolably and reports severe headache
   d. A 40-year-old woman with complaints of severe pain on the left thigh
90. An appropriate instruction to be included in the discharge teaching of a patient following a spinal fusion is?
   a. Don't use the stairs
   b. Don't bend at the waist
   c. Don't walk for long hours
   d. Swimming should be avoided
91. A nurse is preparing to give an IM injection of iron dextran that is irritating to the subcutaneous tissue. To prevent irritation to the tissue, what is the best action to be taken?
   a. Apply ice over the injection site
   b. Administer drug at a 45 degree angle
   c. Use a 24-gauge needle
   d. Use the z-track technique

92. What should a nurse do prior to taking the patient's history?
   a. Offer the patient a glass of water
   b. Establish rapport
   c. Ask the patient to disrobe and put on gown
   d. Ask pertinent information for insurance purposes
93. A pregnant woman is admitted with pre-eclampsia. The nurse would include in the health teaching that magnesium will be part of the medical management to accomplish the following?
   a. Control seizures
   b. promote renal perfusion
   c. To decrease sustained contractions
   d. Maintain intrauterine homeostasis
94. A nurse is going to administer ear drops to a 4-year-old child. What is the correct way of instilling the medicine after tilting the patient's head sidewards?
   a. Pull the pinna back then downward
   b. Pull the pinna back then upward
   c. Pull the pinna up then backward
   d. Pull the pinna down then backward
95. A nursing student was intervened by the clinical instructor if which of the following is observed?
   a. Inserting a nasogastric tube
   b. Positioning the infant in a "sniffing "position
   c. Suctioning first the mouth, then the nose
   d. Squeezing the bulb syringe to suction mouth
96. Choose amongst the options illustrated below that best describes the angle for an intradermal injection?

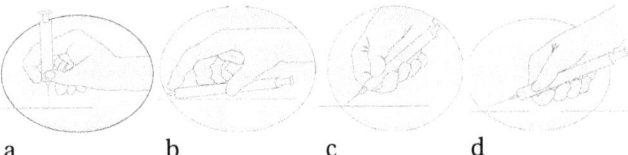

a   b   c   d

97. During a basic life support class, the instructor said that blind finger sweeping is not advisable for infants. Which among the following could be the reason?
   a. The mouth is still too small
   b. The object may be pushed deeper into the throat
   c. Sharp fingernails might injure the victim
   d. The infant might bite
98. A nurse enters a room and finds a patient lying on the floor. Which of the following actions should the nurse perform first?
   a. Call for help
   b. Establish responsiveness of patient
   c. Ask the patient what happened
   d. Assess vital signs

99. A patient with complaints of chest pain was rushed to the emergency department. Which priority action should the nurse do first?
    a. Administer morphine sulfate intravenously
    b. Initiate venous access by performing venipunture
    c. Administer oxygen via nasal cannula
    d. Complete physical assessment and patient history

100. A rehabilitation nurse reviews a post-stroke patient's immunization history. Which immunization is a priority for a 72-year-old patient?
    a. Hepatitis A vaccine
    b. Hepatitis B vaccine
    c. Rotavirus Vaccine
    d. Pneumococcal vaccine

Answers (Part 2)

1. Ans. is (c) Open the airway
2. Ans. is (a) Do vaginal examination to evaluate the presenting part
3. Ans. is (b) Work with lifting up to 7 kg
4. Ans. is (c) A health care facility must provide a patient informational material advising them of their rights to declare their desires concerning treatment decisions.
5. Ans. is (d) High in calories
6. Ans. is (d) Pain control
7. Ans. is (b) Use moisturizing lotion on dry skin
8. Ans. is (b) Heel stick blood glucose
9. Ans. is (a) Inspects facial features
10. Ans. is (a) Irrigate the tube with cola
11. Ans. is (a) Apical pulse
12. Ans. is (c) Raised 30 degree
13. Ans. is (b) Hypersalivation
14. Ans. is (a) Hydrocephalus
15. Ans. is (b) I should avoid anyone with cold symptoms
16. Ans. is (a) Reflexes
17. Ans. is (c) To assess if the nurse fit to practice
18. Ans. is (d) Digoxin
19. Ans. is (c) Morphine and oxygen
20. Ans. is (a) Restlessness
21. Ans. is (b) Vitamin B12
22. Ans. is (a) 0.9 sodium chloride with 70% albumin solution
23. Ans. is (c) Apply ice to the affected eye
24. Ans. is (c) Encourage the client to chew food thoroughly
25. Ans. is (c) Nonhairy.
26. Ans. is (b) The client who has been treated for Crohn's disease for 20 years
27. Ans. is (c) Monitor Ms. McNamara for the return of the gag reflex
28. Ans. is (d) Applying gentle finger pressure to the client's inner canthus for one or two minutes after administration.
29. Ans. is (d) Contact the physical therapy department again and repeat the order
30. Ans. is (e) Both b and c
31. Ans. is (a) Skin has a purple/bluish color
32. Ans. is (c) More insulin
33. Ans. is (c) Intramuscular
34. Ans. is (b) Pericardial tamponade
35. Ans. is (b) Mutual pretense
36. Ans. is (c) Make frequent round for patients
37. Ans. is (a) 500 calories
38. Ans. is (a) I will mix the medication with food
39. Ans. is (a) Elevate HOB at least 30
40. Ans. is (d) HbA1c
41. Ans. is (b) Dryness of the mouth
42. Ans. is (c) Semi Fowler
43. Ans. is (a) Give 1000 cc regulate at 83 cc/hr then replace after 12 hrs

    What mL/hour setting on the pump will you use to run an IV for 24 hours and infuse 2000 mL?

    $24x = 2000$

    $x = 2000/24$

    $= 83$ mL/hour

    Note: The answer is 83.333, but you must round to a whole number for the pump setting.

44. Ans. is (c) 40 years old with severe headache, vomiting and stiff neck
45. Ans. is (d) Breastfeeding is contraindicated for HIV-positive mothers

46. Ans. is (c) Bring both parties together to discuss underlying issues of conflict
47. Ans. is (d) Enlarged lymph nodes
48. Ans. is (d) Breast self-examination is not necessary if I get regular mammograms
49. Ans. is (d) Diameter >6 mm
50. Ans. is (b) Draining wound
51. Ans. is (b) Cluster headache
52. Ans. is (d) Prolonged bleeding
53. Ans. is (c) Spontaneous abortion
54. Ans. is (a) Elevate HOB at least 30
55. Ans. is (a) The process is focused on the patient
56. Ans. is (c) O+ baby
57. Ans. is (d) MMR
58. Ans. is (a) Multi bedroom with another child
59. Ans. is (c) Immune response
60. Ans. is (a) Stop – discontinue – dialysis
61. Ans. is (a) Sitting position (upright position)
62. Ans. is (c) Metabolic acidosis
63. Ans. is (a) Dextrose 5% water
64. Ans. is (d) Peptic ulcer disease. The peptic ulcer results in bleeding and thereby leads to melena or tarry color stools
65. Ans. is (a) Circulating nurse
66. Ans. is (a) Hypotonic
67. Ans. is (b) Explain that the pain will subside after the first few exchanges.
68. Ans. is (c) Prolonged QT interval
69. Ans. is (a) Hypovolemic shock
70. Ans. is (c) Full-thickness or third degree burn
71. Ans. is (d) Vomiting patient on brachytherapy
72. Ans. is (b) Fluid administration
73. Ans. is (a) Oxytocin
74. Ans. is (d) Hypotonic
75. Ans. is (a) Sickle cell
76. Ans. is (a) Serum arginine vasopressin (AVP)
77. Ans. is (c) Pulmonary function test
78. Ans. is (d) Oranges and green leafy vegetables

    Dark green leafy vegetables are good sources of iron. Oranges are good sources of vitamin C that enhances iron absorption in the small intestines.
79. Ans. is (b) Acute hemolytic anemia

    Individuals with G6PD may exhibit hemolytic anemia when exposed to infection, certain medications or chemicals. Salicylates, such as Aspirin damages plasma membranes of erythrocytes, leading to hemolytic anemia.
80. Ans. is (b) Metabolic acidosis

    Lower GI fluids are alkaline in nature and can be lost via ileostomy. Thus, loss of HCO_3, results to metabolic acidosis.
81. Ans. is (c) Respiratory rate of 30 beats/min

    Initially, respiratory system will try to compensate metabolic acidosis. Patients with metabolic acidosis have high respiratory rate.
82. Ans. is (a) Signs of tetany

    Normal phosphorus level is 2.5-4.5 mg/dL. The level reflects hyperphosphatemia which is inversely proportional to calcium. Client should be assessed for tetany which is a prominent symptom of hypocalcemia.
83. Ans. is (c) Projectile vomiting

    Clinical manifestations of pyloric Stenosis include projectile vomiting, irritability, constipation, and signs of dehydration, including a decrease in urine output.
84. Ans. is (a, e, f, c, b, d)

    In accordance with the new guidelines, remembers **AB-CABS**. **A**—airway **B**—breathing normally? **C**—chest compression, **A**—airway open, **B**—breathing for patient, **S**—serious bleeding, shock, spinal injury. The nurse should first assess consciousness of the patient. Next, open patient's airway to check for breathing. When there is no breathing, immediately perform chest compression then give 2 breaths, do the cycle of care over. Finally, check for serious bleeding, shock, and spinal injury.
85. Ans. is (d) Air leak in the system

    Continuous bubbling seen in water-seal bottle/chamber indicates an air leak or loose connection, and air is sucked continuously into the closed chest drainage system.
86. Ans. is (c) 20-year-old with undescended testis

    Testicular cancer is most likely to affect males in late adolescence. Undescended testis is also one major risk for testicular cancer.
87. Ans. is (d) Laryngospasm

    Hypocalcemia occurs when there is accidental removal or destruction of parathyroid tissue during surgical removal of the thyroid gland. Laryngospasm is one of the clinical manifestations of tetany, an indicator of hypocalcemia.
88. Ans. is (a) The child appears to be a normal toddler

    It's normal for a toddler to have bowlegs and a protruding belly. The head still appears somewhat large in proportion from the rest of the body.

89. **Ans. is (a) A 15-year-old girl, with burns on the face and chest, reports hoarseness of the voice**

    Burns on the face and neck can cause swelling of the respiratory mucosa that can lead to airway obstruction manifested by hoarseness of voice and difficulty in breathing. Maintaining an airway patency is the main concern.

90. **Ans. is (b) Don't bend at the waist**

    There is 6-8 months activity restriction following a spinal fusion. Sitting, lying, standing, normal stair climbing, walking, and gentle swimming is allowed. Bending and twisting at the waist should be avoided, along with lifting more than 10 lbs.

91. **Ans. is (d) Use the Z-track technique**

    Z-track technique is used to administer drugs especially irritating to the subcutaneous tissue. This method promotes absorption of the drug by preventing drug leakage into the subcutaneous layer.

92. **Ans. is (b) Establish rapport**

    Establishing rapport is a way to gain trust that will lead for a patient to relax. You can get more insights and information from a patient when rapport is established.

93. **Ans. is (a) Control seizures**

    Low magnesium (hypomagnesemia) produces clinical manifestations like increased reflexes, tremors, and seizures. Magnesium sulfate is the drug of choice to prevent seizures in pre-eclampsia and eclampsia.

94. **Ans. is (c) Pull the pinna up then backward**

    Ear canal of children ages 3 years and above can be straightened by pulling the pinna up then backward. For children below 3 years of age, the ear canal can be straightened by pulling the pinna down then backward.

95. **Ans. is (a) Inserting a nasogastric tube**

    Infants are nose breathers. A gastric tube may be inserted to facilitate lung expansion and stomach decompression, but not a nasogastric tube as it can occlude the nares of nose, thus, making breathing difficult for the infant.

96. **Ans. is (b).**

97. **Ans. is (b) The object may be pushed deeper into the throat**

    Blind finger sweeps are not recommended in all CPR cases especially for infants and children because the foreign object may be pushed back into the airway.

98. **Ans. is (b) Establish responsiveness of patient**

    First step in cardiopulmonary resuscitation (CPR) is assessing responsiveness of the patient.

99. **Ans. is (c) Administer oxygen via nasal cannula**

    Priority nursing action is to administer oxygen to patients with chest pain. Chest pain is caused by insufficient myocardial oxygenation.

100. **Ans. is (d) Pneumococcal vaccine**

    Pneumococcal vaccine is a priority immunization for the elderly. Seniors, ages 65 years old and above, have higher risk for serious pneumococcal infection and likely have low immunity. This is administered every 5 years.

Part 3

1. An unconscious patient with multiple injuries arrives in the emergency room. Which nursing intervention receives the highest priority?
   a. Establishing an airway
   b. Replacing blood loss
   c. Stopping bleeding from open wound
   d. Check for a neck fracture

2. What should the nurse do first when a client with a head injury begins to have clear drainage from the nose?
   a. Compress the nose
   b. Tilt the head back
   c. Give client a white pad to collect the fluid
   d. Administer an antihistamine

3. The nurses administer mannitol to the client with increased ICP. Which parameters require close monitoring?
   a. Muscle relaxation
   b. Intake and output
   c. Widening the pulse pressure
   d. Pupil dilation

4. Which activity would the nurse encourage the client to avoid when there is a risk for increased ICP?
   a. Deep breathing
   b. Turning
   c. Coughing
   d. Passive range of motion exercise

5. A client with Parkinson's disease is prescribed levodopa therapy. Which of the following effective therapy indicates improvement?
   a. Mood
   b. Muscle rigidity
   c. Appetite
   d. Alertness

6. Which of the following nursing intervention would promotes effective airway clearance in a client with acute respiratory distress?
   a. Administering the oxygen every 2 hours
   b. Turning the client every 4 hours
   c. Administering sedatives to promote rest
   d. Suctioning if cough is ineffective

7. A 21 years old male client is transported by the ambulance to the emergency department after a serious automobile accident. He complains of severe pain in his right chest where he struck the steering wheel. What is the primary client goal at this time?
   a. Reduce the client's anxiety
   b. Maintain adequate oxygenation
   c. Decrease chest pain
   d. Maintain adequate circulatory volume

8. A client is admitted with pheochromocytoma. The nurse assess the client's BP frequently. This is based on the knowledge that pheochromocytoma of the adrenal medulla releases excessive amount of:
   a. Renin
   b. Aldosterone
   c. Catecholamine
   d. Glucocorticoids

9. A chest tube is just inserted for a client aged 18 years, an important nursing action is to
   a. Place a hemostat nearby in case of an air leak
   b. Check the chest tubes every 2 hours for air leak
   c. Coil the tube carefully to prevent kinking, which could result in air leak
   d. Keep the client flat to avoid leaks in tubing

10. A nursing instructor is conducting lecture and is reviewing the functions of the female reproductive system. She asks mark to describe the follicle-stimulating hormone (FSH) and the luteinizing hormone (LH). Mark accurately responds by stating that:
    a. FSH and LH are released from the anterior pituitary gland
    b. FSH and LH are secreted by the corpus luteum of the ovary
    c. FSH and LH are secreted by the adrenal glands
    d. FSH and LH stimulate the formation of milk during pregnancy.

11. A nurse is describing the process of fetal circulation to a client during a prenatal visit. The nurse accurately tells the client that fetal circulation consists of:
    a. Two umbilical veins and one umbilical artery
    b. Two umbilical arteries and one umbilical vein
    c. Arteries carrying oxygenated blood to the fetus
    d. Veins carrying deoxygenated blood to the fetus

12. During a prenatal visit at 38 weeks, a nurse assesses the fetal heart rate. The nurse determines that the fetal heart rate is normal if which of the following is noted?
    a. 80 BPM
    b. 100 BPM
    c. 150 BPM
    d. 180 BPM

13. A client arrives at a prenatal clinic for the first prenatal assessment. The client tells a nurse that the first day of her last menstrual period was September 19th, 2013. Using Naegele's rule, the nurse determines the estimated date of confinement as:
    a. July 26, 2013
    b. June 12, 2014
    c. June 26, 2014
    d. July 12, 2014

14. A nurse is collecting data during an admission assessment of a client who is pregnant with twins. The client has a healthy 5-year-old child that was delivered at 37 weeks and tells the nurse that she doesn't have any history of abortion or fetal demise. The nurse would document the GTPAL for this client as:
    a. G = 3, T = 2, P = 0, A = 0, L = 1
    b. G = 2, T = 0, P = 1, A = 0, L = 1
    c. G = 1, T = 1. P = 1, A = 0, L = 1
    d. G = 2, T = 0, P = 0, A = 0, L = 1

15. A nurse is performing an assessment of a primipara who is being evaluated in a clinic during her second trimester of pregnancy. Which of the following indicates an abnormal physical finding necessitating further testing?
    a. Consistent increase in fundal height
    b. Fetal heart rate of 180 BPM
    c. Braxton hicks contractions
    d. Quickening

16. A nurse is reviewing the record of a client who has just been told that a pregnancy test is positive. The physician has documented the presence of a Goodell's sign. The nurse determines this sign indicates:
    a. A softening of the cervix
    b. A soft blowing sound that corresponds to the maternal pulse during auscultation of the uterus
    c. The presence of hCG in the urine
    d. The presence of fetal movement

17. A nursing instructor asks a nursing student who is preparing to assist with the assessment of a pregnant client to describe the process of quickening. Which of the following statements if made by the student indicates an understanding of this term?
    a. It is the irregular, painless contractions that occur throughout pregnancy.
    b. It is the soft blowing sound that can be heard when the uterus is auscultated.
    c. It is the fetal movement that is felt by the mother.
    d. It is the thinning of the lower uterine segment.

18. A nurse midwife is performing an assessment of a pregnant client and is assessing the client for the presence of ballottement. Which of the following would the nurse implement to test for the presence of ballottement?
    a. Auscultating for fetal heart sounds
    b. Palpating the abdomen for fetal movement
    c. Assessing the cervix for thinning
    d. Initiating a gentle upward tap on the cervix

19. A nurse is assisting in performing an assessment on a client who suspects that she is pregnant and is checking the client for probable signs of pregnancy. *Select all* probable signs of pregnancy.
    a. Uterine enlargement
    b. Fetal heart rate detected by nonelectric device
    c. Outline of the fetus via radiography or ultrasound
    d. Chadwick's sign
    e. Braxton Hicks contractions
    f. Ballottement

20. A pregnant client calls the clinic and tells a nurse that she is experiencing leg cramps and is awakened by the cramps at night. To provide relief from the leg cramps, the nurse tells the client to:
    a. Dorsiflex the foot while extending the knee when the cramps occur
    b. Dorsiflex the foot while flexing the knee when the cramps occur
    c. Plantar flex the foot while flexing the knee when the cramps occur
    d. Plantar flex the foot while extending the knee when the cramps occur

21. A nurse is providing instructions to a client in the first trimester of pregnancy regarding measures to assist in reducing breast tenderness. The nurse tells the client to:
    a. Avoid wearing a bra
    b. Wash the nipples and areola area daily with soap, and massage the breasts with lotion.
    c. Wear tight-fitting blouses or dresses to provide support
    d. Wash the breasts with warm water and keep them dry

22. A pregnant client in the last trimester has been admitted to the hospital with a diagnosis of severe preeclampsia. Nurse monitors for complications associated with the diagnosis and assess the client for:
    a. Any bleeding, such as in the gums, petechiae, and purpura
    b. Enlargement of the breasts
    c. Periods of fetal movement followed by quiet periods
    d. Complaints of feeling hot when the room is cool

23. A client in the first trimester of pregnancy arrives at a health care clinic and reports that she has been experiencing vaginal bleeding. A threatened abortion is suspected, and the nurse instructs the client regarding management of care. Which statement, if made by the client, indicates a need for further education?
    a. I will maintain strict bed rest throughout the remainder of pregnancy.
    b. I will avoid sexual intercourse until the bleeding has stopped, and for 2 weeks following the last evidence of bleeding.
    c. I will count the number of perineal pads used on a daily basis and note the amount and color of blood on the pad.
    d. I will watch for the evidence of the passage of tissue.

24. A prenatal nurse is providing instructions to a group of pregnant client regarding measures to prevent toxoplasmosis. Which statement if made by one of the clients indicates a need for further instructions?
    a. I need to cook meat thoroughly
    b. I need to avoid touching mucous membranes of the mouth or eyes while handling raw meat

c. I need to drink unpasteurized milk only
d. I need to avoid contact with materials that are possibly contaminated with cat feces

25. A homecare nurse visits a pregnant client who has a diagnosis of mild Preeclampsia and who is being monitored for pregnancy-induced hypertension (PIH). Which assessment finding indicates a worsening of the preeclampsia and the need to notify the physician?
    a. Blood pressure reading is at the prenatal baseline
    b. Urinary output has increased
    c. The client complains of a headache and blurred vision
    d. Dependent edema has resolved

26. A nurse implements a teaching plan for a pregnant client who is newly diagnosed with gestational diabetes. Which statement if made by the client indicates a need for further education?
    a. I need to stay on the diabetic diet
    b. I will perform glucose monitoring at home
    c. I need to avoid exercise because of the negative effects of insulin production
    d. I need to be aware of any infections and report signs of infection immediately to my health care provider.

27. A primigravida is receiving magnesium sulfate for the treatment of pregnancy-induced hypertension (PIH). The nurse who is caring for the client is performing assessments every 30 minutes. Which assessment finding would be of most concern to the nurse?
    a. Urinary output of 20 ml since the previous assessment
    b. Deep tendon reflexes of 2+
    c. Respiratory rate of 10 BPM
    d. Fetal heart rate of 120 BPM

28. A nurse is caring for a pregnant client with preeclampsia. The nurse prepares a plan of care for the client and documents in the plan that if the client progresses from preeclampsia to eclampsia, the nurse's first action is to:
    a. Administer magnesium sulfate intravenously
    b. Assess the blood pressure and fetal heart rate
    c. Clean and maintain an open airway
    d. Administer oxygen by face mask

29. A nurse is monitoring a pregnant client with pregnancy-induced hypertension who is at risk for preeclampsia. The nurse checks the client for which specific signs of preeclampsia (select all that apply)?
    a. Elevated blood pressure
    b. Negative urinary protein
    c. Facial edema
    d. Increased respirations

30. Rho (D) immune globulin (RhoGAM) is prescribed for a woman following delivery of a newborn infant and the nurse provides information to the woman about the purpose of the medication. The nurse determines that the woman understands the purpose of the medication if the woman states that it will protect her next baby from which of the following?
    a. Being affected by Rh incompatibility
    b. Having Rh positive blood
    c. Developing a rubella infection
    d. Developing physiological jaundice

31. A pregnant client is receiving magnesium sulfate for the management of preeclampsia. A nurse determines the client is experiencing toxicity from the medication if which of the following is noted on assessment?
    a. Presence of deep tendon reflexes
    b. Serum magnesium level of 6 mEq/L
    c. Proteinuria of +3
    d. Respirations of 10 per minute

32. A woman with preeclampsia is receiving magnesium sulfate. The nurse assigned to care for the client determines that the magnesium therapy is effective if:
    a. Ankle clonus in noted
    b. The blood pressure decreases
    c. Seizures do not occur
    d. Scotomas are present

33. A nurse is caring for a pregnant client with severe preeclampsia who is receiving IV magnesium sulfate. Select *all* nursing interventions that apply in the care for the client.
    a. Monitor maternal vital signs every 2 hours
    b. Notify the physician if respirations are less than 18 per minute.
    c. Monitor renal function and cardiac function closely
    d. Keep calcium gluconate on hand in case of a magnesium sulfate overdose
    e. Monitor deep tendon reflexes hourly
    f. Monitor I and Os hourly
    g. Notify the physician if urinary output is less than 30 ml per hour.

34. In the 12th week of gestation, a client completely expels the products of conception. Because the client is Rh negative, the nurse must:
    a. Administer RhoGAM within 72 hours

b. Make certain she receives RhoGAM on her first clinic visit
c. Not give RhoGAM, since it is not used with the birth of a stillborn
d. Make certain the client does not receive RhoGAM, since the gestation only lasted 12 weeks.

35. In a lecture on sexual functioning, the nurse plans to include the fact that ovulation occurs when the:
   a. Oxytocin is too high
   b. Blood level of LH is too high
   c. Progesterone level is high
   d. Endometrial wall is sloughed off

36. The chief function of progesterone is the:
   a. Development of the female reproductive system
   b. Stimulation of the follicles for ovulation to occur
   c. Preparation of the uterus to receive a fertilized egg
   d. Establishment of secondary male sex characteristics

37. The developing cells are called a fetus from the:
   a. Time the fetal heart is heard
   b. Eighth week to the time of birth
   c. Implantation of the fertilized ovum
   d. End of the send week to the onset of labor

38. After the first four months of pregnancy, the chief source of estrogen and progesterone is the:
   a. Placenta
   b. Adrenal cortex
   c. Corpus luteum
   d. Anterior hypophysis

39. The nurse recognizes that an expected change in the hematologic system that occurs during the 2nd trimester of pregnancy is:
   a. A decrease in WBCs
   b. In increase in hematocrit
   c. An increase in blood volume
   d. A decrease in sedimentation rate

40. The nurse is aware than an adaptation of pregnancy is an increased blood supply to the pelvic region that results in a purplish discoloration of the vaginal mucosa, which is known as:
   a. Ladin's sign
   b. Hegar's sign
   c. Goodell's sign
   d. Chadwick's sign

41. A pregnant client is making her first Antepartum visit. She has a two years old son born at 40 weeks, a 5 years old daughter born at 38 weeks, and 7 years old twin daughters born at 35 weeks. She had a spontaneous abortion 3 years ago at 10 weeks. Using the GTPAL format, the nurse should identify that the client is:
   a. G4 T3 P2 A1 L4
   b. G5 T2 P2 A1 L4
   c. G5 T2 P1 A1 L4
   d. G4 T3 P1 A1 L4

42. An expected cardiopulmonary adaptation experienced by most pregnant women is:
   a. Tachycardia
   b. Dyspnea at rest
   c. Progression of dependent edema
   d. Shortness of breath on exertion

43. Nutritional planning for a newly pregnant woman of average height and weighing 145 pounds should include:
   a. A decrease of 200 calories a day
   b. An increase of 300 calories a day
   c. An increase of 500 calories a day
   d. A maintenance of her present caloric intake per day

44. During a prenatal examination, the nurses' draws blood from a young Rh negative client and explain that an indirect Coombs test will be performed to predict whether the fetus is at risk for:
   a. Acute hemolytic disease
   b. Respiratory distress syndrome
   c. Protein metabolic deficiency
   d. Physiologic hyperbilirubinemia

45. When involved in prenatal teaching, the nurse should advise the clients that an increase in vaginal secretions during pregnancy is called leukorrhea and is caused by increased:
   a. Metabolic rates
   b. Production of estrogen
   c. Functioning of the Bartholin glands
   d. Supply of sodium chloride to the cells of the vagina

46. A 26-year-old multigravida is 14 weeks' pregnant and is scheduled for an alpha-fetoprotein test. She asks the nurse, "What does the alpha-fetoprotein test indicate?" The nurse bases a response on the knowledge that this test can detect:
   a. Kidney defects
   b. Cardiac defects
   c. Neural tube defects
   d. Urinary tract defects

47. At a prenatal visit at 36 weeks' gestation, a client complains of discomfort with irregularly occurring contractions. The nurse instructs the client to:
   a. Lie down until they stop
   b. Walk around until they subside

c. Time contraction for 30 minutes
d. Take 10 grains of aspirin for the discomfort

48. The nurse teaches a pregnant woman to avoid lying on her back. The nurse has based this statement on the knowledge that the supine position can:
    a. Unduly prolong labor
    b. Cause decreased placental perfusion
    c. Lead to transient episodes of hypotension
    d. Interfere with free movement of the coccyx

49. The pituitary hormone that stimulates the secretion of milk from the mammary glands is:
    a. Prolactin
    b. Oxytocin
    c. Estrogen
    d. Progesterone

50. Which of the following symptoms occurs with a hydatidiform mole?
    a. Heavy, bright red bleeding every 21 days
    b. Fetal cardiac motion after 6 weeks gestation
    c. Benign tumors found in the smooth muscle of the uterus
    d. "Snowstorm" pattern on ultrasound with no fetus or gestational sac

51. Which of the following terms applies to the tiny, blanched, slightly raised end arterioles found on the face, neck, arms, and chest during pregnancy?
    a. Epulis
    b. Linea nigra
    c. Striae gravidarum
    d. Telangiectasias

52. Which of the following conditions is common in pregnant women in the 2nd trimester of pregnancy?
    a. Mastitis
    b. Metabolic alkalosis
    c. Physiologic anemia
    d. Respiratory acidosis

53. A 21-year-old client, 6 weeks' pregnant is diagnosed with hyperemesis gravidarum. This excessive vomiting during pregnancy will often result in which of the following conditions?
    a. Bowel perforation
    b. Electrolyte imbalance
    c. Miscarriage
    d. Pregnancy-induced hypertension (PIH)

54. Clients with gestational diabetes are usually managed by which of the following therapies?
    a. Diet
    b. NPH insulin (long-acting)
    c. Oral hypoglycemic drugs
    d. Oral hypoglycemic drugs and insulin

55. The antagonist for magnesium sulfate should be readily available to any client receiving IV magnesium. Which of the following drugs is the antidote for magnesium toxicity?
    a. Calcium gluconate
    b. Hydralazine (Apresoline)
    c. Narcan
    d. RhoGAM

56. Which of the following answers best describes the stage of pregnancy in which maternal and fetal blood are exchanged?
    a. Conception
    b. 9 weeks' gestation, when the fetal heart is well developed
    c. 32–34 weeks gestation
    d. Maternal and fetal blood are never exchanged

57. Gravida refers to which of the following descriptions?
    a. A serious pregnancy
    b. Number of times a female has been pregnant
    c. Number of children a female has delivered
    d. Number of term pregnancies a female has had.

58. A pregnant woman at 32 weeks' gestation complains of feeling dizzy and lightheaded while her fundal height is being measured. Her skin is pale and moist. The nurse's initial response would be to:
    a. Assess the woman's blood pressure and pulse
    b. Have the woman breathe into a paper bag
    c. Raise the woman's legs
    d. Turn the woman on her side.

59. A pregnant woman's last menstrual period began on April 8, 2005, and ended on April 13. Using Naegele's rule her estimated date of birth would be:
    a. January 15, 2006
    b. January 20, 2006
    c. July 1, 2006
    d. November 5, 2005

60. A primiparous client, who has just delivered a healthy term neonate after 12 hrs of labor, holds and looks at her neonate and begins to cry. The nurse correctly interprets this behaviors as a sign of which of the following?
    a. Disappointment in the baby's gender.
    b. Grief over the ending of the pregnancy
    c. A normal response to the birth
    d. Indication of postpartum "blues".

61. When developing a teaching plan for a childbirth education class for a group of primigravid clients about pain during labor and delivery, which of the following would the nurse expect to discuss

as the primary cause of pain in the first stage of labor?
a. Dilation of the uterine blood vessels.
b. Hypoxia to the uterine muscle fibers
c. Distention of the upper uterine segment
d. Status of the amniotic membranes

62. When caring for a term neonate during the first hour after birth, the nurse expects to assess the neonate's blood glucose level, obtaining the blood sample from the neonate foot near which of the following area?
a. Lateral aspect of the heel
b. Middle of the heel
c. Middle of the foot
d. Base of the toes

63. The parents of a 9-month-old bring the infant to the clinic for a regular checkup. The infant has received no immunizations which of the following would be appropriate for the nurse to administer at this visit?
a. DTaP, Hib, IPN and PPD
b. DTaP, Hib, OPV and MMR
c. PPD, MMR, Hep B and OPV
d. HEPB, IPV, Hib and varicella

64. When developing the ongoing plan of care for the parents whose infant died of SIDS, the community health nurse would expect to accomplish which of the following on the second home visit.
a. Allow the parents to express their feelings
b. Have the parents gain an understanding of the disease
c. Assess the impact of the infant's death on their other children.
d. Deal with issues such as having other children

65. A client has the following Arterial Blood Gas values PH—7.52, PaO$_2$—50 mm Hg, PaCO$_2$, 28 mm Hg. HCO$_3$ 24 MEq/L. The nurse determines that which of the following is a possible cause for these findings?
a. Chronic obstructive pulmonary disease (COPD)
b. Diabetic ketoacidosis with Kussmaul's respiration
c. Myocardial infarction
d. Pulmonary embolism

66. To help minimize the risk of postoperative respiratory complications after a hypophysectomy the nurse would focus the clients preoperative teaching on the importance of:
a. Using blow bottles
b. Making frequent position changes
c. Deep breathing
d. Coughing

67. A client with chronic renal failure has asked to be evaluated for a home continuous—ambulatory peritoneal dialysis (CAPD) program. The nurse should explain that the major advantage of this approach in that it.
a. Is relatively low in cost
b. Allows the client to be more independent
c. Is faster and more efficient than standard peritoneal dialysis
d. Have fewer potential complications than standard peritoneal dialysis.

68. Which of the following positions would be best for a clients rights arm when she returns to her room after a right modified radical mastectomy with multiple lymph mode excisions?
a. Across her chest wall
b. At her side at the same level as her body.
c. In the position that affords her the greatest comfort without placing pressure on the incision
d. On pillows with her hand higher than her elbow and her elbow higher than her shoulder.

69. What is a priority nursing assessment in the first 24 hrs after admission of the client with a thrombotic CVA?
a. Cholesterol level
b. Pupil size and papillary response
c. Bowel sound
d. Echocardiogram

70. An agitated, confused female client arrives in the emergency department. Her history includes type 1 diabetes mellitus, hypertension, and angina pectoris. Assessment reveals pallor, diaphoresis, headache, and intense hunger. Blood glucose sample measures 42 mg/dl, and the client is treated for an acute hypoglycemic reaction. After recovery, the nurse teaches the client to treat hypoglycemia by ingesting:
a. 2 to 5 g of a simple carbohydrate
b. 10 to 15 g of a simple carbohydrate
c. 18 to 20 g of a simple carbohydrate
d. 25 to 30 g of a simple carbohydrate

71. A female adult client with a history of chronic hyperparathyroidism admits to being noncompliant. Based on initial assessment findings, the nurse formulates the nursing diagnosis of Risk for injury. To complete the nursing diagnosis statement for this client, which "related-to" phrase should the nurse add?
a. Related to bone demineralization resulting in pathologic fractures
b. Related to exhaustion secondary to an accelerated metabolic rate

c. Related to edema and dry skin secondary to fluid infiltration into the interstitial spaces
d. Related to tetany secondary to a decreased serum calcium level

72. Nurse Joey is assigned to care for a postoperative male client who has diabetes mellitus. During the assessment interview, the client reports that he's impotent and says he's concerned about its effect on his marriage. In planning this client's care, the most appropriate intervention would be to:
   a. Encourage the client to ask questions about personal sexuality.
   b. Provide time for privacy.
   c. Provide support for the spouse or significant other.
   d. Suggest referral to a sex counselor or other appropriate professional.

73. During a class on exercise for diabetic clients, a female client asks the nurse educator how often to exercise. The nurse educator advises the clients to exercise how often to meet the goals of planned exercise?
   a. At least once a week
   b. At least three times a week
   c. At least five times a week
   d. Every day

74. Nurse oliver should expect a client with hypothyroidism to report which health concerns?
   a. Increased appetite and weight loss
   b. Puffiness of the face and hands
   c. Nervousness and tremors
   d. Thyroid gland swelling

75. A female client with hypothyroidism (myxedema) is receiving levothyroxine (Synthroid), 25 mcg P.O. daily. Which finding should nurse Hans recognize as an adverse drug effect?
   a. Dysuria
   b. Leg cramps
   c. Tachycardia
   d. Blurred vision

76. A 76-year-old male client has been complaining of sleeping more, increased urination, anorexia, weakness, irritability, depression, and bone pain that interferes with her going outdoors. Based on these assessment findings, Nurse Richard would suspect which of the following disorders?
   a. Diabetes mellitus
   b. Diabetes insipidus
   c. Hypoparathyroidism
   d. Hyperparathyroidism

77. When caring for a male client with diabetes insipidus, nurse Juliet expects to administer:
   a. Vasopressin (Pitressin Synthetic)
   b. Furosemide (Lasix)
   c. Regular insulin
   d. 10% dextrose

78. The nurse is aware that the following is the most common cause of hyperaldosteronism?
   a. Excessive sodium intake
   b. A pituitary adenoma
   c. Deficient potassium intake
   d. An adrenal adenoma

79. A male client with type 1 diabetes mellitus has a highly elevated glycosylated hemoglobin (Hb) test result. In discussing the result with the client, nurse would be most accurate in stating:
   a. The test needs to be repeated following a 12-hour fast.
   b. It looks like you aren't following the prescribed diabetic diet.
   c. It tells us about your sugar control for the last 3 months.
   d. Your insulin regimen needs to be altered significantly.

80. Following a unilateral adrenalectomy, nurse Josmy would assess for hyperkalemia shown by which of the following?
   a. Muscle weakness
   b. Tremors
   c. Diaphoresis
   d. Constipation

81. Nurse Louie is developing a teaching plan for a male client diagnosed with diabetes insipidus. The nurse should include information about which hormone lacking in clients with diabetes insipidus?
   a. Antidiuretic hormone (ADH)
   b. Thyroid-stimulating hormone (TSH)
   c. Follicle-stimulating hormone (FSH)
   d. Luteinizing hormone (LH)

82. Early this morning, a female client had a subtotal thyroidectomy. During evening rounds, nurse Tina assesses the client, who now has nausea, a temperature of 105°F (40.5°C), tachycardia, and extreme restlessness. What is the most likely cause of these signs?
   a. Diabetic ketoacidosis
   b. Thyroid crisis
   c. Hypoglycemia
   d. Tetany

83. For a male client with hyperglycemia, which assessment finding best supports a nursing diagnosis of deficient fluid volume?
   a. Cool, clammy skin

b. Distended neck veins
c. Increased urine osmolarity
d. Decreased serum sodium level

84. When assessing a male client with pheochromocytoma, a tumor of the adrenal medulla that secretes excessive catecholamine, nurse April is most likely to detect:
   a. A blood pressure of 130/70 mm Hg
   b. A blood glucose level of 130 mg/dl
   c. Bradycardia
   d. A blood pressure of 176/88 mm Hg

85. A male client is admitted for treatment of the syndrome of inappropriate antidiuretic hormone (SIADH). Which nursing intervention is appropriate?
   a. Infusing IV fluids rapidly as ordered
   b. Encouraging increased oral intake
   c. Restricting fluids
   d. Administering glucose-containing IV fluids as ordered

86. A female client has a serum calcium level of 7.2 mg/dl. During the physical examination, nurse Noah expects to assess:
   a. Trousseau's sign
   b. Homans' sign
   c. Hegar's sign
   d. Goodell's sign

87. Which outcome indicates that treatment of a male client with diabetes insipidus has been effective?
   a. Fluid intake is less than 2,500 ml/day
   b. Urine output measures more than 200 ml/hour
   c. Blood pressure is 90/50 mm Hg
   d. The heart rate is 126 beats/minute

88. Jemma, who weighs 210 lb (95 kg) and has been diagnosed with hyperglycemia tells the nurse that her husband sleeps in another room because her snoring keeps him awake. The nurse notices that she has large hands and a hoarse voice. Which of the following would the nurse suspect as a possible cause of the client's hyperglycemia?
   a. Acromegaly
   b. Type 1 diabetes mellitus
   c. Hypothyroidism
   d. Deficient growth hormone

89. Nurse Kate is providing dietary instructions to a male client with hypoglycemia. To control hypoglycemic episodes, the nurse should recommend:
   a. Increasing saturated fat intake and fasting in the afternoon.
   b. Increasing intake of vitamins B and D and taking iron supplements.
   c. Eating a candy bar if lightheadedness occurs.
   d. Consuming a low-carbohydrate, high-protein diet and avoiding fasting.

90. An incoherent female client with a history of hypothyroidism is brought to the emergency department by the rescue squad. Physical and laboratory findings reveal hypothermia, hypoventilation, respiratory acidosis, bradycardia, hypotension, and non pitting edema of the face and pretibial area. Knowing that these findings suggest severe hypothyroidism, nurse Libby prepares to take emergency action to prevent the potential complication of:
   a. Thyroid storm
   b. Cretinism
   c. Myxedema coma
   d. Hashimoto's thyroiditis

91. A male client with type 1 diabetes mellitus asks the nurse about taking an oral antidiabetic agent. Nurse Jack explains that these medications are only effective if the client:
   a. Prefers to take insulin orally
   b. Has type 2 diabetes
   c. Has type 1 diabetes
   d. Is pregnant and has type 2 diabetes

92. When caring for a female client with a history of hypoglycemia, nurse Ruby should avoid administering a drug that may potentiate hypoglycemia. Which drug fits this description?
   a. Sulfisoxazole (Gantrisin)
   b. Mexiletine (Mexitil)
   c. Prednisone (Orasone)
   d. Lithium carbonate (Lithobid)

93. After taking glipizide (Glucotrol) for 9 months, a male client experiences secondary failure. Which of the following would the nurse expect the physician to do?
   a. Initiate insulin therapy
   b. Switch the client to a different oral antidiabetic agent
   c. Prescribe an additional oral antidiabetic agent
   d. Restrict carbohydrate intake to less than 30% of the total caloric intake

94. During preoperative teaching for a female client who will undergo subtotal thyroidectomy, the nurse should include which statement?
   a. The head of your bed must remain flat for 24 hours after surgery.
   b. You should avoid deep breathing and coughing after surgery.
   c. You won't be able to swallow for the first day or two.

d. You must avoid hyperextending your neck after surgery.

95. Nurse Ronn is assessing a client with possible Cushing's syndrome. In a client with Cushing's syndrome, the nurse would expect to find:
    a. Hypotension
    b. Thick, coarse skin
    c. Deposits of adipose tissue in the trunk and dorsocervical area
    d. Weight gain in arms and legs

96. A male client with primary diabetes insipidus is ready for discharge on desmopressin (DDAVP). Which instruction should nurse Lima provide?
    a. Administer desmopressin while the suspension is cold.
    b. Your condition isn't chronic, so you won't need to wear a medical identification bracelet.
    c. You may not be able to use desmopressin nasally if you have nasal discharge or blockage.
    d. You won't need to monitor your fluid intake and output after you start taking desmopressin.

97. Nurse Wayne is aware that a positive Chvostek's sign indicate?
    a. Hypocalcemia
    b. Hyponatremia
    c. Hypokalemia
    d. Hypermagnesemia

98. In a 29-year-old female client who is being successfully treated for Cushing's syndrome, nurse Lyzette would expect a decline in:
    a. Serum glucose level
    b. Hair loss
    c. Bone mineralization
    d. Menstrual flow

99. A male client has recently undergone surgical removal of a pituitary tumor. Dr. Wong prescribes corticotropin (Acthar), 20 units I.M. q.i.d. as a replacement therapy. What is the mechanism of action of corticotropin?
    a. It decreases cyclic adenosine monophosphate (cAMP) production and affects the metabolic rate of target organs.
    b. It interacts with plasma membrane receptors to inhibit enzymatic actions.
    c. It interacts with plasma membrane receptors to produce enzymatic actions that affect protein, fat, and carbohydrate metabolism.
    d. It regulates the threshold for water resorption in the kidneys.

100. Capillary glucose monitoring is being performed every 4 hours for a female client diagnosed with diabetic ketoacidosis. Insulin is administered using a scale of regular insulin according to glucose results. At 2 pm, the client has a capillary glucose level of 250 mg/dl for which he receives 8 U of regular insulin. Nurse Vince should expect the doses:
    a. Onset to be at 2 pm and its peak to be at 3 pm
    b. Onset to be at 2:15 pm and its peak to be at 3 pm
    c. Onset to be at 2:30 pm and its peak to be at 4 pm
    d. Onset to be at 4 pm and its peak to be at 6 pm

Answers (Part 3)

1. **Ans. is (a) Establishing an airway**
   The highest priority for a client with multiple injuries is to establish an open airway for effective ventilation and oxygenation.

2. **Ans. is (c) Give client a white pad to collect the fluid**
   The clear drainage must be analyzed to determine whether it is a nasal discharge of CSF.

3. **Ans. is (b) Intake and output**
   After administering mannitol, the nurse closely monitor intake and output because mannitol promotes diuresis and give primarily to pull water from the extracellular fluid of the edematous brain.

4. **Ans. is (c) Coughing**
   Coughing is contraindicated for a client because it may increase ICP.

5. **Ans. is (b) Muscle rigidity**
   Levodopa is prescribed to decrease the severe muscle rigidity.

6. **Ans. is (d) Suctioning if cough is ineffective**
   The nurse should suction the client if the client is not able to cough up secretion and clear the airway.

7. **Ans. is (b) Maintain adequate oxygenation**
   Blunt chest trauma may leads to respiratory failure and maintain adequate oxygenation is the priority nursing care for the client.

8. **Ans. is (c) Catecholamine**

   Pheochromocytoma releases catecholamine, epinephrine and norepinephrine. The excessive hormone secretion can be constant or episodic.

9. **Ans. is (a) Place a hemostat nearby in case of an air leak**

10. **Ans. is (a) FSH and LH are released from the anterior pituitary gland**

    FSH and LH, when stimulated by gonadotropin-releasing hormone from the hypothalamus, are released from the anterior pituitary gland to stimulate follicular growth and development, growth of the Graafian follicle, and production of progesterone.

11. **Ans. is (b) Two umbilical arteries and one umbilical vein**

    Blood pumped by the embryo's heart leaves the embryo through two umbilical arteries. Once oxygenated, the blood then is returned by one umbilical vein. Arteries carry deoxygenated blood and waste products from the fetus, and veins carry oxygenated blood and provide oxygen and nutrients to the fetus.

12. **Ans. is (c) 150 BPM**

    The fetal heart rate depends in gestational age and ranges from 160-170 BPM in the first trimester but slows with fetal growth to 120-160 BPM near or at term. At or near term, if the fetal heart rate is less than 120 or more than 160 BPM with the uterus at rest, the fetus may be in distress.

13. **Ans. is (c) June 26, 2014**

    Accurate use of Naegele's rule requires that the woman have a regular 28-day menstrual cycle. Add 7 days to the first day of the last menstrual period, subtract three months, and then add one year to that date.

14. **Ans. is (b) G = 2, T = 0, P = 1, A = 0, L = 1**

    Pregnancy outcomes can be described with the acronym GTPAL.
    - "G" is Gravidity, the number of pregnancies.
    - "T" is term births, the number of born at term (38 to 41 weeks).
    - "P" is preterm births, the number born before 38 weeks gestation.
    - "A" is abortions or miscarriages, included in "G" if before 20 weeks gestation, included in parity if past 20 weeks AOE.
    - "L" is live births, the number of births of living children.

    Therefore, a woman who is pregnant with twins and has a child has a gravida of 2. Because the child was delivered at 37 weeks, the number of preterm births is 1, and the number of term births is 0. The number of abortions is 0, and the number of live births is 1.

15. **Ans. is (b) Fetal heart rate of 180 BPM**

    The normal range of the fetal heart rate depends on gestational age. The heart rate is usually 160-170 BPM in the first trimester and slows with fetal growth, near and at term, the fetal heart rate ranges from 120-160 BPM. The other options are expected.

16. **Ans. is (a) A softening of the cervix**

    In the early weeks of pregnancy, the cervix becomes softer as a result of increased vascularity and hyperplasia, which causes the Goodell's sign.

17. **Ans. is (c) It is the fetal movement that is felt by the mother**

    Quickening is fetal movement and may occur as early as the 16th and 18th week of gestation, and the mother first notices subtle fetal movements that gradually increase in intensity. Braxton Hicks contractions are irregular, painless contractions that may occur throughout the pregnancy. A thinning of the lower uterine segment occurs about the 6th week of pregnancy and is called Hegar's sign.

18. **Ans. is (d) Initiating a gentle upward tap on the cervix**

    Ballottement is a technique of palpating a floating structure by bouncing it gently and feeling it rebound. In the technique used to palpate the fetus, the examiner places a finger in the vagina and taps gently upward, causing the fetus to rise. The fetus then sinks, and the examiner feels a gentle tap on the finger.

19. **Ans. is (a, d, e, f)**

    The probable signs of pregnancy include:
    - Uterine enlargement
    - Hegar's sign or softening and thinning of the uterine segment that occurs at week 6.
    - Goodell's sign or softening of the cervix that occurs at the beginning of the 2nd month.
    - Chadwick's sign or bluish coloration of the mucous membranes of the cervix, vagina and vulva. Occurs at week 6.
    - Ballottement or rebounding of the fetus against the examiner's fingers of palpation
    - Braxton-Hicks contractions
    - Positive pregnancy test measuring for hCG.

    Positive signs of pregnancy include:

- Fetal heart rate detected by electronic device (Doppler) at 10–12 weeks
- Fetal heart rate detected by nonelectronic device (fetoscope) at 20 weeks AOG
- Active fetal movement palpable by the examiners
- Outline of the fetus via radiography or ultrasound

20. **Ans. is (a) Dorsiflex the foot while extending the knee when the cramps occur**

    Legs cramps occur when the pregnant woman stretches the leg and plantar flexes the foot. Dorsiflexion of the foot while extending the knee stretches the affected muscle, prevents the muscle from contracting, and stops the cramping.

21. **Ans. is (d) Wash the breasts with warm water and keep them dry**

    The pregnant woman should be instructed to wash the breasts with warm water and keep them dry. The woman should be instructed to avoid using soap on the nipples and areola area to prevent the drying of tissues. Wearing a supportive bra with wide adjustable straps can decrease breast tenderness. Tight-fitting blouses or dresses will cause discomfort.

22. **Ans. is (a) Any bleeding, such as in the gums, petechiae, and purpura**

    Severe preeclampsia can trigger disseminated intravascular coagulation because of the widespread damage to vascular integrity. Bleeding is an early sign of DIC and should be reported to the MD.

23. **Ans. is (a) "I will maintain strict bed rest throughout the remainder of pregnancy**

    Strict bed rest throughout the remainder of pregnancy is not required. The woman is advised to curtail sexual activities until the bleeding has ceased, and for 2 weeks following the last evidence of bleeding or as recommended by the physician. The woman is instructed to count the number of perineal pads used daily and to note the quantity and color of blood on the pad. The woman also should watch for the evidence of the passage of tissue.

24. **Ans. is (c) I need to drink unpasteurized milk only**

    All pregnant women should be advised to do the following to prevent the development of toxoplasmosis. Women should be instructed to cook meats thoroughly, avoid touching mucous membranes and eyes while handling raw meat; thoroughly wash all kitchen surfaces that come into contact with uncooked meat, wash the hands thoroughly after handling raw meat; avoid uncooked eggs and unpasteurized milk; wash fruits and vegetables before consumption, and avoid contact with materials that possibly are contaminated with cat feces, such as cat litter boxes, sandboxes, and garden soil.

25. **Ans. is (c) The client complains of a headache and blurred vision**

    If the client complains of a headache and blurred vision, the physician should be notified because these are signs of worsening preeclampsia.

26. **Ans. is (c) I need to avoid exercise because of the negative effects of insulin production**

    Exercise is safe for the client with gestational diabetes and is helpful in lowering the blood glucose level.

27. **Ans. is (c) Respiratory rate of 10 BPM**

    Magnesium sulfate depresses the respiratory rate. If the respiratory rate is less than 12 breaths per minute, the physician or other health care provider needs to be notified, and continuation of the medication needs to be reassessed. A urinary output of 20 ml in a 30 minutes period is adequate; less than 30 ml in one hour needs to be reported. Deep tendon reflexes of 2+ are normal. The fetal heart rate is WNL for a resting fetus.

28. **Ans. is (c) Clean and maintain an open airway**

    The immediate care during a seizure (eclampsia) is to ensure a patent airway. The other options are actions that follow or will be implemented after the seizure has ceased.

29. **Ans. is (a) Elevated blood pressure**

    Elevated blood pressure and 3 facial edemas. The three classic signs of preeclampsia are hypertension, generalized edema, and proteinuria. Increased respirations are not a sign of preeclampsia.

30. **Ans. is (a) Being affected by Rh incompatibility**

    Rh incompatibility can occur when an Rh-negative mom becomes sensitized to the Rh antigen. Sensitization may develop when an Rh-negative woman becomes pregnant with a fetus who is Rh positive. During pregnancy and at delivery, some of the baby's Rh-positive blood can enter the maternal circulation, causing the woman's immune system to form antibodies against Rh-positive blood. Administration of Rho(D) immune globulin prevents the woman from developing antibodies against Rh-positive blood by providing passive antibody protection against the Rh antigen.

31. **Ans. is (d) Respirations of 10 per minute**

    Magnesium toxicity can occur from magnesium sulfate therapy. Signs of toxicity relate to the central nervous system depressant effects of the medication and include respiratory depression, loss of deep tendon reflexes, and a sudden drop in the fetal heart rate and maternal heart rate and blood pressure. Therapeutic levels of magnesium are 4-7 mEq/L. Proteinuria of +3 would be noted in a client with preeclampsia.

32. **Ans. is (c) Seizures do not occur**

    For a client with preeclampsia, the goal of care is directed at preventing eclampsia (seizures). Magnesium sulfate is an anticonvulsant, not an antihypertensive agent. Although a decrease in blood pressure may be noted initially, this effect is usually transient. Ankle clonus indicated hyperreflexia and may precede the onset of eclampsia. Scotomas are areas of complete or partial blindness. Visual disturbances, such as scotomas, often precede an eclamptic seizure.

33. **Ans. is (c, d, e, f, g)**

    When caring for a client receiving magnesium sulfate therapy, the nurse would monitor maternal vital signs, especially respirations, every 30-60 minutes and notify the physician if respirations are less than 12, because this would indicate respiratory depression. Calcium gluconate is kept on hand in case of magnesium sulfate overdose, because calcium gluconate is the antidote for magnesium sulfate toxicity. Deep tendon reflexes are assessed hourly. Cardiac and renal function is monitored closely. The urine output should be maintained at 30 ml per hour because the medication is eliminated through the kidneys.

34. **Ans. is (a) Administer RhoGAM within 72 hours**

    RhoGAM is given within 72 hours postpartum if the client has not been sensitized already.

35. **Ans. is (b) Blood level of LH is too high**

    It is the surge of LH secretion in mid cycle that is responsible for ovulation.

36. **Ans. is (c) Preparation of the uterus to receive a fertilized egg**

    Progesterone stimulates differentiation of the endometrium into a secretory type of tissue.

37. **Ans. is (b) Eighth week to the time of birth**

    In the first 7-14 days, the ovum is known as a blastocyst; it is called an embryo until the eighth week; the developing cells are then called a fetus until birth.

38. **Ans. is (a) Placenta**

    When placental formation is complete, around the 16th week of pregnancy; it produces estrogen and progesterone.

39. **Ans. is (c) An increase in blood volume**

    The blood volume increases by approximately 40-50% during pregnancy. The peak blood volume occurs between 30 and 34 weeks of gestation. The hematocrit decreases as a result of the increased blood volume.

40. **Ans. is (d) Chadwick's sign**

    A purplish color results from the increased vascularity and blood vessel engorgement of the vagina.

41. **Ans. is (c) G5 T2 P1 A1 L4**

    5 pregnancies; 2 term births; twins count as 1; one abortion; 4 living children.

42. **Ans. is (d) Shortness of breath on exertion**

    This is an expected cardiopulmonary adaptation during pregnancy; it is caused by an increased ventricular rate and elevated diaphragm.

43. **Ans. is (b) An increase of 300 calories a day**

    This is the recommended caloric increase for adult women to meet the increased metabolic demands of pregnancy.

44. **Ans. is (a) Acute hemolytic disease**

    When an Rh negative mother carries an Rh positive fetus, there is a risk for maternal antibodies against Rh-positive blood; antibodies cross the placenta and destroy the fetal RBCs.

45. **Ans. is (b) Production of estrogen**

    The increase of estrogen during pregnancy causes hyperplasia of the vaginal mucosa, which leads to increased production of mucus by the endocervical glands. The mucus contains exfoliated epithelial cells.

46. **Ans. is (c) Neural tube defects**

    The alpha-fetoprotein test detects neural tube defects and Down syndrome.

47. **Ans. is (b) Walk around until they subside**

    Ambulation relieves Braxton Hicks.

48. **Ans. is (b) Cause decreased placental perfusion**

    This is because impedance of venous return by the gravid uterus, which causes hypotension and decreased systemic perfusion.

49. **Ans. is (a) Prolactin**

    Prolactin is the hormone from the anterior pituitary gland that stimulates mammary gland secretion.

Oxytocin, a posterior pituitary hormone, stimulates the uterine musculature to contract and causes the "let down" reflex.

50. **Ans. is (d) "Snowstorm" pattern on ultrasound with no fetus or gestational sac**

    The chorionic villi of a molar pregnancy resemble a snowstorm pattern on ultrasound. Bleeding with a hydatidiform mole is often dark brown and may occur erratically for weeks or months.

51. **Ans. is (d) Telangiectasias**

    The dilated arterioles that occur during pregnancy are due to the elevated level of circulating estrogen. The linea nigra is a pigmented line extending from the symphysis pubis to the top of the fundus during pregnancy.

52. **Ans. is (c) Physiologic anemia**

    Hemoglobin and hematocrit levels decrease during pregnancy as the increase in plasma volume exceeds the increase in red blood cell production.

53. **Ans. is (b) Electrolyte imbalance**

    Excessive vomiting in clients with hyperemesis gravidarum often causes weight loss and fluid, electrolyte, and acid-base imbalances.

54. **Ans. is (a) Diet**

    Clients with gestational diabetes are usually managed by diet alone to control their glucose intolerance. Oral hypoglycemic agents are contraindicated in pregnancy. NPH is not usually needed for blood glucose control for GDM.

55. **Ans. is (a) Calcium gluconate**

    Calcium gluconate is the antidote for magnesium toxicity. Ten ml of 10% calcium gluconate is given IV push over 3–5 minutes. Hydralazine is given for sustained elevated blood pressures in preeclamptic clients.

56. **Ans. is (d) Maternal and fetal blood are never exchanged**

    Only nutrients and waste products are transferred across the placenta. Blood exchange only occurs in complications and some medical procedures accidentally.

57. **Ans. is (b) Number of times a female has been pregnant**

    Gravida refers to the number of times a female has been pregnant, regardless of pregnancy outcome or the number of neonates delivered.

58. **Ans. is (d) Turn the woman on her side**

    During a fundal height measurement, the woman is placed in a supine position. This woman is experiencing supine hypotension as a result of uterine compression of the vena cava and abdominal aorta. Turning her on her side will remove the compression and restore cardiac output and blood pressure. Then vital signs can be assessed. Raising her legs will not solve the problem since pressure will still remain on the major abdominal blood vessels, thereby continuing to impede cardiac output. Breathing into a paper bag is the solution for dizziness related to respiratory alkalosis associated with hyperventilation.

59. **Ans. is (a) January 15, 2006**

    Naegele's rule requires subtracting 3 months and adding 7 days and 1 year if appropriate to the first day of a pregnant woman's last menstrual period. When this rule, is used with April 8, 2005, the estimated date of birth is January 15, 2006.

60. **Ans. is (c) A normal response to the birth**

    Child birth is a very emotional experience. An expression of happiness with tears is a normal reaction. Cultural factors, exhaustion and anxieties over the new role can all affect maternal responses. So, the name must be sensitive to the client's emotional expressions.

61. **Ans. is (b) Hypoxia to the uterine muscle fibers**

    Pain during the first stage of labor is primarily caused by hypoxia of the uterine and cervical muscle cells during contraction, stretching of the lower uterine segment, dilation of the cervix and perineum, and pressure on adjacent structures.

62. **Ans. is (a) Lateral aspect of the heel**

    In a neonate, the lateral aspect of the heel is the most appropriate site for obtaining a blood specimen. Using this area, prevents damage to the calcaneus bone, which is located in the middle of the heel.

63. **Ans. is (a) DTaP, Hib, IPN and PPD**

    The American Academy of Pediatrics recommends that infants who are delayed in receiving their immunizations or have not started their series by 9 months of age begin with DTap, IPV, Hib and PPD. oral polio vaccine is not used because cases of polio have been reported with use of the vaccine.

64. **Ans. is (a) Allow the parents to express their feelings**

    The goal of the second home visit is to help the parents express their feelings more openly. Many parents are reluctant to express their grief and need help.

65. **Ans. is (d) Pulmonary embolism**

    $PaCO_2$ of 28 mm Hg and PaO_2 of 50 mm Hg are both abnormal. The PaO_2 of 50 mm Hg signifies acute respiratory failure. In evaluating possible causes for this disorder, the nurse should consider conditions that lead to hypoxia and hyperventilation, such as pulmonary embolism. COPD is typically associated with respiratory acidosis and elevated $PaCO_2$.

66. **Ans. is (c) Deep breathing**

    Deep breathing is the best choice for helping to prevent atelectasis. The client should be placed in the semi Fowler's position and taught deep breathing and how to avoid coughing.

67. **Ans. is (b) Allows the client to be more independent**

    The major benefit of CAPD is that it frees the client from daily dependence on dialysis centers, health care personnel, and machines for life-sustaining treatment.

68. **Ans. is (d) On pillows with her hand higher than her elbow and her elbow higher than her shoulder**

    Lymph nodes can be removed from the auxiliary area when a modified radical mastectomy is done and biopsy is performed. To facilitate drainage from the arm on the affected side, the clients arm should be elevated on pillows her elbow higher than her shoulder.

69. **Ans. is (b) Pupil size and papillary response**

    It is crucial to monitor the pupil size and pupillary response to indicate changes around the cranial nerves.

70. **Ans. is (b) 10 to 15 g of a simple carbohydrate**

    To reverse hypoglycemia, the American Diabetes Association recommends ingesting 10 to 15 g of a simple carbohydrate, such as three to five pieces of hard candy, two to three packets of sugar (4 to 6 tsp), or 4 oz of fruit juice. If necessary, this treatment can be repeated in 15 minutes. Ingesting only 2 to 5 g of a simple carbohydrate may not raise the blood glucose level sufficiently. Ingesting more than 15 g may raise it above normal, causing hyperglycemia.

71. **Ans. is (a) Related to bone demineralization resulting in pathologic fractures**

    Poorly controlled hyperparathyroidism may cause an elevated serum calcium level. This, in turn, may diminish calcium stores in the bone, causing bone demineralization and setting the stage for pathologic fractures and a risk for injury. Hyperparathyroidism doesn't accelerate the metabolic rate. A decreased thyroid hormone level, not an increased parathyroid hormone level, may cause edema and dry skin secondary to fluid infiltration into the interstitial spaces. Hyperparathyroidism causes hypercalcemia, not hypocalcemia; therefore, it isn't associated with tetany.

72. **Ans. is (d) Suggest referral to a sex counselor or other appropriate professional**

    The nurse should refer this client to a sex counselor or other professional. Making appropriate referrals is a valid part of planning the client's care. The nurse doesn't normally provide sex counseling.

73. **Ans. is (b) At least three times a week**

    Diabetic clients must exercise at least three times a week to meet the goals of planned exercise—lowering the blood glucose level, reducing or maintaining the proper weight, increasing the serum high-density lipoprotein level, decreasing serum triglyceride levels, reducing blood pressure, and minimizing stress. Exercising once a week wouldn't achieve these goals. Exercising more than three times a week, although beneficial, would exceed the minimum requirement.

74. **Ans. is (b) Puffiness of the face and hands**

    Hypothyroidism (myxedema) causes facial puffiness, extremity edema, and weight gain. Signs and symptoms of hyperthyroidism (Graves' disease) include an increased appetite, weight loss, nervousness, tremors, and thyroid gland enlargement (goiter).

75. **Ans. is (c) Tachycardia**

    Levothyroxine, a synthetic thyroid hormone, is given to a client with hypothyroidism to simulate the effects of thyroxine. Adverse effects of this agent include tachycardia. The other options aren't associated with levothyroxine.

76. **Ans. is (d) Hyperparathyroidism**

    Hyperparathyroidism is most common in older women and is characterized by bone pain and weakness from excess parathyroid hormone (PTH). Clients also exhibit hypercalciuria-causing polyuria. While clients with diabetes mellitus and diabetes insipidus also have polyuria, they don't have bone pain and increased sleeping. Hypoparathyroidism is characterized by urinary frequency rather than polyuria.

77. **Ans. is (a) Vasopressin (Pitressin synthetic)**

    Because diabetes insipidus results from decreased antidiuretic hormone (vasopressin) production, the nurse should expect to administer synthetic vasopressin for hormone replacement therapy. Frusemide, a diuretic, is contraindicated because a client with diabetes insipidus experiences polyuria. Insulin and dextrose are used to treat diabetes mellitus and its complications, not diabetes insipidus.

78. **Ans. is (d) An adrenal adenoma**

    An autonomous aldosterone-producing adenoma is the most common cause of hyperaldosteronism. Hyperplasia is the second most frequent cause. Aldosterone secretion is independent of sodium and potassium intake as well as of pituitary stimulation.

79. **Ans. is (c) It tells us about your sugar control for the last 3 months**

    The glycosylated Hb test provides an objective measure of glycemic control over a 3-month period. The test helps identify trends or practices that impair glycemic control, and it doesn't require a fasting period before blood is drawn. The nurse can't conclude that the result occurs from poor dietary management or inadequate insulin coverage.

80. **Ans. is (a) Muscle weakness**

    Muscle weakness, bradycardia, nausea, diarrhea, and paresthesia of the hands, feet, tongue, and face are findings associated with hyperkalemia, which is transient and occurs from transient hypoaldosteronism when the adenoma is removed. Tremors, diaphoresis, and constipation aren't seen in hyperkalemia.

81. **Ans. is (a) Antidiuretic hormone (ADH)**

    ADH is the hormone clients with diabetes insipidus lack. The client's TSH, FSH, and LH levels won't be affected.

82. **Ans. is (b) Thyroid crisis**

    Thyroid crisis usually occurs in the first 12 hours after thyroidectomy and causes exaggerated signs of hyperthyroidism, such as high fever, tachycardia, and extreme restlessness. Diabetic ketoacidosis is more likely to produce polyuria, polydipsia, and polyphagia; hypoglycemia, to produce weakness, tremors, profuse perspiration, and hunger. Tetany typically causes uncontrollable muscle spasms, stridor, cyanosis, and possibly asphyxia.

83. **Ans. is (c) Increased urine osmolarity**

    In hyperglycemia, urine osmolarity (the measurement of dissolved particles in the urine) increases as glucose particles move into the urine. The client experiences glucosuria and polyuria, losing body fluids and experiencing fluid volume deficit. Cool, clammy skin; distended neck veins; and a decreased serum sodium level are signs of fluid volume excess, the opposite imbalance.

84. **Ans. is (d) A blood pressure of 176/88 mm Hg**

    Pheochromocytoma, a tumor of the adrenal medulla that secretes excessive catecholamine, causes hypertension, tachycardia, hyperglycemia, hypermetabolism, and weight loss. It isn't associated with the other options.

85. **Ans. is (c) Restricting fluids**

    To reduce water retention in a client with the SIADH, the nurse should restrict fluids. Administering fluids by any route would further increase the client's already heightened fluid load.

86. **Ans. is (a) Trousseau's sign**

    This client's serum calcium level indicates hypocalcemia, an electrolyte imbalance that causes Trousseau's sign (carpopedal spasm induced by inflating the blood pressure cuff above systolic pressure). Homans' sign (pain on dorsiflexion of the foot) indicates deep vein thrombosis. Hegar's sign (softening of the uterine isthmus) and Goodell's sign (cervical softening) are probable signs of pregnancy.

87. **Ans. is (d) The heart rate is 126 beats/minute**

    Diabetes insipidus is characterized by polyuria (up to 8 L/day), constant thirst, and an unusually high oral intake of fluids. Treatment with the appropriate drug should decrease both oral fluid intake and urine output. A urine output of 200 ml/hour indicates continuing polyuria. A blood pressure of 90/50 mm Hg and a heart rate of 126 beats/minute indicate compensation for the continued fluid deficit, suggesting that treatment hasn't been effective.

88. **Ans. is (a) Acromegaly**

    Acromegaly, which is caused by a pituitary tumor that releases excessive growth hormone, is associated with hyperglycemia, hypertension, diaphoresis, peripheral neuropathy, and joint pain. Enlarged hands and feet are related to lateral bone growth, which is seen in adults with this disorder. The accompanying soft tissue swelling causes hoarseness and often sleep apnea. Type 1 diabetes is usually seen in children, and newly diagnosed persons are usually very ill and thin. Hypothyroidism isn't associated with hyperglycemia, nor is growth hormone deficiency.

89. **Ans. is (d) Consuming a low-carbohydrate, high-protein diet and avoiding fasting**

    To control hypoglycemic episodes, the nurse should instruct the client to consume a low-carbohydrate, high-protein diet, avoid fasting, and avoid simple sugars. Increasing saturated fat intake and increasing vitamin supplementation wouldn't help control hypoglycemia.

90. **Ans. is (c) Myxedema coma**

    Severe hypothyroidism may result in myxedema coma, in which a drastic drop in the metabolic rate causes decreased vital signs, hypoventilation (possibly leading to respiratory acidosis), and nonpitting edema. Thyroid storm is an acute complication of hyperthyroidism. Cretinism is a form of hypothyroidism that occurs in infants. Hashimoto's thyroiditis is a common chronic inflammatory disease of the thyroid gland in which autoimmune factors play a prominent role.

91. **Ans. is (b) Has type 2 diabetes**

    Oral antidiabetic agents are only effective in adult clients with type 2 diabetes. Oral antidiabetic agents aren't effective in type 1 diabetes. Pregnant and lactating women aren't prescribed oral antidiabetic agents because the effect on the fetus is uncertain.

92. **Ans. is (a) Sulfisoxazole (Gantrisin)**

    Sulfisoxazole and other sulfonamides are chemically related to oral antidiabetic agents and may precipitate hypoglycemia. Mexiletine, an antiarrhythmic, is used to treat refractory ventricular arrhythmias; it doesn't cause hypoglycemia. Prednisone, a corticosteroid, is associated with hyperglycemia. Lithium may cause transient hyperglycemia, not hypoglycemia.

93. **Ans. is (b) Switch the client to a different oral antidiabetic agent**

    Many clients (25% to 60%) with secondary failure respond to a different oral antidiabetic agent. Therefore, it wouldn't be appropriate to initiate insulin therapy at this time. However, if a new oral antidiabetic agent is unsuccessful in keeping glucose levels at an acceptable level, insulin may be used in addition to the antidiabetic agent.

94. **Ans. is (d) You must avoid hyperextending your neck after surgery**

    To prevent undue pressure on the surgical incision after subtotal thyroidectomy, the nurse should advise the client to avoid hyperextending the neck. The client may elevate the head of the bed as desired and should perform deep breathing and coughing to help prevent pneumonia. Subtotal thyroidectomy doesn't affect swallowing.

95. **Ans. is (c) Deposits of adipose tissue in the trunk and dorsocervical area**

    Because of changes in fat distribution, adipose tissue accumulates in the trunk, face (moonface), and dorsocervical areas (buffalo hump). Hypertension is caused by fluid retention. Skin becomes thin and bruises easily because of a loss of collagen. Muscle wasting causes muscle atrophy and thin extremities.

96. **Ans. is (c) You may not be able to use desmopressin nasally if you have nasal discharge or blockage**

    Desmopressin may not be absorbed if the intranasal route is compromised. Although diabetes insipidus is treatable, the client should wear medical identification and carry medication at all times to alert medical personnel in an emergency and ensure proper treatment. The client must continue to monitor fluid intake and output and receive adequate fluid replacement.

97. **Ans. is (a) Hypocalcemia**

    Chvostek's sign is elicited by tapping the client's face lightly over the facial nerve, If the client's facial muscles twitch, it indicates hypocalcemia. Hyponatremia is indicated by weight loss, abdominal cramping, muscle weakness, headache, and postural hypotension. Hypokalemia causes paralytic ileus and muscle weakness. Clients with hypermagnesemia exhibit a loss of deep tendon reflexes, coma, or cardiac arrest.

98. **Ans. is (a) Serum glucose level**

    Hyperglycemia, which develops from glucocorticoid excess, is a manifestation of Cushing's syndrome. With successful treatment of the disorder, serum glucose levels decline. Hirsutism is common in Cushing's syndrome; therefore, with successful treatment, abnormal hair growth also declines. Osteoporosis occurs in Cushing's syndrome; therefore, with successful treatment, bone mineralization increases. Amenorrhea develops in Cushing's syndrome. With successful treatment, the client experiences a return of menstrual flow, not a decline in it.

99. **Ans. is (c) It interacts with plasma membrane receptors to produce enzymatic actions that affect protein, fat, and carbohydrate metabolism**

    Corticotropin interacts with plasma membrane receptors to produce enzymatic actions that affect protein, fat, and carbohydrate metabolism. It doesn't decrease cAMP production. The posterior pituitary hormone, antidiuretic hormone, regulates the threshold for water resorption in the kidneys.

100. **Ans. is (c) Onset to be at 2:30 pm, and its peak to be at 4 pm**

    Regular insulin, which is a short-acting insulin, has an onset of 15 to 30 minutes and a peak of 2 to 4 hours. Because the nurse gave the insulin at 2 pm, the expected onset would be from 2:15 pm to 2:30 pm and the peak from 4 pm to 6 pm.

Part 4

1. Once a nurse assesses a client's condition and identifies appropriate nursing diagnoses as:
   a. Plan is developed for nursing care.
   b. Physical assessment begins
   c. List of priorities is determined.
   d. Review of the assessment is conducted with other team members.

2. Planning is a category of nursing behaviors in which:
   a. The nurse determines the health care needed for the client.
   b. The physician determines the plan of care for the client.
   c. Client-centered goals and expected outcomes are established.
   d. The client determines the care needed.

3. Priorities are established to help the nurse anticipate and sequence nursing interventions when a client has multiple problems or alterations. Priorities are determined by the clients:
   a. Physician
   b. Non emergent, nonlife-threatening needs
   c. Future well-being
   d. Urgency of problems

4. A client centered goal is a specific and measurable behavior or response that reflects a clients:
   a. Desire for specific health care interventions
   b. Highest possible level of wellness and independence in function
   c. Physician's goal for the specific client
   d. Response when compared to another client with a like problem.

5. For clients to participate in goal setting, they should be:
   a. Alert and have some degree of independence
   b. Ambulatory and mobile
   c. Able to speak and write
   d. Able to read and write

6. The nurse writes an expected outcome statement in measurable terms. An example is:
   a. Client will have less pain
   b. Client will be pain free
   c. Client will report pain acuity less than 4 on a scale of 0-10
   d. Client will take pain medication every 4 hours around the clock

7. As goals, outcomes, and interventions are developed, the nurse must:
   a. Be in charge of all care and planning for the client.
   b. Be aware of and committed to accepted standards of practice from nursing and other disciples.
   c. Not change the plan of care for the client.
   d. Be in control of all interventions for the client.

8. When establishing realistic goals, the nurse:
   a. Bases the goals on the nurse's personal knowledge.
   b. Knows the resources of the health care facility, family, and the client.
   c. Must have a client who is physically and emotionally stable.
   d. Must have the client's cooperation.

9. To initiate an intervention the nurse must be competent in three areas, which include:
   a. Knowledge, function, and specific skills
   b. Experience, advanced education, and skills
   c. Skills, finances, and leadership
   d. Leadership, autonomy, and skills

10. Collaborative interventions are therapies that require:
    a. Physician and nurse interventions
    b. Nurse and client interventions
    c. Client and physician intervention
    d. Multiple health care professionals

11. Well formulated, client-centered goals should:
    a. Meet immediate client needs
    b. Include preventative health care
    c. Include rehabilitation needs
    d. All of the above

12. The following statement appears on the nursing care plan for an immunosuppressed client: The client will remain free from infection throughout hospitalization. This statement is an example of a (an):
    a. Nursing diagnosis
    b. Short-term goal
    c. Long-term goal
    d. Expected outcome

13. The following statements appear on a nursing care plan for a client after a mastectomy: Incision site approximated; absence of drainage or prolonged erythema at incision site; and client remains afebrile. These statements are examples of:
    a. Nursing interventions

b. Short-term goals
c. Long-term goals
d. Expected outcomes

14. The planning step of the nursing process includes which of the following activities?
    a. Assessing and diagnosing
    b. Evaluating goal achievement
    c. Performing nursing actions and documenting them
    d. Setting goals and selecting interventions.

15. The nursing care plan is:
    a. A written guideline for implementation and evaluation.
    b. A documentation of client care.
    c. A projection of potential alterations in client behaviors
    d. A tool to set goals and project outcomes.

16. After determining a nursing diagnosis of acute pain, the nurse develops the following appropriate client-centered goal:
    a. Encourage client to implement guided imagery when pain begins
    b. Determine effect of pain intensity on client function
    c. Administer analgesic 30 minutes before physical therapy treatment
    d. Pain intensity reported as a 3 or less during hospital stay

17. When developing a nursing care plan for a client with a fractured right tibia, the nurse includes in the plan of care independent nursing interventions, including:
    a. Apply a cold pack to the tibia.
    b. Elevate the leg 5 inches above the heart.
    c. Perform range of motion to right leg every 4 hours.
    d. Administer aspirin 325 mg every 4 hours as needed.

18. Which of the following nursing interventions are written correctly? (Select all that apply):
    a. Apply continuous passive motion machine during day
    b. Perform neurovascular checks
    c. Elevate head of bed 30 degree before meals
    d. Change dressing once a shift

19. A client's wound is not healing and appears to be worsening with the current treatment. The nurse first considers:
    a. Notifying the physician
    b. Calling the wound care nurse
    c. Changing the wound care treatment
    d. Consulting with another nurse

20. When calling the nurse consultant about a difficult client-centered problem, the primary nurse is sure to report the following:
    a. Length of time the current treatment has been in place
    b. The spouse's reaction to the client's dressing change
    c. Client's concern about the current treatment
    d. Physician's reluctance to change the current treatment plan

21. The primary nurse asked a clinical nurse specialist (CNS) to consult on a difficult nursing problem. The primary nurse is obligated to:
    a. Implement the specialist's recommendations
    b. Report the recommendations to the primary physician
    c. Clarify the suggestions with the client and family members
    d. Discuss and review advised strategies with CNS.

22. After assessing the client, the nurse formulates the following diagnoses. Place them in order of priority, with the most important (classified as high) listed first.
    a. Constipation
    b. Anticipated grieving
    c. Ineffective airway clearance
    d. Ineffective tissue perfusion

23. The nurse is reviewing the critical paths of the clients on the nursing unit. In performing a variance analysis, which of the following would indicate the need for further action and analysis?
    a. A client's family attending a diabetic teaching session
    b. Canceling physical therapy sessions on the weekend
    c. Normal vital signs and absence of wound infection in a postoperative client
    d. A client demonstrating accurate medication administration following teaching

24. The RN has received her client assignment for the day-shift. After making the initial rounds and assessing the clients, which client would the RN need to develop a care plan first?
    a. A client who is ambulatory
    b. A client, who has a fever, is diaphoretic and restless
    c. A client scheduled for operation theater at 13:00
    d. A client who just had an appendectomy and has just received pain medication

25. A female client with Cushing's syndrome is admitted to the medical-surgical unit. During the admission assessment, nurse Tizzy notes that the client is agitated and irritable, has poor memory, reports loss of appetite, and appears disheveled. These findings are consistent with which problem?
    a. Depression
    b. Neuropathy
    c. Hypoglycemia
    d. Hyperthyroidism
26. Nurse Ruth is assessing a client after a thyroidectomy. The assessment reveals muscle twitching and tingling, along with numbness in the fingers, toes, and mouth area. The nurse should suspect which complication?
    a. Tetany
    b. Hemorrhage
    c. Thyroid storm
    d. Laryngeal nerve damage
27. After undergoing a subtotal thyroidectomy, a female client develops hypothyroidism. Dr. Smith prescribes levothyroxine (Levothroid), 25 mcg P.O. daily. For which condition is levothyroxine, the preferred agent?
    a. Primary hypothyroidism
    b. Graves' disease
    c. Thyrotoxicosis
    d. Euthyroidism
28. Which of these signs suggests that a male client with the syndrome of inappropriate antidiuretic hormone (SIADH) secretion is experiencing complications?
    a. Tetanic contractions
    b. Neck vein distention
    c. Weight loss
    d. Polyuria
29. A female client with a history of pheochromocytoma is admitted to the hospital in an acute hypertensive crisis. To reverse hypertensive crisis caused by pheochromocytoma, Nurse Linda expects to administer:
    a. Phentolamine (Regitine)
    b. Methyldopa (Aldomet)
    c. Mannitol (Osmitrol)
    d. Felodipine (Plendil)
30. A male client with a history of hypertension is diagnosed with primary hyperaldosteronism. This diagnosis indicates that the client's hypertension is caused by excessive hormone secretion from which of the following glands?
    a. Adrenal cortex
    b. Pancreas
    c. Adrenal medulla
    d. Parathyroid
31. Nurse Roy is aware that the most appropriate for a client with Addison's disease?
    a. Risk for infection
    b. Excessive fluid volume
    c. Urinary retention
    d. Hypothermia
32. Acarbose (Precose), an alpha-glucosidase inhibitor, is prescribed for a female client with type 2 diabetes mellitus. During discharge planning, nurse jose would be aware of the client's need for additional teaching when the client states:
    a. If I have hypoglycemia, I should eat some sugar, not dextrose.
    b. The drug makes my pancreas release more insulin.
    c. I should never take insulin while I'm taking this drug.
    d. It's best if I take the drug with the first bite of a meal.
33. A female client whose physical findings suggest a hyperpituitary condition undergoes an extensive diagnostic workup. Test results reveal a pituitary tumor, which necessitates a transsphenoidal hypophysectomy. The evening before the surgery, Nurse Jacob reviews preoperative and postoperative instructions given to the client earlier. Which postoperative instruction should the nurse emphasize?
    a. You must lie flat for 24 hours after surgery.
    b. You must avoid coughing, sneezing, and blowing your nose.
    c. You must restrict your fluid intake.
    d. You must report ringing in your ears immediately.
34. Dr Kennedy prescribes glipizide (Glucotrol), an oral antidiabetic agent, for a male client with type 2 diabetes mellitus who has been having trouble controlling the blood glucose level through diet and exercise. Which medication instruction should the nurse provide?
    a. Be sure to take glipizide 30 minutes before meals.
    b. Glipizide may cause a low serum sodium level, so make sure you have your sodium level checked monthly.
    c. You won't need to check your blood glucose level after you start taking glipizide.
    d. Take glipizide after a meal to prevent heartburn.

35. For a diabetic male client with a foot ulcer, the physician orders bed rest, a wet-to-dry dressing change every shift, and blood glucose monitoring before meals and bedtime. Why are wet-to-dry dressings used for this client?
    a. They contain exudate and provide a moist wound environment
    b. They protect the wound from mechanical trauma and promote healing
    c. They debride the wound and promote healing by secondary intention
    d. They prevent the entrance of microorganisms and minimize wound discomfort

36. When instructing the female client diagnosed with hyperparathyroidism about diet, nurse Gina should stress the importance of which of the following?
    a. Restricting fluids
    b. Restricting sodium
    c. Forcing fluids
    d. Restricting potassium

37. Which nursing diagnosis takes highest priority for a female client with hyperthyroidism?
    a. Risk for imbalanced nutrition: More than body requirements related to thyroid hormone excess
    b. Risk for impaired skin integrity related to edema, skin fragility, and poor wound healing
    c. Body image disturbance related to weight gain and edema
    d. Imbalanced nutrition: Less than body requirements related to thyroid hormone excess

38. A male client with a tentative diagnosis of hyperosmolar hyperglycemic nonketotic syndrome (HHNS) has a history of type 2 diabetes that is being controlled with an oral diabetic agent, tolazamide (Tolinase). Which of the following is the most important laboratory test for confirming this disorder?
    a. Serum potassium level
    b. Serum sodium level
    c. Arterial blood gas (ABG) values
    d. Serum osmolarity

39. A male client has just been diagnosed with type 1 diabetes mellitus. When teaching the client and family how diet and exercise affect insulin requirements, Nurse Joy should include which guideline?
    a. You'll need more insulin when you exercise or increase your food intake
    b. You'll need less insulin when you exercise or reduce your food intake
    c. You'll need less insulin when you increase your food intake
    d. You'll need more insulin when you exercise or decrease your food intake

40. Nurse Salomi administers glucagon to her diabetic client, then monitors the client for adverse drug reactions and interactions. Which type of drug interacts adversely with glucagon?
    a. Oral anticoagulants
    b. Anabolic steroids
    c. Beta-adrenergic blockers
    d. Thiazide diuretics

41. Which instruction about insulin administration should Nurse Kate give to a client?
    a. Always follow the same order when drawing the different insulins into the syringe.
    b. Shake the vials before withdrawing the insulin
    c. Store unopened vials of insulin in the freezer at temperatures well below freezing
    d. Discard the intermediate-acting insulin if it appears cloudy

42. Nurse Perry is caring for a female client with type 1 diabetes mellitus who exhibits confusion, light-headedness, and aberrant behavior. The client is still conscious. The nurse should first administer:
    a. IM or subcutaneous glucagon
    b. IV bolus of dextrose 50%
    c. 15 to 20 g of a fast-acting carbohydrate such as orange juice
    d. 10 U of fast-acting insulin

43. For the first 72 hours after thyroidectomy surgery, nurse Jamie would assess the female client for Chvostek's sign and Trousseau's sign because they indicate which of the following?
    a. Hypocalcemia
    b. Hypercalcemia
    c. Hypokalemia
    d. Hyperkalemia

44. The Nurse is aware that the ability to enter into the life of another person and perceive his current feelings and their meaning is known:
    a. Belongingness
    b. Genuineness
    c. Empathy
    d. Respect

45. The termination phase of the nurse-patient relationship is best described one of the following:
    a. Review progress of therapy and attainment of goals
    b. Exploring the client's thoughts, feelings and concerns
    c. Identifying and solving patients problem
    d. Establishing rapport

46. During the process of cocaine withdrawal, the physician orders which of the following:
    a. Haloperidol (Haldol)
    b. Imipramine (Tofranil)
    c. Benztropine (Cogentin)
    d. Diazepam (Valium)
47. The nurse is aware that cocaine is classified as:
    a. Hallucinogen
    b. Psycho stimulant
    c. Anxiolytic
    d. Narcotic
48. In community health nursing, which is the most important risk factor in the development of mental illness?
    a. Separation of parents
    b. Political problems
    c. Poverty
    d. Sexual abuse
49. All of the following are characteristics of crisis except:
    a. The client may become resistive and active in stopping the crisis
    b. It is self-limiting for 4-6 weeks
    c. It is unique in every individual
    d. It may also affect the family of the client
50. Freud states that temper tantrums is observed in which of the following:
    a. Oral
    b. Anal
    c. Phallic
    d. Latency
51. The nurse is aware that ego development begins during:
    a. Toddler period
    b. Preschool age
    c. School age
    d. Infancy
52. A 19-year-old nursing student has lost 36 lbs for 4 weeks. Her parents brought her to the hospital for medical evaluation. The diagnosis was ANOREXIA NERVOSA. The primary gain of a client with anorexia nervosa is:
    a. Weight loss
    b. Weight gain
    c. Reduce anxiety
    d. Attractive appearance
53. The nurse is aware that the primary nursing diagnosis for the client is:
    a. Altered nutrition: Less than body requirement
    b. Altered nutrition: More than body requirement
    c. Impaired tissue integrity
    d. Risk for malnutrition
54. After 14 days in the hospital, which finding indicates that her condition in improving?
    a. She tells the nurse that she had no idea that she is thin
    b. She arrives earlier than scheduled time of group therapy
    c. She tells the nurse that she eat 3 times or more in a day
    d. She gained 4 lbs in two weeks
55. The nurse is aware that ataractics or psychic energizers are also known as:
    a. Antimanic
    b. Antidepressants
    c. Antipsychotics
    d. Antianxiety
56. Which is known as mood elevators:
    a. Antidepressants
    b. Antipsychotics
    c. Antimanic
    d. Antianxiety
57. The priority of care for a client with Alzheimer's disease is:
    a. Help client develop coping mechanism
    b. Encourage to learn new hobbies and interest
    c. Provide him stimulating environment
    d. Simplify the environment to eliminate the need to make chores
58. Autism is diagnosed at:
    a. Infancy
    b. 3 years old
    c. 5 years old
    d. School age
59. The common characteristic of autism child is:
    a. Impulsivity
    b. Self destructiveness
    c. Hostility
    d. Withdrawal
60. The nurse is aware that the most common indication in using ECT is:
    a. Schizophrenia
    b. Bipolar
    c. Anorexia Nervosa
    d. Depression
61. A therapy that focuses on here and now principle to promote self-acceptance?
    a. Gestalt therapy
    b. Cognitive therapy
    c. Behavior therapy
    d. Personality therapy
62. A client has many irrational thoughts. The goal of therapy is to change her:
    a. Personality
    b. Communication

c. Behavior
d. Cognition

63. The appropriate nutrition for Bipolar I disorder, in manic phase is:
   a. Low fat, low sodium
   b. Low calorie, high fat
   c. Finger foods, high in calorie
   d. Small frequent feedings

64. Which of the following activity would be best for a depressed client?
   a. Chess
   b. Basketball
   c. Swimming
   d. Finger painting

65. The nurse is aware that clients with severe depression possess which defense mechanism:
   a. Introjection
   b. Suppression
   c. Repression
   d. Projection

66. Nurse John is aware that self mutilation among Bipolar disorder patients is a means of:
   a. Overcoming fear of failure
   b. Overcoming feeling of insecurity
   c. Relieving depression
   d. Relieving anxiety

67. Which of the following may cause an increase in the cystitis symptoms?
   a. Water
   b. Orange juice
   c. Coffee
   d. Mango juice

68. In caring for clients with renal calculi, which is the priority nursing intervention?
   a. Record vital signs
   b. Strain urine
   c. Limit fluids
   d. Administer analgesics as prescribed

69. In patient with renal failure, the diet should be:
   a. Low protein, low sodium, low potassium
   b. Low protein, high potassium
   c. High carbohydrate, low protein
   d. High calcium, high protein

70. Which of the following cannot be corrected by dialysis?
   a. Hypernatremia
   b. Hyperkalemia
   c. Elevated creatinine
   d. Decreased hemoglobin

71. Tony with infection is receiving antibiotic therapy. Later the client complaints of ringing in the ears. This Ototoxicity is damage to:
   a. 4th CN
   b. 8th CN
   c. 7th CN
   d. 9th CN

72. Nurse Emma provides teaching to a patient with recurrent urinary tract infection includes the following:
   a. Increase intake of tea, coffee and colas
   b. Void every 6 hours per day
   c. Void immediately after intercourse
   d. Take tub bath everyday

73. Which assessment finding indicates circulatory constriction in a male client with a newly applied long leg cast?
   a. Blanching or cyanosis of legs
   b. Complaints of pressure or tightness
   c. Inability to move toes
   d. Numbness of toes

74. During acute gout attack, the nurse administers which of the following drug:
   a. Prednisone (deltasone)
   b. Colchicines
   c. Aspirin
   d. Allopurinol (zyloprim)

75. Information in the patients chart is inadmissible in court as evidence when:
   a. The client objects to its use
   b. Handwriting is not legible
   c. It has too many unofficial abbreviations
   d. The clients parents refuses to use it

76. Nurse Karen is revising a client plan of care. During which step of the nursing process does such revision take place?
   a. Planning
   b. Implementation
   c. Diagnosing
   d. Evaluation

77. When examining a client with abdominal pain, Nurse Hazel should assess:
   a. Symptomatic quadrant either second or first
   b. The symptomatic quadrant last
   c. The symptomatic quadrant first
   d. Any quadrant

78. How long will Nurse John obtain an accurate reading of temperature via oral route?
   a. 3 minutes
   b. 1 minute
   c. 8 minutes
   d. 15 minutes

79. The one filing the criminal care against an accused party is said to be the?
   a. Guilty
   b. Accused

c. Plaintiff
d. Witness

80. A male client has a standing DNR order. He then suddenly stopped breathing and you are at his bedside. You would:
   a. Call the physician
   b. Stay with the client and do nothing
   c. Call another nurse
   d. Call the family

81. The ANA recognized nursing informatics heralding its establishment as a new field in nursing during what year?
   a. 1994
   b. 1992
   c. 2000
   d. 2001

82. When is the first certification of nursing informatics given?
   a. 1990-1993
   b. 2001-2002
   c. 1994-1996
   d. 2005-2008

83. The nurse is assessing a female client with possible diagnosis of osteoarthritis. The most significant risk factor for osteoarthritis is:
   a. Obesity
   b. Race
   c. Job
   d. Age

84. A male client complains of vertigo. Nurse Bea anticipates that the client may have a problem with which portion of the ear?
   a. Tympanic membranes
   b. Inner ear
   c. Auricle
   d. External ear

85. When performing Weber's test, Nurse Rose expects that this client will hear:
   a. On unaffected side
   b. Longer through bone than air conduction
   c. On affected side by bone conduction
   d. By neither bone or air conduction

86. Roy with a tentative diagnosis of myasthenia gravis is admitted for diagnostic check up. Myasthenia gravis can confirm by:
   a. Kernig's sign
   b. Brudzinski's sign
   c. A positive sweat chloride test
   d. A positive edrophonium (Tensilon) test

87. A male client is hospitalized with Guillain-Barre syndrome. Which assessment finding is the most significant?
   a. Even, unlabored respirations
   b. Soft, nondistended abdomen
   c. Urine output of 50 ml/hr
   d. Warm skin

88. For a female client with suspected intracranial pressure (ICP), a most appropriate respiratory goal is:
   a. Maintain partial pressure of arterial oxygen (PaO$_2$) above 80 mm Hg
   b. Promote elimination of carbon dioxide
   c. Lower the PH
   d. Prevent respiratory alkalosis

89. Which nursing assessment would identify the earliest sign of ICP?
   a. Change in level of consciousness
   b. Temperature of over 103°F
   c. Widening pulse pressure
   d. Unequal pupils

90. The greatest danger of an uncorrected atrial fibrillation for a male patient will be which of the following:
   a. Pulmonary embolism
   b. Cardiac arrest
   c. Thrombus formation
   d. Myocardial infarction

91. Linda, A 30 years old posthysterectomy client has visited the health center. She inquired about BSE and asked the nurse when BSE should be performed. You answered that the BSE is best performed:
   a. 7 days after menstruation
   b. At the same day each month
   c. During menstruation
   d. Before menstruation

92. An infant is ordered to receive 500 ml of D5NSS for 24 hours. The Intravenous drip is running at 60 gtts/min. How many drops per minute should the flow rate be?
   a. 60 gtts/min
   b. 21 gtts/min
   c. 30 gtts/min
   d. 15 gtts/min

93. Mr. Gutierrez is to receive 1 liter of D5RL to run for 12 hours. The drop factor of the IV infusion set is 10 drops per minute. Approximately, how many drops per minutes should the IV be regulated?
   a. 13-14 drops
   b. 17-18 drops
   c. 10-12 drops
   d. 15-16 drops

94. Which of the following is formal continuing education?
   a. Conference

b. Enrollment in graduate school
c. Refresher course
d. Seminar

95. The BSN (Bachelor of Science in Nursing) curriculum prepares the graduates to become?
   a. Nurse generalist
   b. Nurse specialist
   c. Primary health nurse
   d. Clinical instructor

96. Disposal of medical records in government hospital/institutions must be done in close coordination with what agency?
   a. Department of Health
   b. Records Management Archives Office
   c. Metro Manila Development Authority
   d. Bureau of Internal Revenue

97. Nurse Jolina must see to it that the written consent of mentally ill patients must be taken from:
   a. Nurse
   b. Priest
   c. Family lawyer
   d. Parents/legal guardians

98. When Nurse Clarence respects the client's self-disclosure, this is a gauge for the nurses':
   a. Respectfulness
   b. Loyalty
   c. Trustworthiness
   d. Professionalism

99. The Nurse is aware that the following tasks can be safely delegated by the nurse to a non-nurse health worker except:
   a. Taking vital signs
   b. Change IV infusions
   c. Transferring the client from bed to chair
   d. Irrigation of NGT

100. During the evening round, Nurse Tina saw Mr. Torralba meditating and afterward started singing prayerful hymns. What would be the best response of Nurse Tina?
   a. Call the attention of the client and encourage to sleep
   b. Report the incidence to head nurse
   c. Respect the client's action
   d. Document the situation

Answers (Part 4)

1. Ans. is (a) Plan is developed for nursing care
2. Ans. is (b) The physician determines the plan of care for the patient
3. Ans. is (d) Urgency of problems
4. Ans. is (b) Highest possible level of wellness and independence in function
5. Ans. is (a) Alert and have some degree of independence
6. Ans. is (c) Client will report pain acuity less than 4 on a scale of 0 to 10
7. Ans. is (b) Be aware of and committed to accept standards of practice from nursing and other disciples
8. Ans. is (b) Knows the resources of the health care facility, family and the client
9. Ans. is (a) Knowledge, function and specific skills
10. Ans. is (d) Multiple health care professionals
11. Ans. is (d) All of the above
12. Ans. is (b) Short-term goal
13. Ans. is (d) Expected outcomes
14. Ans. is (d) Setting goals and selecting interventions
15. Ans. is (a) A written guideline for implementation and evaluation
16. Ans. is (d) Pain intensity reported as a 3 or less during hospital stay

   This is measurable and objective in the pain scale (VAS scale or visual analogue scale) numbered from 0 to 10.

17. Ans. is (b) Elevate the leg 5 inches above the heart

   This does not require a physician's order (A&D require an order; C is not appropriate for a fractured tibia).

18. Ans. is (c) Elevate head of bed 30 degree before meals

   It is specific in what to do and when (it is performed in case of tube feeding) and all others are not a specific nursing intervention.

19. Ans. is (b) Calling the wound care nurse

   Calling in the wound care nurse as a consultant is appropriate because he or she is a specialist in the area of wound management. Professional and competent nurses recognize limitations and seek appropriate consultation (a. This might be appropriate after deciding on a plan of action with the wound care nurse specialist. The nurse may need to obtain orders for special wound care products. c. Unless the nurse is knowledgeable in wound management, this could delay wound healing. Also, the current wound management plan could have been ordered by the physician. d. Another nurse most likely will not be knowledgeable about wounds, and the primary nurse would know the history of the wound management plan.).

20. **Ans. is (a) Length of time the current treatment has been in place**

    This gives the consulting nurse facts that will influence a new plan (b, c, and d. These are all subjective and emotional issues/conclusions about the current treatment plan and may cause a bias in the decision of a new treatment plan by the nurse consultant.).

21. **Ans. is (d) Discuss and review advised strategies with CNS**

    Because the primary nurse requested the consultation, it is important that they communicate and discuss recommendations. The primary nurse can then accept or reject the CNS recommendations (a. Some of the recommendations may not be appropriate for this client. The primary nurse would know this information. A consultation requires review of the recommendations, but not immediate implementation. b. This would be appropriate after first talking with the CNS about recommended changes in the plan of care and the rationale. Then the primary nurse should call the physician. c. The client and family do not have the knowledge to determine whether new strategies are appropriate or not. Better to wait until the new plan of care is agreed upon by the primary nurse and physician before talking with the client and/or family.).

22. **Ans. is (c, d, a, b)**

23. **Ans. is (b) Canceling physical therapy sessions on the weekend**

24. **Ans. is (b) A client, who has a fever, is diaphoretic and restless**

    This client's needs are a priority.

25. **Ans. is (a) Depression**

    Agitation, irritability, poor memory, loss of appetite, and neglect of one's appearance may signal depression, which is common in clients with Cushing's syndrome. Neuropathy affects clients with diabetes mellitus—not Cushing's syndrome. Although hypoglycemia can cause irritability, it also produces increased appetite, rather than loss of appetite. Hyperthyroidism typically causes such signs as goiter, nervousness, heat intolerance, and weight loss despite increased appetite.

26. **Ans. is (a) Tetany**

    Tetany may result if the parathyroid glands are excised or damaged during thyroid surgery. Hemorrhage is a potential complication after thyroid surgery but is characterized by tachycardia, hypotension, frequent swallowing, feelings of fullness at the incision site, choking, and bleeding. Thyroid storm is another term for severe hyperthyroidism—not a complication of thyroidectomy. Laryngeal nerve damage may occur postoperatively, but its signs include a hoarse voice and, possibly, acute airway obstruction.

27. **Ans. is (a) Primary hypothyroidism**

    Levothyroxine is the preferred agent to treat primary hypothyroidism and cretinism, although it also may be used to treat secondary hypothyroidism. It is contraindicated in Graves' disease and thyrotoxicosis because these conditions are forms of hyperthyroidism. Euthyroidism, a term used to describe normal thyroid function, wouldn't require any thyroid preparation.

28. **Ans. is (b) Neck vein distention**

    SIADH secretion causes antidiuretic hormone overproduction, which leads to fluid retention. Severe SIADH can cause such complications as vascular fluid overload, signaled by neck vein distention. This syndrome isn't associated with tetanic contractions. It may cause weight gain and fluid retention (secondary to oliguria).

29. **Ans. is (a) Phentolamine (Regitine)**

    Pheochromocytoma causes excessive production of epinephrine and norepinephrine, natural catecholamines that raise the blood pressure. Phentolamine, an alpha-adrenergic blocking agent given by IV bolus or drip, antagonizes the body's response to circulating epinephrine and norepinephrine, reducing blood pressure quickly and effectively. Although methyldopa is an antihypertensive agent available in parenteral form, it isn't effective in treating hypertensive emergencies. Mannitol, a diuretic, isn't used to treat hypertensive emergencies. Felodipine, an antihypertensive agent, is available only in extended-release tablets and therefore doesn't reduce blood pressure quickly enough to correct hypertensive crisis.

30. **Ans. is (a) Adrenal cortex**

    Excessive secretion of aldosterone in the adrenal cortex is responsible for the client's hypertension. This hormone acts on the renal tubule, where it promotes reabsorption of sodium and excretion of potassium and hydrogen ions. The pancreas mainly secretes hormones involved in fat metabolism. The adrenal medulla secretes the catecholamines—epinephrine and norepinephrine. The parathyroids secrete parathyroid hormone.

31. **Ans. is (a) Risk for infection**

    Addison's disease decreases the production of all adrenal hormones, compromising the body's normal stress response and increasing the risk of infection. Other appropriate nursing diagnoses for a client with Addison's disease include Deficient fluid volume and Hyperthermia. Urinary retention isn't appropriate because Addison's disease causes polyuria.

32. **Ans. is (a) If I have hypoglycemia, I should eat some sugar, not dextrose**

    Acarbose delays glucose absorption, so the client should take an oral form of dextrose rather than a product containing table sugar when treating hypoglycemia. The alpha-glucosidase inhibitors work by delaying the carbohydrate digestion and glucose absorption. It's safe to be on a regimen that includes insulin and an alpha-glucosidase inhibitor. The client should take the drug at the start of a meal, not 30 minutes to an hour before.

33. **Ans. is (b) You must avoid coughing, sneezing, and blowing your nose**

    After a transsphenoidal hypophysectomy, the client must refrain from coughing, sneezing, and blowing the nose for several days to avoid disturbing the surgical graft used to close the wound. The head of the bed must be elevated, not kept flat, to prevent tension or pressure on the suture line. Within 24 hours after a hypophysectomy, transient diabetes insipidus commonly occurs; this calls for increased, not restricted, fluid intake. Visual, not auditory, changes are a potential complication of hypophysectomy.

34. **Ans. is (a) Be sure to take glipizide 30 minutes before meals**

    The client should take glipizide twice a day, 30 minutes before a meal, because food decreases its absorption. The drug doesn't cause hyponatremia and therefore doesn't necessitate monthly serum sodium measurement. The client must continue to monitor the blood glucose level during glipizide therapy.

35. **Ans. is (c) They debride the wound and promote healing by secondary intention**

    For this client, wet-to-dry dressings are most appropriate because they clean the foot ulcer by debriding exudate and necrotic tissue, thus promoting healing by secondary intention. Moist, transparent dressings contain exudate and provide a moist wound environment. Hydrocolloid dressings prevent the entrance of microorganisms and minimize wound discomfort. Dry sterile dressings protect the wound from mechanical trauma and promote healing.

36. **Ans. is (c) Forcing fluids**

    The client should be encouraged to force fluids to prevent renal calculi formation. Sodium should be encouraged to replace losses in urine. Restricting potassium isn't necessary in hyperparathyroidism.

37. **Ans. is (d) Imbalanced nutrition: Less than body requirements related to thyroid hormone excess**

    In the client with hyperthyroidism, excessive thyroid hormone production leads to hypermetabolism and increased nutrient metabolism. These conditions may result in a negative nitrogen balance, increased protein synthesis and breakdown, decreased glucose tolerance, and fat mobilization and depletion. This puts the client at risk for marked nutrient and calorie deficiency, making imbalanced nutrition: Less than body requirements the most important nursing diagnosis. Options B and C may be appropriate for a client with hypothyroidism, which slows the metabolic rate.

38. **Ans. is (d) Serum osmolarity**

    Serum osmolarity is the most important test for confirming HHNS; it's also used to guide treatment strategies and determine evaluation criteria. A client with HHNS typically has a serum osmolarity of more than 350 mOsm/L. Serum potassium, serum sodium, and ABG values are also measured, but they aren't as important as serum osmolarity for confirming a diagnosis of HHNS. A client with HHNS typically has hypernatremia and osmotic diuresis. ABG values reveal acidosis, and the potassium level is variable.

39. **Ans. is (b) You'll need less insulin when you exercise or reduce your food intake**

    Exercise, reduced food intake, hypothyroidism, and certain medications decrease the insulin requirements. Growth, pregnancy, greater food intake, stress, surgery, infection, illness, increased insulin antibodies, and certain medications increase the insulin requirements.

40. **Ans. is (a) Oral anticoagulants**

    As a normal body protein, glucagon only interacts adversely with oral anticoagulants, increasing the anticoagulant effects. It doesn't interact adversely with anabolic steroids, beta-adrenergic blockers, or thiazide diuretics.

41. **Ans. is (a) Always follow the same order when drawing the different insulins into the syringe**

    The client should be instructed always to follow the same order when drawing the different insulin into the syringe. Insulin should never be shaken because the resulting froth prevents withdrawal of an accurate dose and may damage the insulin protein molecules. Insulin also should never be frozen because the insulin protein molecules may be damaged. Intermediate-acting insulin is normally cloudy.

42. **Ans. is (c) 15 to 20 g of a fast-acting carbohydrate, such as orange juice**

    This client is having a hypoglycemic episode. Because the client is conscious, the nurse should first administer a fast-acting carbohydrate, such as orange juice, hard candy, or honey. If the client has lost consciousness, the nurse should administer either I.M. or subcutaneous glucagon or an I.V. bolus of dextrose 50%. The nurse shouldn't administer insulin to a client who's hypoglycemic; this action will further compromise the client's condition.

43. **Ans. is (a) Hypocalcemia**

    The client who has undergone a thyroidectomy is at risk for developing hypocalcemia from inadvertent removal or damage to the parathyroid gland. The client with hypocalcemia will exhibit a positive Chvostek's sign (facial muscle contraction when the facial nerve in front of the ear is tapped) and a positive Trousseau's sign (carpal spasm when a blood pressure cuff is inflated for a few minutes). These signs aren't present with hypercalcemia, hypokalemia, or hyperkalemia.

44. **Ans. is (c) Empathy**
45. **Ans. is (a) Review progress of therapy and attainment of goals.**
46. **Ans. is (d) Diazepam (valium)**
47. **Ans. is (b) Psychostimulant**
48. **Ans. is (c) Poverty**
49. **Ans. is (a) The client may become resistive and active in stopping the crisis**
50. **Ans. is (b) Anal**
51. **Ans. is (d) Infancy**
52. **Ans. is (c) Reduce anxiety**
53. **Ans. is (a) Altered nutrition: Less than body requirement**
54. **Ans. is (d) She gained 4 lbs in two weeks.**
55. **Ans. is (c) Antipsychotics**
56. **Ans. is (a) Antidepressants**
57. **Ans. is (d) Simplify the environment to eliminate the need to make chores.**
58. **Ans. is (b) 3 years old**
59. **Ans. is (d) Withdrawal**
60. **Ans. is (d) Depression**
61. **Ans. is (a) Gestalt therapy**
62. **Ans. is (d) Cognition**
63. **Ans. is (c) Finger foods high in calories**
64. **Ans. is (d) Finger painting**
65. **Ans. is (a) Introjection**
66. **Ans. is (b) Overcoming feeling of insecurity**
67. **Ans. is (c) Coffee**
68. **Ans. is (d) Administer analgesics as prescribed**
69. **Ans. is (a) Low protein, low sodium, low potassium**
70. **Ans. is (d) Decreased hemoglobin**
71. **Ans. is (b) 8th CN**
72. **Ans. is (c) Void immediately after intercourse**
73. **Ans. is (a) Blanching or cyanosis of legs**
74. **Ans. is (b) Colchicines**
75. **Ans. is (a) The client objects to its use**
76. **Ans. is (d) Evaluation**
77. **Ans. is (b) Symptomatic quadrant last**
78. **Ans. is (a) 3 minutes**
79. **Ans. is (c) Plaintiff**
80. **Ans. is (b) Stay with the client and do nothing**
81. **Ans. is (a) 1994**
82. **Ans. is (b) 2001–2002**
83. **Ans. is (d) Age**
84. **Ans. is (b) Inner ear**
85. **Ans. is (c) On affected site by bone conduction**
86. **Ans. is (d) A positive edrophonium (Tensilon) test**
87. **Ans. is (a) Even, unlabored respirations**
88. **Ans. is (b) Promote elimination of carbon dioxide**

89. Ans. is (a) Change in level of consciousness
90. Ans. is (c) Thrombus formation
91. Ans. is (b) At the same day each month
92. Ans. is (b) 21 gtts/min
93. Ans. is (a) 13–14 drops
94. Ans. is (b) Enrollment in graduate school
95. Ans. is (c) Primary health nurse
96. Ans. is (a) Department of health
97. Ans. is (d) Parents/legal guardians
98. Ans. is (c) Trustworthiness
99. Ans. is (b) Change IV infusions
100. Ans. is (c) Respect the client's action

Part 5

1. Which of the following conditions would a nurse recognized as contributing to the development of respiratory alkalosis?
    a. Chronic obstructive pulmonary disease (COPD)
    b. Episodes of hyperventilation
    c. Frequent loose stool
    d. Hiatal hernia

2. When planning preoperative care for a child suspected of having WILMS tumor, the nurse should recognized that which of the following interventions places the child at risk for complications?
    a. Palpating the child's abdomen every 8 hrs
    b. Measuring the child's temperature rectally
    c. Monitoring the child's blood pressure every 4 hrs
    d. Monitoring the child's intake and output

3. Which of the following comments by a patient should indicate to a nurse that the patient has ideas of reference?
    a. Those other nurses are talking about me
    b. The nurse explained how my medication works
    c. Does the entire nurse here have a college degree?
    d. Will a nurse lead group therapy today?

4. Which of the following conditions would a nurse recognize as contributing to development of respiratory acidosis?
    a. Emphysema
    b. Hyperventilation
    c. Diarrhea
    d. Achalasia

5. A woman who is 24 hrs postpartum and who has an episiotomy would be instructed to report which of the following findings immediately?
    a. Decrease in urine output
    b. Absence of a daily bowel movement
    c. Presence of lochia rubra
    d. Increase in perineal pain sensation

6. A nurse is counseling a parent of a 6 months old infant about beginning solid foods in the infant's diet. Which of the following should the nurse recommend be introduced initially:
    a. Poached egg
    b. Strained peaches
    c. Pureed peas
    d. Rice cereal

7. A nurse observes a nurse's aide taking all of the following measures when caring for a patient in postoperative period following a pneumonectomy. Which measures would require immediate intervention by the nurse?
    a. Assisting the patient to ambulate in the hall
    b. Positioning the patient on the unoperated side
    c. Placing elastic stockings on the patient's legs
    d. Splinting the patient's chest during coughing

8. Which of the following pulmonary findings would a nurse expect to assess in a patient who has lower lobe pneumonia?
    a. Paradoxical chest movement
    b. Eupnea
    c. Bronchial breath sounds
    d. Kussmaul respirations

9. A nurse would assess a patient who has peripheral vascular disease of which of the following venous insufficiencies?
    a. Paresthesias
    b. Bounding pedal pulses

c. Intermittent claudication
d. Edematous ankles

10. A young boy who is receiving chemotherapy develops alopecia and says to the nurse, "I've lost all my hair." Which of the following responses would be appropriate for the nurse to make to the child?
    a. Did you know that because your hair fell out, we know that the medicine is working to make you better?
    b. Would you like to see some pictures of famous men who are bald?
    c. You can wear a baseball cap until your hair grows back.

11. A patient expresses many physical complaints during the first 2 weeks on the alcohol rehabilitation unit. The results of physical examination have been negative. The patient frequently approaches staff members to request medication for her discomfort. Based on the patient's behavior, which of the following interpretations is correct?
    a. The patient is trying to make the staff feel guilty
    b. The patient is attempting to relieve her anxiety
    c. The patient is experiencing organic pain from alcohol withdrawal
    d. The patient is using a more mature way of meeting her needs than alcohol

12. Which of the following foods should be removed from the dietary tray of a patient who has hepatic encephalopathy?
    a. Pasta
    b. Spinach
    c. Fresh fruit
    d. Eggs

13. A patient who had a tonsillectomy reports spitting up copious amounts of blood at home 10 days after the operation. Which of the following actions would the nurse instruct the patient to take first?
    a. Take nothing by mouth and go to the emergency room
    b. Gargle with warm saline solution
    c. Drink ice cold water
    d. Apply direct pressure to the carotid artery

14. Intravenous heparin therapy is prescribed for a client. While implementing the order a nurse should ensure that which of the following medication is available on the nursing unit?
    a. Protamine sulfate
    b. Potassium chloride
    c. Aminocaproic acid
    d. Vitamin K

15. The male client has a tentative diagnosis of urethritis. The nurses assess the client for which of the following manifestations of the disorder.
    a. Hematuria and pyuria
    b. Dysuria and proteinuria
    c. Hematuria and urgency
    d. Dysuria and penile discharge

16. Which of the following behaviors would indicated the greatest improvement in a patient who was admitted to the hospital with a diagnosis of hyperactivity?
    a. The patient completes an assigned task
    b. The patient frequently apologizes for his behavior
    c. The patient takes naps during the day
    d. The patient is on the unit

17. When admitting a 4 days old hispanic infant to the pediatric unit, the nurse notes irregular bluish discoloration over the infant's sacrum and buttocks. The nurse should recognize that this is a?
    a. Sign of child abuse and is reportable
    b. Manifestation of a rare bleeding disorder
    c. Normal variation in the skin assessment of a newborn
    d. Result of a traumatic birth injury

18. The nurse assessing a toddler who has an acute upper respiratory infection notes that the child has been vomiting. The nurse correctly interprets the vomiting as:
    a. An indication that the child also has a gastrointestinal infection
    b. A sign that the child is unable to mobilize secretions in the lungs
    c. A common manifestation of fever in young children
    d. A common manifestation of respiratory illness in young children

19. A patient in the recovery room complains of incisional pain. Which of the following nursing interventions would be most appropriate?
    a. Give meperidine (Demerol) 50 mg, IM, as ordered
    b. Encourage deep breathing exercises
    c. Place the patient in a prone position
    d. Give acetaminophen (Tylenol), 2 tablets as ordered

20. Which of the following nursing measures would be most appropriate in the care of a patient who has acute epistaxis?
    a. Tilt the patient's head back
    b. Place the patient's head between his legs

c. Pinch the nose and have the patient lean forward
d. Place warm compresses on the patient's nasal bridge

21. Which of the following questions is most important for a nurse to ask when taking a history from a patient who presents with symptoms of peripheral arterial occlusive disease?
   a. Do your legs hurt while walking?
   b. Do you notice swelling in your legs at night?
   c. Do you have calf pain when you flex your foot?
   d. Do your feet feel warm after exercise?

22. When assessing a woman who is 6 days postpartum following a vaginal delivery, a nurse would expect to describe the lochia in which of the following ways?
   a. Red in color with occasional small clots
   b. Brown in color without clots
   c. Pink in color with occasional small clots
   d. White in color without clots

23. A nurse would assess a patient who has adrenal insufficiency for signs of Addison's disease which include:
   a. Striae on the abdomen
   b. Acne lesions on the face
   c. Bronzed appearance of the skin
   d. Buffalo hump on the shoulders

24. To which of the following nursing diagnosis would a nurse give priority when caring for a patient who has septic shock?
   a. Initiating a bowel program
   b. Encouraging deep breathing
   c. Increasing sensory stimulation
   d. Promoting fluid intake

25. Which of these findings should a nurse expect to identify when assessing a patient who is receiving radiation therapy for cancer of the esophagus?
   a. Peripheral neuropathy
   b. Gingival hyperplasia
   c. Alopecia
   d. Hypersalivation

26. When taking the history of a patient who has multiple myeloma, a nurse would expect the patient to report which of the following symptoms?
   a. Back pain
   b. Blurred vision
   c. Hair loss
   d. Cloudy urine

27. A nurse would recognize that adolescents perceive which of the following issues as being a priority?
   a. Nutrition
   b. Safety
   c. Education
   d. Privacy

28. A 7 yrs old girl is to begin her first immunization schedule. According to recommended guidelines, which of the following vaccines is not needed?
   a. Polio
   b. Measles
   c. Pertussis
   d. Mumps

29. An elderly widow who has dementia of the Alzheimer type says to the nurse who offers her breakfast, "Oh no, honey. I have to wait until my husband gets here." The nurse should say to the woman.
   a. Your husband died 6 yrs ago. Let me put milk on your cereal for you.
   b. I've told you several times that your husband is dead. It's time to eat now.
   c. You're going to have to wait a long time. Your food will get cold.
   d. Why do you think he's alive? Why can't you just eat your breakfast?

30. Which of the following findings would a nurse identify as indicative of septic shock in a patient?
   a. Bradycardia
   b. Flushed appearance
   c. Cool, clammy skin
   d. S3 gallop

31. The nurse should instruct a patient who is to receive Digoxin (lanoxin) to report development of which of the following side effects?
   a. Ringing in the ears
   b. Loss of appetite
   c. Signs of bruising
   d. Sensitivity to sunlight

32. A 16 yrs old female who has cystic fibrosis and is sexually active asks a nurse, "Can I get pregnant?" The nurse's response would be based on the understanding that cystic fibrosis:
   a. Causes sterility in females
   b. Leads to a higher incidence of spontaneous abortion
   c. May results in problems with infertility in females
   d. Does not affect the reproductive system

33. Which of the following instructions should a nurse give to a patient who has history of venous leg ulcers in order to prevent recurrence?
   a. Sit with your legs dependent whenever possible
   b. Use warm compresses on your legs in the evening

c. Examine your legs for areas of redness everyday
d. Keep your legs flexed when standing for long periods

34. A woman, who is 30 weeks pregnant and attending the prenatal clinic, has symptoms of pregnancy-induced hypertension. Which of the following findings is indicative of this condition?
   a. The woman has been getting short of breath when climbing the second flight of stairs to her family's apartment.
   b. The woman has had a craving for salty foods lately
   c. The woman has a blood pressure of 124/80 mm Hg, compared with 90/60 mm Hg a months ago
   d. The woman has gained 3 lbs (1.4 kgs) during the past months

35. Which of the following responses of a female patient who is co-dependent and has low self esteem indicates that nursing interventions have been successful?
   a. The patient encourages her 16 yrs old daughter to prepare her own breakfast
   b. The patient regularly prepares refreshments for her reading club
   c. The patient refuses help from her child with meal preparation
   d. The patient seeks other family member's approval prior to preparing meals

36. A 4 months old infant who has acquired immune deficiency syndrome (AIDS) and is living with the biological mother would receive the injectable form of polio vaccine for which of the following reasons?
   a. Improve absorption
   b. Improve immunity
   c. Decreased viral shedding
   d. Decreased risk of anaphylaxis

37. Which of the following parameters should be given priority when caring for a patient with hypoadrenalism (Addison's disease)?
   a. Evaluating pulmonary function
   b. Monitoring blood sugar
   c. Measuring blood pressure
   d. Assessing neurological status

38. Which of the following comments, if made by the spouse of a patient who has been newly diagnosed with schizophrenia, would indicate that the spouse has a correct understanding of the disorder?
   a. I can't wait for these illness-related problems to disappear.
   b. My spouse and I will need ongoing psychiatric support in the community.
   c. I'll be glad when my spouse becomes the person I married again.
   d. My spouse will no longer live with me because permanent hospitalization is necessary

39. A physician has written all of the following orders for a patient who has a diagnosis of septic shock. Which order should the nurse carry out first?
   a. Obtain culture specimens
   b. Initiate antibiotic therapy
   c. Insert indwelling urinary (Foley) catheter
   d. Apply antiembolism stocking

40. A child present with periorbital edema, dark-colored urine and decreased urine output. A priority question for the nurse to ask when obtaining the history from the parent is:
   a. Has your children diagnosed recently with strep throat?
   b. Does your child get short of breath when playing?
   c. Is there any history of liver disease in the family?
   d. Does your child seem to be more tired than usual?

41. When assessing a 14 yrs old girl who has mittelschmerz, a nurse would expect the girl to have which of the following symptoms?
   a. Nausea and vomiting
   b. Heavy menstrual flow
   c. Low grade fever and malaise
   d. Lower abdominal pain

42. A 30 yrs old primigravida at 38 weeks gestation is admitted to the hospital in labor. The woman and her husband both attended education for childbirth classes. In the labor room, the husband is timing the frequency of his wife's contractions. If he is timing the frequency accurately he is noting the time from.
   a. The beginning of one contraction to the beginning of the next contraction
   b. The beginning of one contraction to the end of that contraction
   c. The end of one contraction to the beginning of the next contraction
   d. The end of one contraction to the peak of the next contraction

43. Because a woman is planning to breast-feed her infant, measures to prevent her nipples from

becoming sore are discussed with her. Which of the following comments, if made by the woman, would indicate that she understood the instruction?
  a. I'll use a nipple shield with every other breastfeed during my first postpartum week
  b. I'll cleanse my nipples with soap and water before each feeding
  c. I'll expose my nipples to the air several times a day
  d. I'll apply an antiseptic cream to my nipples after each feeding

44. Which of the following laboratory result, if identified in a patient who is experiencing vomiting and diarrhea, is most suggestive of hypovolemic shock?
  a. Potassium, 5.6 mEq/L
  b. Hematocrit, 58%
  c. Hemoglobin, 11 g/dL
  d. Calcium, 6 mEq/L

45. Nursing care for a patient who has polycythemia vera would focus on preventing:
  a. Dysrhythmias
  b. Hypotension
  c. Thrombosis
  d. Decubitus ulcer

46. Which of the following concepts should a nurse emphasize when conducting a community education program on reducing the risk of rape?
  a. Rape rarely occurs in rural areas
  b. The very young and the very old are usually safe from rape
  c. People who walk in groups are less likely to be raped
  d. Rape is a response to sexual needs

47. A child who has sickle cell disease should eat foods rich in folic acid. Which of the following foods would a nurse encourage the child to eat?
  a. Peas
  b. Spinach
  c. Squash
  d. Carrots

48. Which of the following instructions regarding skin care should a nurse give to a patient who is receiving radiation therapy?
  a. Cover the irradiated area with a light gauze dressing
  b. Rinse the irradiated area with normal saline solution
  c. Apply petroleum-based ointment to the treatment area
  d. Use a mild soap to cleanse the affected area

49. The family you are caring for had difficult labor and an unexpected cesarean delivery. They voice their displeasure with the way the situation was handled and are threatening to sue. As the nurse caring for this family, you will.
  a. Carefully document your care on the patient's chart
  b. Delegate routine care to other personnel
  c. Go into the room only when called, to allow for privacy
  d. Contact the hospital legal advisor prior to giving care

50. An infant is born at 34 weeks gestation is at risk for respiratory syncytial virus (RSV). When teaching the family about health care promotion, what primary recommendation should the nurse make to the parents?
  a. Avoid group settings of other children if at all possible
  b. Limit visitation of the infant by anyone who has cold
  c. Use good handwashing techniques
  d. Keep the baby out of drafts

51. A nurse is assessing a patient who presents with manifestations of leukemia. Which of the following blood test results would support this diagnosis?
  a. Platelets, 150,000/mm
  b. WBC, 150,000/mm
  c. Hematocrit, 40%
  d. Hemoglobin, 18.0 g/dL

52. A patient who has a diagnosis of metastatic cancer of the kidney is told by the physician that the kidney needs to be removed. The patient asks the nurse. "What should I do?" Which of the following responses by the nurse would be most therapeutic?
  a. Let's talk about your options
  b. You need to follow the doctor's advice
  c. What does your family want you to do?
  d. I wouldn't have the surgery done without a second opinion

53. An adolescent who has sickle cell disease is planning to go camping. A nurse would advise the child that a crisis might be precipitated by:
  a. Walking in the woods
  b. Fishing in a cold water stream
  c. Canoeing on a lake
  d. Cycling up mountain trails

54. A patient who has peptic ulcer disease is receiving sucralfate (Carafate). The nurse should instruct the patient to take the medication:

a. 1 hr after meals
b. Only at bedtime
c. With meals
d. Up to one hour before meals

55. **A patient diagnosed with post-traumatic stress disorder is troubled by frequent nightmares. The patient asks the nurse, "What's wrong with me?" Which of the following responses by the nurse would be most therapeutic?**
    a. Many people experience intense reactions following a frightening experience
    b. Nightmares are a means of working off psychic energy
    c. Nothing is wrong with you
    d. Why do you think there's something wrong with you?

56. **Which of the following statements, if made by a patient who is being discharged with a posterior nasal pack, indicates that the patient needs further instruction?**
    a. I will irrigate the packing daily
    b. I will change the packing every 2 days
    c. I will cough and deep breathe 4 × a day
    d. I will take antibiotics until the packing is removed

57. **A nurse observes a colleague taking all of the following actions when caring for a patient who has a leakage of cerebrospinal fluid from the nose. Which action would require further discussion?**
    a. Placing the patient in low-Fowler's position
    b. Assisting the patient to void on a bedpan
    c. Inserting gauze packing into the patient's nose
    d. Shining a penlight into the patient's eye

58. **To which of the following nursing diagnosis would a nurse give priority for a patient whose blood test reveals a white blood cell count of 3000 mm?**
    a. Risk for activity intolerance
    b. Impaired gas exchange
    c. Impaired tissue integrity
    d. Risks for infection

59. **A patient is to receive an intramuscular injection of iron dextran (INFeD). Which of the following steps should a nurse take before giving the injection?**
    a. Rotate the medication vial for one minute prior to drawing the medication into the syringe
    b. Pull the skin to one side prior to inserting the needle
    c. Apply ice to the site prior to plunging the needle
    d. Change to a 25-gauge needle prior to administering the medication

60. **A nurse would expect a typical preschool-age child to display which of the following behaviors?**
    a. Responding to requests by frequently using the term "no"
    b. Making change for a quarter
    c. Imitating behavior of significant adults during play
    d. Readily accepting a substitute babysitter

61. **Test results indicate that your patient is HIV positive. The patient has stated that her choice of infant feeding is breast milk. Your postpartum plan of care should be based on the knowledge that:**
    a. Breastfeeding should be encouraged for all new mothers to foster maternal child bonding.
    b. Formula feeding should be encouraged because the mother is not likely to live long enough to successfully breastfeed the infant
    c. The mother's HIV status should not influence her decision on how to feed her infant
    d. Breastfeeding is contraindicated for HIV-positive mothers

62. **A nursing assistant tells the charge nurse that another nursing assistant never cleans up the utility room at the end of the shift. The most effective approach to resolving the conflict would be to:**
    a. Acknowledge that the nursing assistant who is supposed to clean the utility room may feel overworked.
    b. Tell the nursing assistant who never helps clean that she needs to help
    c. Bring both parties together to discuss underlying issues of conflict
    d. Develop a schedule for rotating responsibility for the department's utility room

63. **A patient is admitted to the unit with a tentative diagnosis of Hodgkin's disease. Which of the following findings are most significant in supporting this diagnosis?**
    a. Change in mental status
    b. Dependent edema
    c. Distended abdomen
    d. Enlarged lymph nodes

64. **Which of the following statements, if made by a 44 yrs old female, would support a nursing diagnosis of knowledge deficit early detection of breast cancer?**
    a. I should not examine my breast or have mammogram during my menstrual period.
    b. I include the underarm area when I examine my breasts

c. Women who practice regular breast examination find breast lumps earlier than women who do not
d. Breast self-examination is not necessary if I get regular mammograms

65. Which of the following measures is most important when providing nursing care for a patient who has disseminated intravascular coagulation (DIC)?
a. Avoiding intramuscular injections
b. Limiting green, leafy vegetables
c. Using automatic blood pressure cuffs
d. Providing meticulous oral care

66. A patient does not swallow medication, but hold the tablet in her mouth until she is able to expectorate. The nurse should:
a. Discuss with the physician the use of aversion therapy to promote patient compliance
b. Ask the physician for an order to change to an intramuscular form of the medication
c. Discuss with the physician the use of a liquid instead of a tablet
d. Ask the physician for an order to discontinue the medication

67. A child has just undergone a shunting procedure for hydrocephalus. A nurse should question the placement of which of the following patients in the child's room?
a. A child who has acute glomerulonephritis
b. A child who has viral pneumonia
c. A child who has infantile eczema
d. A child who has undergone an appendectomy

68. A nurse should include which of the following strategies in the care plan of a child who is receiving cyclophosphamide (CYTOXAN) for treatment of Hodgkin's disease?
a. Monitor the child's intake and output
b. Assess the child's apical heart rate
c. Place a footboard at the end of the child's bed
d. Evaluate the child's hemoglobin level

69. A nurse teaches self-care management to a teenaged patient who is being treated for scoliosis using a Milwaukee brace. Which of the statements, if made by the patient, indicates a correct understanding of the instructions?
a. I can swim for 1 hr without brace
b. I must wear the brace over my jacket
c. I can remove the brace for sleeping
d. I must give up driving my car

70. A patient who has disseminated intravascular coagulation (DIC) is administered heparin sodium. Which of the following responses, identified in the patient, would indicate that the heparin is effective?
a. Breath sounds clear to auscultation
b. Stools negative for occult blood
c. Pupils equal and reactive to light
d. Oral mucosa pink and moist

71. Which of the following manifestations would a nurse expect to identify when assessing a patient who has atrial fibrillation?
a. Bounding headache
b. Visual disturbances
c. Irregular radial pulse
d. Elevated blood pressure

72. A nurse should inform a patient who is taking hydrochlorothiazide (hydrodiuril) that it is important to make which of the following dietary changes?
a. Limit green, leafy vegetables
b. Drink plenty of tomato juice
c. Decrease ingestion of red meat
d. Increase intake of oranges

73. Which of the following findings, if identified in a patient who is administered procainamide hydrochloride (Procan SR), would indicate that the patient is experiencing an adverse effect of the medication?
a. Butterfly rash on the face
b. Blurring of visual fields
c. dryness of the mouth
d. Ringing in the ears

74. Which of the following actions would a nurse take first when caring for a patient experiencing a cardiac arrest?
a. Initiate cardiac monitoring
b. Provide intravenous access
c. Establish an open airway
d. Obtain a pulse oximetry reading

75. Which of the following comments by a nurse would be most effective in dealing with a patient who has a diagnosis of severe (+3) anxiety?
a. Call me when you are calm enough to sit down
b. Sit in this chair
c. Where would you like to sit?
d. How would you feel about sitting down?

76. At 33 weeks of pregnancy, a woman who has been treated for pregnancy-induced hypertension is admitted to the hospital because her condition has not improved. She is placed on bed rest and

started on magnesium sulfate therapy. Which of the following assessment is essential for the nurse to make?
   a. Obtaining the woman's weight daily
   b. Assessing the woman's abdominal circumference
   c. Observing the woman for jaundice
   d. Checking the equality of the woman's femoral pulses

77. An infant has a temperature of 104 F (40.0°C) which of the following interventions would be most effective in reducing the infant's fever?
   a. Placing the infant in a cooling blanket
   b. Putting the infant in a tub of tepid water
   c. Administering the prescribed antipyretic to the infant
   d. Sponging the infant with alcohol

78. Which of the following comments by the spouse of a patient who abuses alcohol indicates a correct understanding of the term "Blockouts" as applied to alcoholism?
   a. My spouse only drinks after work
   b. My spouse drinking causes him to forget some event
   c. My spouse becomes angry when he's drinking
   d. My spouse's employer doesn't know he drinks

79. A nurse should assess a patient who has had a recent myocardial infarction for which of the following symptoms of pericarditis?
   a. Dull pain while sitting
   b. Burning pain in the chest
   c. Throbbing pain radiating to the jaw
   d. Sharp pain on inspiration

80. Which expected outcome should be given priority in the nursing care plan for a patient with adult respiratory distress syndrome (ARDS)?
   a. Systolic blood pressure greater than 90 mm Hg
   b. Oxygen saturation greater than 95%
   c. Respiration rate less than 20/min
   d. Heart rate less than 100/min

81. A patient who is connected to a cardiac monitor develops a heart rate of 40 beat/mt. Which of the following actions should a nurse take first?
   a. Establish intravenous access
   b. Call the physicians
   c. Check the patient's blood pressure
   d. Position the patient flat in bed

82. A patient is brought to the emergency department following a severe automobile accident. By the time the patient's spouse arrives, the patient has died. The spouse demands to see the body. Which of the following responses should a nurse make?
   a. It would be best for you to talk to the doctor first
   b. Your really don't want to see your spouse. The injuries are too severe
   c. If you wish, I will stay with you while you are with your spouse
   d. You might want to talk to your children before you see your spouse

83. A community health nurse teaches a mother comfort measures for her 6 yrs old child who has varicella zoster. Which of the following actions, if taken by the mother, requires further intervention?
   a. Applying a cortisone-based cream to the child's lesions
   b. Patting the child's lesions with calamine lotion
   c. Bathing the child in a tepid oatmeal bath
   d. Trimming the child's fingernails very short

84. Before administering the measles, mumps and rubella (MMR) vaccine to a 12 yrs old child, it is essential that a nurse assess for an allergy to:
   a. Peanuts
   b. Eggs
   c. Seafood
   d. Milk

85. A nurse is caring for a patient on a mechanical ventilator with positive end-expiratory pressure (PEED).
   a. Increase pulmonary vascular permeability
   b. Increase intrathoracic pressure
   c. Improve pulmonary tidal volume
   d. Maximize alveolar gas diffusion

86. A nurse is planning a community education presentation on domestic violence. Which of the following factors should the nurse include?
   a. Instructions on harmonious living with a spouse
   b. The telephone number of the local safe house
   c. Ways to include the extended family
   d. Assertiveness training

87. A nurse is caring for a patient who has just had an endotracheal tube inserted. Which of the following actions would the nurse take first?
   a. Inflate the cuff with appropriate volume
   b. Auscultate for bilateral breath sounds
   c. Tape the tube securely in place
   d. Suction for pulmonary secretions

88. When caring for a patient who is on a mechanical ventilator, the nurse should monitor the patient for which of the following complications?
   a. Flail chest
   b. Pleural effusion
   c. Pneumothorax
   d. Pulmonary embolus

89. Which of the following nursing interventions would be most effective in helping a parent who is grieving the loss of a young child?
    a. Schedule times to discuss family pictures with the parent
    b. Encourage the parent to have another child as soon as possible
    c. Recommend frequent periods of sleep during the day
    d. Distract the parent from thinking about the child

90. Which of the following nursing actions should be carried out first when a patient requires tracheostomy care?
    a. Cleansing around the tracheostomy tube stoma
    b. Deflating the tracheostomy tube cuff
    c. Removing the inner cannula from the tracheostomy
    d. Suctioning the tracheostomy tube

91. A nurse caring for a patient from a different culture notices that the patient did not eat the food on the meal tray. Which of the following comments by the nurse demonstrate an understanding of cultural diversity?
    a. What foods do you eat at home?
    b. You need to eat to keep up your strength
    c. You will lose weight if you do not eat
    d. Why didn't you tell me you don't like hospital food?

92. A 6 weeks old infant who has complex congenital heart defect is hospitalized and awaiting surgery. The infant experiences a hypercyanotic episode. Which of the following actions would the nurse take first?
    a. Suction the infant
    b. Place infant in knee-chest position
    c. Hyperextend the infant's neck
    d. Take a pulse oximetry reading on the infant

93. Which of the following suggestions should a nurse make to a known poly-substance-abusing woman who is 18 weeks pregnant?
    a. If you cannot stop taking drugs, you might consider terminating the pregnancy
    b. You should stop using all drugs immediately before your baby develops birth defects
    c. If you enter the drug treatment program now, your baby will be born healthy
    d. It may not be possible for you to stop drugs completely, but you should consider limiting the drugs you use during pregnancy

94. Which of the following complications are most likely to develop in a patient who is undergoing mechanical ventilation?
    a. Stress ulcers
    b. Paralytic ileus
    c. Urinary retention
    d. Peripheral neuropathy

95. Which of the following statements, if made by a patient who is being discharged following a lumbar laminectomy, would indicate a correct understanding of the discharge instructions?
    a. I will clean my incision daily with peroxide
    b. I will only sit for short periods of time
    c. I will eat foods that are low in fiber
    d. I will wear an abdominal binder for support

96. A 2 yrs old is being discharged from the ambulatory surgery center 10 hrs after undergoing a tonsillectomy. Which of the following findings would prompt the nurse to delay discharge?
    a. Complaints of pain
    b. Frequent swallowing
    c. Refusing to speak
    d. Continual mouth breathing

97. To which of the following nursing diagnosis should a nurse give priority when planning care for a patient who is in cardiogenic shock?
    a. Risk for infection
    b. Altered nutrition: less than body requirements
    c. Altered tissue perfusion: peripheral
    d. Fluid volume deficit

98. A nurse observes a colleague performing an assessment of a child who has a head injury by using the Glasgow coma scale. Which of the following assessments, if performed by the colleague, indicates the colleague needs instruction regarding the use of this scale?
    a. Motor response
    b. Deep tendon reflexes
    c. Verbal ability
    d. Eye opening

99. Which of the following statements, if made by a patient who has had a basal cell carcinoma removed, would indicate to the nurse the need for further instruction?
    a. I will use sunscreen with at least a sun protection factor (SPF) of 15
    b. I will use tanning booths rather than sunbathing from now on
    c. I will stay out of the sun between 10:00 am and 2:00 pm

d. I will wear a broad-brimmed hat when I am in the sun

100. To which of the following nursing diagnosis would a nurse give priority in the care of a patient whose blood test reveals a red blood cell count of 3.0 million/mm?
    a. Risk for activity intolerance
    b. Risk for fluid volume deficit
    c. Risk for impaired skin integrity
    d. Risk for infection

101. A man who has suicidal thoughts and dissatisfaction with his job is admitted to a psychiatric unit. Which of the following approaches would be most likely to elicit his involvement in scheduled activities?
    a. Working with him during activities
    b. Asking him if he would like to participate in activities
    c. Waiting for him to show interest in activities
    d. Telling him the therapeutic importance of activities

Answers (Part 5)

1. **Ans. is (b) Episodes of hyperventilation**

   Respiratory alkalosis is due to hyperventilation, which causes excessive "blowing off" of carbon dioxide and hence, a decrease in plasma carbonic acid concentration.

2. **Ans. is (a) Palpating the child's abdomen every 8 hrs**

   Wilms tumor, or neuroblastoma, is the most frequent intra-abdominal tumor of childhood and the most common type of cancer. Preoperatively, it is important that the tumor is not palpated unless absolutely necessary, since manipulation of the tumor may case dissemination of cancer cells so to adjacent and distal sites.

3. **Ans. is (a) Those other nurses are talking about me**

   Patient experiencing ideas of reference frequently misinterpret the messages of the others or give meaning of the communications of the others. Patient believe that certain events, situations or interactions are directly related to them.

4. **Ans. is (a) Emphysema**

   Chronic respiratory acidosis occurs with pulmonary disease, such as chronic emphysema and bronchitis, obstructive sleep apnea and obesity.

5. **Ans. is (d) Increase in perineal pain sensation**

   Signs of an infected episiotomy include pain, redness, warmth, swelling and discharge.

6. **Ans. is (d) Rice cereal**

   Rice cereal is usually introduced first, at 5 to 6 months of age, because of its low allergic potential. Wheat products should be avoided for the first 12 months of life.

7. **Ans. is (b) Positioning the patient on the unoperated side**

   The post-pneumonectomy position is on the back or operated side only. The patient is not allowed to lie with the operated side uppermost because the bronchial stump might open, causing fluid to drain into the unoperated side. Lying on the back or operated side also allows for maximum expansion of the unaffected lungs. The nurse should intervene if the aide is positioning the patient incorrectly.

8. **Ans. is (c) Bronchial breath sounds**

   Bronchial and bronchovesicular sounds that are audible in the lungs signify pathology. Usually they indicate consolidated areas in the lungs (e.g. pneumonia, heart failure) and necessitate further evaluation.

9. **Ans. is (d) Edematous ankles**

   There is moderate to severe edema in venous insufficiency. The patient would exhibit edema of the ankles

10. **Ans. is (c) You can wear a baseball cap until your hair grows back**

    This response encourages the teenager to elaborate about his body image.

11. **Ans. is (b) The patient is attempting to relieve her anxiety**

    The patient detoxifying from alcohol and other drugs experiences anxiety because the patient's usual coping mechanism is removed. Consequently, the patient will often use any method to obtain a drug, include feigning illness. When the patient complains, he/she should be assesses for the presence of a physical illness. In the absence of illness, the patient's behavior can be seen as an attempt to control the anxiety.

12. **Ans. is (d) Eggs**

    Patient with hepatic encephalopathy is on a very low protein or no protein diet. Food high in protein, such as eggs, need to be restricted.

13. **Ans. is (a) Take nothing by mouth and go to the emergency room**

    Hemorrhage may occur up to 10 days after surgery as a result of tissue sloughing from the healing process. Any sign of bleeding warrants immediate medical attention.

14. **Ans. is (a) Protamine sulfate**

    Protamine sulfate, it's the antidote for heparin.

15. **Ans. is (d) Dysuria and penile discharge**

16. **Ans. is (a) The patient completes an assigned task**

    Completing an assigned task indicates that the patients anxiety is under greater control, that his concentration has improved, and that he can tolerate focusing on an activity.

17. **Ans. is (c) Normal variation in the skin assessment of a newborn**

    Irregular bluish discoloration over the infant's sacrum and buttocks is normal in dark skinned infants. It is called the Mongolian spot.

18. **Ans. is (d) A common manifestation of respiratory illness in young children**

    Vomiting commonly occur in conjunction with respiratory illness in young children.

19. **Ans. is (a) Give meperidine (Demerol) 50 mg, IM, as ordered**

    Intramuscular pain medication should be administered as ordered in the immediate postoperative period, so that the pain does not become severe and interfere with recovery.

20. **Ans. is (c) Pinch the nose and have the patient lean forward**

    Initial treatment of epistaxis includes applying direct pressure by pinching the soft, outer portion of the nose against the midline septum.

21. **Ans. is (a) Do your legs hurt while walking?**

    Pain while walking is a sign of intermittent claudication and arterial insufficiency.

22. **Ans. is (b) Brown in color without clots**

    Lochia serosa (pink or brown) begins three to four days after childbirth and continues to about 10 days, when it changes to lochia alba, a yellow to white discharge.

23. **Ans. is (c) Bronzed appearance of the skin**

    Patient with primary adrenal hypo perfusion (Addison's disease) have elevated levels of plasma adrenal corticotropic hormones (ACTH) and melanocyte-stimulating hormone which can result in areas of increase pigmentation.

24. **Ans. is (d) Promoting fluid intake**

    Interventions of patients experiencing septic shock include correcting the conditions contributing to the shock and preventing complications. Increasing IV fluids will help to control the fluid volume deficit associated with septic shock.

25. **Ans. is (d) Hypersalivation**

    Side effects of radiation to the upper and middle thirds of the esophagus include retrosternal discomfort, pain on swallowing, increased salivation and nausea.

26. **Ans. is (a) Back pain**

    The nurse should assess the patient with multiple myeloma for pathologic fracture of the ribs and weight-bearing bones and compression fractures of the spine due to osteoporosis. These may be evidenced by sudden, severe pain usually related to bending or lifting.

27. **Ans. is (d) Privacy**

    Boundaries around confidentiality and privacy should be established at the beginning of the interview so that adolescents feel that they can discuss sensitive topics. Ensuring confidentiality is one of the most essential ingredients for establishing a trusting relationship. This is particularly essential in sensitive situations such as that involving substance use, sexual concerns or abuse.

28. **Ans. is (c) Pertussis**

    Pertussis vaccine is not given to children seven years of age or older because the risk related to receiving the vaccine increases as the incidence, severity and fatality of the disease decrease.

29. **Ans. is (a) "Your husband died 6 yrs ago. Let me put milk on your cereal for you**

    The nurse should orient the patient reality by reminding the patient that her husband died six years ago. The nurse should then move on to the activity at hand.

30. **Ans. is (b) Flushed appearance**

    Warm, flushed skin is an integumentary finding of septic shock.

31. **Ans. is (b) Loss of appetite**

    The dose of digoxin should be withheld and the doctor notified if the patients pulse if <60 or >110, or if the patient experiences anorexia, nausea, vomiting, sudden weight gain or edema. Blurred vision and seeing green or yellow halos around objects should be reported.

32. **Ans. is (c) May results in problems with infertility in females**

    Women with cystic fibrosis may have lessened fertility from the inability of sperm to migrate through viscid cervical mucus. Other reasons for possible infertility are malnutrition and chronic infection.

33. **Ans. is (c) Examine your legs for areas of redness everyday**

    Instruct the patient and the family to observe the skin daily for changes and to maintain good foot care.

34. **Ans. is (c) The woman has a blood pressure of 124/80 mm Hg, compared with 90/60 mmHg a months ago**

    A rise of 30 mm Hg in systolic blood pressure or a diastolic increase of 15 mm Hg is cause for concern by the nurse. These changes are associated with mild preeclampsia.

35. **Ans. is (a) The patient encourages her 16 yrs old daughter to prepare her own breakfast**

    Co-dependents try to control events and people around them. The fact that the women is encouraging her daughter to make her own breakfast, rather than making it for her, shows that the interventions have been successful.

36. **Ans. is (c) Decreased viral shedding**

    Increased protection against wild polio virus by oral polio virus vaccine (OPV) occurs because this vaccine immunizes the gastrointestinal tract. Shedding of OPV is danger to contacts that are immune-compromised, such as patients with AIDS. For this reason, the injectable form of the polio vaccine is given.

37. **Ans. is (c) Measuring blood pressure**

    Careful monitoring of the patients reported symptoms, vital signs, weight and fluid and electrolyte balance is essential to determine the patients progress and return to a pre-crisis state.

38. **Ans. is (b) My spouse and I will need ongoing psychiatric support in the community**

    Information on community resources should be made available to patients and families alike. Family education and family therapy are known to diminish the negative effects of family life on schizophrenia.

39. **Ans. is (a) Obtain culture specimens**

    Septic shock can be caused by any microorganism. Obtaining specimens for culture should be done prior to the administration of antibiotic therapy.

40. **Ans. is (a) Has your children diagnosed recently with strep throat?**

    Manifestation, such as periorbital edema, dark-colored urine and decreased urinary output indicate glomerulonephritis, which occurs after a streptococcal infection.

41. **Ans. is (d) Lower abdominal pain**

    Some women experience a localized lower abdominal pain called mittelschmerz that coincides with ovulation.

42. **Ans. is (a) The beginning of one contraction to the beginning of the next contraction**

    Contractions are timed from the beginning of one contraction to the beginning of the next contraction.

43. **Ans. is (c) I'll expose my nipples to the air several times a day**

    Exposure of nipple to air help to toughen the tissue and decrease the risk of sore nipples.

44. **Ans. is (b) Hematocrit, 58%**

    Hematocrit level above 47% in females and 52% in males are indicative of dehydration that can result from hypovolemic shock.

45. **Ans. is (c) Thrombosis**

    In highly vascular areas, blood flow may become so slow that stasis occurs causing thrombosis in small vessels.

46. **Ans. is (c) People who walk in groups are less likely to be raped**

    Community education should indicate that when walking at night or in an isolated area, the best rape prevention strategy is not to walk alone.

47. **Ans. is (b) Spinach**

    The main sources of folic acid are green leafy vegetables. This includes vegetables, such as spinach, broccoli, kale and turnip, mustard, collard, dandelion and beet greens.

48. **Ans. is (d) Use a mild soap to cleanse the affected area.**

    The irradiated area should be cleansed daily with water, or with a mild soap and water.

49. **Ans. is (a) Carefully document your care on the patient's chart**

All care should be carefully documented on the chart, which becomes a legal document. The chart may be subpoenaed in court and only that care which is documented is considered to have actually been done.

50. **Ans. is (c) Use good handwashing techniques**

    Respiratory syncytial virus is the causative organism in bronchiolitis. Good hand washing techniques are essential to prevent the spread of the virus.

51. **Ans. is (b) WBC, 150,000/mm**

    The WBC count is usually quite high in leukemia. A normal level is 4500–10,000 mm^3

52. **Ans. is (a) Let's talk about your options**

    The nurse should provide an opportunity for the patients to ventilate and to discuss her concern. This response lets the patient know that there are care options and allows for discussion of treatment.

53. **Ans. is (d) Cycling up mountain trails**

    In sickle cell anemia, the goal is to minimize tissue deoxygenation. The adolescents should be instructed to include frequent rest periods during physical activities, avoid contact sports if the spleen is enlarged, avoid environments for low oxygen concentration, such as high altitudes or non-pressurized airplanes and avoid known sources of infection.

54. **Ans. is (d) Up to one hour before meals**

    Carafate should be administered on an empty stomach, one hour before meals and at bedtime.

55. **Ans. is (a) Many people experience intense reactions following a frightening experience.**

    Diagnostic criteria for post-traumatic stress disorder include exposure to a traumatic event in which the person was confronted with actual or threatened death and the person experienced fear helplessness and or horror.

56. **Ans. is (d) I will take antibiotics until the packing is removed.**

    Antibiotics are used to prevent toxic shock syndrome and sinusitis in patients with nasal packing.

57. **Ans. is (c) Inserting gauze packing into the patient's nose**

    The nurse should not insert gauze packing into the nose of a patient. The nurse should further discuss this action with the colleague.

58. **Ans. is (d) Risks for infection**

    The decrease in white blood cells (leucopenia) places the patient at risk for infection. The white blood cells are the first line of defense against invading organisms.

59. **Ans. is (b) Pull the skin to one side prior to inserting the needle**

    The Z-track method of injection is used to administer iron dextran. The skin should be pulled sideways away from the muscles.

60. **Ans. is (c) Imitating behavior of significant adults during play**

    The preschooler characteristically is initiative especially in faithfully reproducing the behavior of significant adults.

61. **Ans. is (d) Breastfeeding is contraindicated for HIV-positive mothers**

    Transmission of HIV to the fetus or neonate can occur transplacentally and less often by blood and vaginal secretions during delivery and or via breast milk.

62. **Ans. is (c) Bring both parties together to discuss underlying issues of conflict**

    Bringing both parties together is the most effective strategy for discussing issues and developing a plan to resolve them. Both parties have an opportunity to express themselves, have the same information from the charge nurse and can be involved in and have responsibility for the resolution.

63. **Ans. is (d) Enlarged lymph nodes**

    Hodgkin's disease usually originates in single lymph node, or a single chain of lymph nodes.

64. **Ans. is (d) Breast self-examination is not necessary if I get regular mammograms**

    Current guidelines include breast self-examination (BSE) starting at 20; physical examination of the breast by a trained professional recovery three years during ages 20 to 40 and every year thereafter; and screening mammography ages 40 to 49 every one to two years and annually thereafter.

65. **Ans. is (a) Avoiding intramuscular injections**

    Patients with disseminated intravascular clotting (DIC) develop a bleeding disorder and may bleed from mucous membranes venipuncture sites and the gastrointestinal and urinary tracts. Intramuscular injection should be avoided.

66. **Ans. is (c) Ask the physician for an order to change to an intramuscular form of the medication**

    The patient should be observed when medication is administered to ensure that the drug is swallowed and not held in the patient's cheek and discharge later. Giving a liquid form of the drug makes it much more difficult of the patient to "cheek" the medication.

67. **Ans. is (b) A child who has viral pneumonia**

    Developing infection is the greatest hazard following a shunting procedure. The nurse should be on the alert for potential source of infection. The patient with a shunt should not be place with a patient who has viral pneumonia.

68. **Ans. is (a) Monitor the child's intake and output**

    Intake and output should be monitored. To prevent the development of hemorrhagic cystitis, fluid intake should be 1000–2000 ml/day.

69. **Ans. is (a) I can swim for 1 hr without brace**

    Swimming strengthens muscles. The brace can be removed for one hour each day for swimming.

70. **Ans. is (b) Stools negative for occult blood**

    Indications of effective treatment with heparin are a return of clotting test to normal and decrease in hemorrhagic manifestations. Stools negative for occult blood is an indication of effectiveness of treatment.

71. **Ans. is (c) Irregular radial pulse**

    Atrial fibrillation is characterized by an irregular atrial and ventricular rhythm.

72. **Ans. is (d) Increase intake of oranges**

    Hydrochlorothiazide can cause hypokalemia. Oranges are a good source of potassium replacement and should not be restricted in the diet.

73. **Ans. is (a) Butterfly rash on the face**

    Development of a butterfly rash is an effect to pronestyl administration.

74. **Ans. is (c) Establish an open airway**

    The initial priority during a cardiac arrest is the maintenance of a patient airway.

75. **Ans. is (b) Sit in this chair**

    The patient experiencing severe anxiety has a narrower range of focus and responds best to simple instructions.

76. **Ans. is (a) Obtaining the woman's weight daily**

    The mother's daily weight is of primary concern because it provides the nurse with a baseline and then a record of increasing weight. Sudden weight gain of four pounds or weight gain of one pound per week in the second and third trimesters are associated with pre-eclampsia.

77. **Ans. is (c) Administering the prescribed antipyretic to the infant**

    Relief measures include pharmacological and or environmental intervention the most effective of which is the use of antipyretics to lower the set points.

78. **Ans. is (b) My spouse drinking causes him to forget some event**

    Blackouts are early symptoms of alcoholism. They are defined as amnesia for short-term memories while remote memory stays intact. For example, after a night of drinking with friends and individual cannot remember how he/she got home the night before.

79. **Ans. is (d) Sharp pain on inspiration**

    Pain associated with pericarditis is classically pleuritic and is aggravated by breathing especially on inspiration.

80. **Ans. is (b) Oxygen saturation greater than 95%**

    The goal of nursing care for the patient with adult respiratory distress syndrome (ARDS) is to monitor the patient's response to the ventilator. This is achieved by monitoring non-invasive respiratory parameters such as pulse oximetry for oxygen saturation levels.

81. **Ans. is (c) Check the patient's blood pressure**

    A patient may be bradycardic and asymptomatic, but treatment is necessary if the patient has symptoms, such as hypotension. The patient should be assessed before any treatment modalities are instituted.

82. **Ans. is (c) If you wish, I will stay with you while you are with your spouse**

    Offering to stay with the spouse is a way of providing support through a difficult event that can be traumatic.

83. **Ans. is (a) Applying a cortisone-based cream to the child's lesions**

    Medications that affect wound healing, such as corticosteroids, impairs phagocytosis inhibit fibroblast proliferation; depress formation of granulation tissue and inhibits wound closure. They should not be used by patients with varicella.

84. **Ans. is (b) Eggs**

    Measles vaccine is contraindicated in patients who have had an allergic reaction to eggs.

85. **Ans. is (d) Maximize alveolar gas diffusion**

    The need for PEEP indicates severe gas exchange disturbance. PEEP prevents alveoli collapse; the lungs are kept partially inflated so that alveolar gas exchanges are facilitated throughout the ventilatory cycle.

86. **Ans. is (b) The telephone number of the local safe house**

   The telephone number of local safe house (a place where battered spouses and children may go) would be most useful in a situation of domestic violence.

87. **Ans. is (b) Auscultate for bilateral breath sounds**

   Immediately after an endotracheal insertion, its placement must be verified. This is done by assessing for bilateral, equal breath sound.

88. **Ans. is (c) Pneumothorax**

   Patients receiving mechanical ventilation can experience barotrauma, or damage to the lungs by positive pressure. Barotraumas include pneumothorax, subcutaneous emphysema, and pneumomediastinum.

89. **Ans. is (a) Schedule times to discuss family pictures with the parent**

   Using memories is positive. This process goes on with great sadness, but is part of resolution of grief. Using family pictures encourages the bereaved to think and talk about numerous memories.

90. **Ans. is (d) Suctioning the tracheostomy tube**

   Tracheostomy care is initiated with suctioning of Tracheostomy tube as needed.

91. **Ans. is (a) What foods do you eat at home?**

   Enquiring as to the types of food eaten at home shows the nurse's awareness of the patient's cultural and dietary norms.

92. **Ans. is (b) Place infant in knee-chest position**

   Hypercyanotic spells also called 'blue' or 'tet' spells are seen in infants with tetralogy of fallot prior to surgical repair. The infant becomes actually cyanotic and hyperpneic because sudden infundibular spasm decreases pulmonary blood flow and increases right to left shunting. Putting the child in knee-chest position reduces the right to left shunting. Oxygen may also be administered.

93. **Ans. is (d) It may not be possible for you to stop drugs completely, but you should consider limiting the drugs you use during pregnancy**

   Women who are drug dependant need nursing support and anticipatory guidance during pregnancy since they have few support systems with which they can discuss their concern and fear. The nurse would encourage the woman to decrease her drug activity during pregnancy.

94. **Ans. is (a) Stress ulcers**

   Stress ulcers occur in approximately 25% of patients receiving mechanical ventilation due to ventilator and lack of food in the stomach.

95. **Ans. is (b) I will only sit for short periods of time**

   Prolonged sitting or standing should be avoided by a patient who had a lumbar laminectomy.

96. **Ans. is (b) Frequent swallowing**

   The nurse should watch for tachycardia pallor and excessive swallowing. Swallowing indicates that blood is trickling down the child's throat. The throat is checked with a flash light to assess for bleeding.

97. **Ans. is (c) Altered tissue perfusion: Peripheral**

   Cardiogenic shock occurs when the contractility of the cardiac muscle is directly impaired. Vasodilatation results in a declining blood pressure and altered tissue perfusion. The priority nursing diagnosis is altered tissue perfusion: peripheral.

98. **Ans. is (b) Deep tendon reflexes**

   The Glasgow coma scale consists of three parts assessment including best verbal response, best motor response and eye opening ability. Deep tendon reflexes are not part of this assessment. The nurse should instruct the colleague in proper use of the scale.

99. **Ans. is (b) I will use tanning booths rather than sunbathing from now on**

   The use of sun lamps or commercial tanning booths should be avoided.

100. **Ans. is (a) Risk for activity intolerance**

   Decreased RBC production can indicate anemia or hemorrhage. In either case, the patient experiences fatigue due to decreased oxygen carrying capacity. Priority should focus on risk for activity intolerance.

101. **Ans. is (a) Working with him during activities**

   Working with the patient provides support and allows for modeling the behavior.

Index

Page numbers followed by *f* refer to figure.

A

Abdomen 150
    regions of 83
Abdominal aneurysm surgery 8
Abdominal aortic aneurysm 65
    management 65
    signs of 65
    symptoms of 65
Abdominoperineal resection 93
Abortion 202
    signs of 202
    symptoms of 202
    types of 202
Abruptio placentae 204
Acid-base imbalances 4, 39
Acne 127
    causes 127
Acquired immune deficiency syndrome 141, 143
    cause 143
Acyanotic heart disorders 157, 157*f*, 158
Addicted newborn 154
Addison's disease 75
    causes of 75
Addisonian crisis 75
    causes 75
Adenocarcinoma 94
Adolescence
    development of 152
    growth of 152
Adrenal gland, disorders of 75
Adrenalectomy 76
Adrenocorticotropic hormones 70
Adventitious 35
Agoraphobia 184
Agranulocytes 120
Air embolism 8, 103
Airway pressure, continuous positive 37
Alarm system 37
    complications 37
Albumin 120
Alcohol-induced
    amnestic disorders 189
    psychiatric disorders 189
Alcoholism 188
    complications 188
Aldosteronism
    causes, primary 76
    primary 76
Allen's test 39
Alpha-fetoprotein screening 202
Altruistic suicide 188

Alzheimer's disease 183
Alzheimer's type, dementia of 183
Ammonia 7
Amniocentesis 201
Amniotic fluid 199
    embolism 208
        management of 209
Amphetamine 190
Amputation 68
Anaerobic exercises 111
Anal stage 170
Anaphylactic shock 131
Android pelvis 197
Anemia 122, 202
    aplastic 123
    causes of 122
    signs of 202
    symptoms of 202
    types of 122
Aneurysms 65
    classification of 65
    dissecting 65
    false 65
    true 65
    types of 65
Angina 56
    causes of 56
    signs of 56
    symptoms of 56
    types of 56
Anomic suicide 188
Anorexia nervosa 187
Anthropoid pelvis 197
Anticathexis 170
Antidiuretic hormone 70
    mechanism 48
Antidouble-stranded DNA blood test 142
Antimanic drugs 181
Antinuclear antibody titer 142
Antipsychotics 180
Anti-TB drugs 41
Anxiety
    disorder 184
    mild 184
    moderate 184
    severe 184
Aorta, coarctation of 158
Aortic stenosis 158
Apgar score 149
Apocrine sweat glands 127
Appendectomy 162
Appendicectomy 162
Appendicitis 8, 162
Aqueous humor 137

Arterial blood gas analysis 38
Arteriosclerosis obliterans 64
    management of 64
    signs of 64
    symptoms of 64
Arterio-venous
    fistula, internal 103
    graft, internal 103
    shunt, external 103
Arthrocentesis 111
Arthroscopy 111
Ascending colon 92
Ascites 89
Aspartate aminotransferase 48
Asterixis 90
Asthma 4, 8, 40
Astigmatism 138
Ataxic cerebral palsy 156
Atelectasis 35
Athetoid cerebral palsy 156
Atrial fibrillation 52, 52*f*
    causes 52
    management 53
Atrial septal defect 157
Atrioventricular septal defect 157
Attention deficit hyperactivity disorder 194
Auditory canal, external 139
Autism 194
Autonomic dysreflexia 8, 30
Autonomic nervous system 24
Autonomy vs shame and doubt 146
Avulsion fracture 116

B

Babinski's reflex 150
Bacterial gingivitis 125
Bacterial vaginosis 205
Barium enema 84
Barlow's sign 164
Barlow's test 164, 165*f*
Bartholin's glands 197
Basal cell carcinoma 128
Basophils 120
Becker muscular dystrophy 166
Bed sore, stages of 130
Behavior therapy 177
Bell's palsy 32
Bishop's score 205
Bladder exstrophy 164
Bland diet 7
Blood 119
    composition of 119
    examination 84, 100

groups 121
pressure, controlling 47
studies 49
sugar 77
    fasting 7
supply to heart 45, 46f
transfusion 122
urea nitrogen 7, 143
Body
    compartments 130
    dysmorphic disorder 186
Bone 108
    flat 108
    formation of new 108
    healing, stages of 108, 109f
    long 108
    marrow 120
        yellow 121
    remodeling occurs 109
    scan 111
    short 108
    types of 108
Bony callus 109
Bowel surgeries 93
Brain 24
    anatomy of 24
    functions of 24
    parts of 24
    structure of 24f
    trauma 4
Brainstem 25
Breast 197, 201
    cancer 134
    changes 209
Breath
    diminished 35
    sounds 34
        abnormal 35
        normal 34
Breathing-related sleep disorder 192
Bronchi
    left 34
    right 34
Bronchial breath sounds 34
Bronchiolitis 157
Bronchogenic carcinoma 42
Bronchoscopy 8, 38
Bronchovesicular sounds 35
Bryant's traction 165f
Buck's traction 113
Buerger's disease 64
    management of 64
    signs of 64
    symptoms of 64
Bulimia nervosa 187
Burns 129
    causes 129
    first degree 129
    full thickness 129
    partial thickness 129
    second degree 129
    stages of 129
    third degree 129
    types of 129

C

Calcium 6, 49
    carbonate 102
Cancer
    signs of 132
    staging of 133
    treatment of 133
    type of 133
Cancer esophagus 87
    causes of 87
Cancer mouth 87
    causes of 87
Cannabis disorders 190
Carbohydrate-rich foods 5
Cardiac arrest 61
    management of 61
    signs of 61
    symptoms of 61
Cardiac arrhythmias 51
Cardiac catheterization 49
Cardiac enzymes 48
Cardiac muscle 109
Cardiac tamponade 62
    causes of 63
    management of 63
    signs of 63
    symptoms of 63
Cardiac troponin 48
Cardiopulmonary resuscitation 61
Cardiovascular changes 209
Cardiovascular system 21, 43, 157, 200
Cardioversion 54
Carditis 159
Carl Jung theory 148
Cartilaginous joints 109
Cataract 138
    causes 138
    surgery 8
    types 138
Cathexis 169
Cecum 83, 92, 162
Celiac disease 160
Cells 120
Cellular immunity 142
Central nervous system 24
Central venous pressure 145
Cerebellum 25
Cerebral
    aneurysm 8, 32
    cortex 25
    palsy 156
        mixed type 156
        spastic 156
        types 156
Cerebrum 25
Cervical cancer 135
Cervical score 205
Cervical traction 113
Cervix, dilation of 206
Cesarean section 207
Chemonucleolysis 118
Chemotherapy 133
    complications of 133
    side effects of 133

Chest 150
    flail 42
    injuries 35
    tube drainage 36
Chickenpox virus 126
Childhood disorders 194
Cholecystitis 91
    acute 91
    causes 91
    chronic 91
Cholecystography 85
Cholesterol 49
Cholinergic crisis 29
Chorea 159
Chorionic villus sampling 201
Choroid 137
Ciliary bodies 137
Circadian rhythms sleep disorder 192
Cirrhosis of liver 89
Clark's formula 8
Clear liquid diet 7
Cleft lip 8, 160
Cleft palate 8, 160
Clitoris 197
Club foot 167
CNS depressants 4
Coagulation disorders 90
Coagulation factors 121
Cocaine use disorders 190
Cognitive evaluation 173
Colon 83
    ascending 83
    cancer 93
        causes 93
Colonoscopy 84
Colostomy 94
    irrigation 7
Comminuted fracture 116
Committing suicide, methods of 188
Communicable hepatitis 96
Community mental health 174
Conduct disorder 194
Congestive cardiac failure 8
Congestive heart failure 59
Conn's syndrome 76
Consciousness, assessment of level of 27
Contraceptives 211
Cornea 137
Coronary
    angiography 58
    arteriography 50
    artery
        bypass grafting 58
        artery disease 56
            causes 56
            signs 56
            symptoms 56
Cranial nerves, assessment of 26
Craniotomy 8
C-reactive protein 48, 111, 142
Crisis intervention 18, 175
    techniques of 19
Crohn's disease 92
    causes 92
Croup syndrome 157

Crutch 112*f*
    gaits, type of 112
Cryptorchidism 164
Cushing's syndrome 75
    causes 75
Cyanotic heart
    disease 7
    disorders 158, 158*f*, 159
Cystic fibrosis 80
    causes 80
Cystitis 104
    causes 104
    signs 104
    symptoms 104
Cystoscopy 101

D

Dawn phenomenon 79
Deep vein thrombosis 67
    signs 67
    symptoms 67
Defense mechanism 176
Defibrillation 54
Dehydration 131
Delegation 17
Delirium 182
    causes 183
    management 183
    tremens 189
Dementia 183
    causes 183
    types 183
Dependence syndrome 190
Depression 181
Dermatitis 127
    causes 127
Dermis 127
Diabetes insipidus 71
    causes 71
Diabetes mellitus 77, 80
    complications of 79
    secondary 78
    types 77
Diabetes, chronic complications of 80
Diabetic coma 77
    ketoacidosis 79
    nephropathy 80
    neuropathy 80
Dialysis encephalopathy 103
Diarrhea 131, 160
Diencephalon 25
Diet
    on basis of consumption, types of 7
    soft 7
Disaster
    impact 15
    management, phases of 15
    man-made 15
    mitigation 16
    nursing 14
        types of 15
    phases of 15
    preparedness 15, 16
    recovery 16
    response 16
Disequilibrium syndrome 103
Disseminated intravascular coagulation 125
Dissociative disorder 186
    types 186
Diverticulosis 93
Diverticulum 93
    inflammation of 93
Dressler's syndrome 57
Drug therapy 62
Duchenne muscular dystrophy 166
Dumping syndrome 7, 95
    causes 95
Duodenal ulcer 88
Duodenum 83
Dysrhythmias 51
Dyssomnias 192
Dysthymic disorder 182
Dystocia 208
    management 208

E

Ear 22, 136, 138, 150
    external 139
    layers of 139
    middle 139
    ossicles 139
    pinna 139
    structure of 138*f*
Eating disorders 187
Eccrine sweat glands 127
Ectopic pregnancy 203
    signs 203
    symptoms 203
Egoistic suicide 188
Electrolytes monitoring 48
Electronic medical record 12
Emphysema 35
Empyema 41
Endocarditis 62
    causes 62
    management 62
    signs 62
    symptoms 62
Endocrine
    glands 70
    system 69, 70*f*, 200
        master gland of 70
End-of-life care 22
Endoscopy 84
Enema 8, 86
    cleansing 86
    types of 86
Enuresis 163
Enzyme-linked immunosorbent assay 143
Eosinophils 120
Epidermis 127
Epiglottis 34
Epiglottitis 156
Epispadias 163
Epistaxis 8
Erythema marginatum 159
Erythroblastosis fetalis 153
Esophageal
    atresia 161
    hernia 97
    ulcer 88
    varices 89, 90
        causes 90
Esophagus 82
Ethambutol 41
Eustachian tube 139
Evidence-based practice 13
Exercise
    active 111
    aerobic 111
    flexibility 111
    passive 111
    type of 111
Exocrine glands 70
Eye 22, 136, 137, 150
    layers of 137
    structure of 137*f*

F

Facioscapulohumeral 166
Fallopian tubes 197
Fallot, tetralogy of 158
Fat-rich diets 5
Female reproductive
    structures 197
    system 197
Femoral
    catheter 103
    hernia 96
Fetal
    circulation 199
    development 200
    distress 208
        causes 208
        management 208
    heart rate 199
Fetor hepaticus 90
Fetus, expulsion of 206
Fibrinogen 120
Fibrocartilage callus 108
Fibrous joints 109
Follicle-stimulating hormone 70
Foreign body in ear 140
Fracture 116
    causes 116
    closed 116
    complicated 116
    compression 116
    leads to pulmonary embolism 66
    open 116
    types 116
Freud's psychosexual development theory 145
Freud's stages of psychosexual development 145
Fundal height, measurement of 201
Fusiform aneurysm 65

G

Gallbladder
    inflammation of 91
    structure of 91*f*

Gastrectomy 88
Gastric
	analysis 84
	cancer 94, 134
	gavage 85
		types 85
	juice 83
	lavage 86
	ulcer 88
		medical management of 88
		surgical management of 88
Gastritis 87
Gastrointestinal system 21, 81, 159, 200
	anatomy of 82f
Gastrostomy tube 86
Gavage 85
Gender identity disorders 193
Genetic screening 201
Genital stage 170
Genitalia 150
Genitourinary system 21, 163
Geriatric 20
	nursing 20
Gestational age, assessment of 149
Gestational diabetes mellitus 78, 203
	signs 203
	symptoms 203
Gestational trophoblastic disorder 203
Gland 69
	adrenal 74, 75
	sweat 127
Glaucoma 138
Glaucoma types 138
Globulin 120
Glomerulonephritis 163
Glucose tolerance test 201
Glucose-6-phosphate-dehydrogenase deficiency 124
Glycosylated hemoglobin count 78
Goiter 72
	causes 72
	diagnosis 72
	types 72
Gout 116
	causes 116
Grading of cancer 132
Granulocytes 120
Grave's disease 73
Great arteries, transposition of 158
Green stick fracture 116
Growth and development, stages of 151f
Guillain-Barré syndrome 32
Gynecoid pelvis 197

H

Haematocrit, normal 7
Haemodialysis, complications of 103
Haemoglobin, normal 7
Hair 127
Hairline fracture 116
Head 150
	injury 31
Healthcare system, ethics in 3
Hearing loss 139
	conductive 139

Heart
	block 45
		second-degree 45
		third degree 45
	catheterization
		left 50f
		right 49f
	chambers of 44
	conduction system of 44, 45f
	failure 59
		management of 60
	failure left side 59
		causes 59
		signs 59
		symptoms 59
	failure, right side 59
		causes 59
		signs 59
		symptoms 59
	layers of 44
	sounds 46
	structure of 44f
	transplantation 61
	valves 46, 46f
Hematological system 119
Hemodialysis 102, 103
Hemolysis reaction 121
Hemolytic
	anemia 123
	reaction 121
Hemophilia 124
	types 124
Hemorrhage
	antepartum 204
	secondary postpartum 209
Hemorrhoids 91
	causes 91
Heparin, classification of 58
Hepatitis 95
	A 96
	B 96
	C 96
	causes 95
	stages of 95
Hernia 96
	causes 96
	diaphragmatic 97
	major sites of 97f
	types of 96
	umbilical 96
Herpes zoster 126, 129
Hiatal hernia 7, 96, 97
	causes of 97
High-protein diet 5
Hip
	contractures, prevent 8
	dislocation, congenital 164
	fracture 117
		causes 117
Hirschsprung's disease 160
Hodgkin's lymphoma 135
Homicidal ideation 173
Homocysteine 48
Hormone 70
	growth 70
	produced by pancreas 77

Hospice care 22
Human
	musculoskeletal system 108
	sexual response cycle 198
Humoral immunity 142
Hydatidiform mole 203
Hydrocephalus 155
Hyperbilirubinemia 154
	types 154
Hyperemesis gravidarum 202
Hyperglycemia 77
	severe 77
Hyperopia 138
Hyperparathyroidism 74
	causes 74
Hyperpituitarism 71
	causes 71
Hypersomnias 192
Hypertension 63
	management 63
	signs 63
	symptoms 63
	types of 63
Hyperthyroidism 73
	causes 73
	diagnosis 73
Hypochondriasis 185
Hypodermis 127
Hypoglycemia 77
	severe 77
Hypoparathyroidism 74
	causes 74
	diagnosis 74
Hypophysectomy 8, 71
	after 71
Hypopituitarism 70
	causes 70
Hypospadias 163
Hypothyroidal dementia 183
Hypothyroidism 72
	causes 72
	diagnosis 73
Hypoventilation 4
Hypovolemic shock 131

I

Icteric stage 95
Idiopathic thrombocytopenic purpura 124
Ileostomy 93, 94
Ileum 83, 92, 162
Immune
	disorders 141
	hemolytic anemia 124
	response 142
	system 141
Immunity 141
	classification of 142
Immunodeficiency 142
Impaired nurse syndrome 172
Incisional hernia 96
Infant
	development of 151
	growth of 151
Infectious hepatitis 96
Infectious mononucleosis 125

Inflammatory bowel disorders, chronic 92
Inflammatory disorders of heart 62
Inguinal hernia 96
Inner ear 139
Insomnia 192
Insulin
    classification of 79
    coma 77
    lipodystrophy 79
    therapy 79
        complications of 79
Integumentary system 126, 201
Intervertebral disc prolapse 117
Intestinal obstruction 92
    causes 92
Intestine
    functions of large 83
    junction of
        large 162
        small 162
    large 83
    small 83
Intoxication, acute 189
Intra-aortic balloon pump 60
Intrapartum period 205
    disorders in 207
Intra-renal cause 101
Intussusception 160
In-vitro hemolysis 121
Involution of uterus 209
Iodine 6
Iron 6
    deficiency anemia 122
    therapy 122
Irreducible hernia 96
Irregular bones 108
Irritable bowel syndrome 162
Isometric exercise 111

J

Jejunostomy tube 86
Jejunum 83
Joints 109
    types of 109

K

Kaposi's sarcoma 141
Kelso's hunchback 107
Kidney 99
    biopsy 8
    cross-section of 100f
    functions of 99
    transplantation 103
Kock pouch 93, 94f
Korsakoff's syndrome 189
Kubler-Ross model 176

L

Labia
    majora 197
    minora 197

Labor 205
    stages of 206
Lactate dehydrogenase 48
Lactose intolerance 161
Laminectomy 118
Laryngeal cancer 42, 134
Laryngectomy 8
Laryngoscopy 38
Larynx 34
Latency stage 170
Lavage 85
Lens 138
Leopold maneuvers 205
Leukemia 135
Lewy body dementia 183
Limb-girdle 166
Liquid diet, full 7
Liver 89
    biopsy 7, 84
    functions of 89
Lobectomy 8
Local allergic reaction 79
Lochia 209
Low-protein diet 5
Lumbar puncture 8, 27
Lung
    biopsy 8, 38
    cancer 133
Luteinizing hormone 70
Lymphocytes 120

M

Macrophages 120
Magnesium 6, 49
Mammary glands, pair of 197
Mania 181
    stages of 181
Mantoux test 38
Marginal placenta previa 204
Maslow's hierarchy 171
Mastectomy 8
Mastitis 210
    management 210
Maternity nursing 196
Mechanical ventilation 37
    modes of 37
    types of 37
Meconium aspiration syndrome 153
Medications, classification of 133
Melanocyte-stimulating hormone 70
Melanoma 128
Memory, short-term 173
Ménière's disease 140
    causes 140
Meninges 25
    layers of 25f
Meningitis 30
Meningocele 155
Menstrual cycle 198
Mental
    health 169
    illness 169
    retardation 194
        causes 194
        management 194

    types 194
    status examination 172, 173
Metabolic
    acidosis 4, 5, 39
    alkalosis 4, 5, 39
Metastasis, route of 132
Milieu therapy 178
Mind, stages of 169
Minerals 6
Monocytes 120
Mononuclear leukocytes 120
Mood disorders 181, 182
Mood stabilizers 181
Moro reflex 150
Motion exercise, range of 111
Mouth 82
    and throat 150
Multi infarct dementia 183
Murphy's sign 91
Muscle 109
    biopsy 111
    movement of 109
    types of 109
Muscular dystrophy 166
Musculoskeletal system 21, 107, 164, 200
    anatomy of 108, 108f
Myasthenia gravis 28
Myasthenic crisis 29
Mycobutol 41
Myeloma, multiple 133
Myelomeningocele 156
Myocardial infarction 57
    acute 57
    causes 57
    signs 57
    symptoms 57
Myopia 138
Myotonic 166
Myxedema coma 73
    causes 73

N

Narcolepsy 192
Nasogastric tube 85, 85f
Nasojejunal tube 85f
Natural disasters 15
Neck 150
Necrotizing enterocolitis 155
Nephron
    function of 100
    structure of 100, 100f
Nephrotic syndrome 163
Nephrotoxic drugs 101
Nervous system, structure of 24f
Neuralgia, trigeminal 32
Neurological assessment 26
Neurological system 21, 23, 155
    anatomy 23
Neuromuscular disorder 28
Neuron 25
    structure of 25f
Neurosis 183
Neurotic disorder 183
Neutrophils 120

Newborn
    assessment 149
    conditions 153
Nightmare disorder 193
Non-Hodgkin's lymphoma 135
Nontherapeutic communication techniques 174
Nose 150
Nostrils 34
Nurse
    and co-workers 3
    and people 3
    and practice 3
    and profession 3
    characteristics 13
    in disaster management, role of 16
    in geriatrics, role of 22
    in psychotherapy, role of 176
    in research, roles of 13
    manager, role of 17
    role of 11, 14
    unique function of 1
Nursing 1
    barrier 18
    care 4, 19, 37
        delivery, modes of 10
        preoperative 74, 76
    ethical issues 2
    functional 10
    fundamentals 1
    innovations 11
    issues in 2
    legal
        issues 3
        liability in 3
    modular 11
    primary 10
    process 2
        assessment 2
        diagnosis 2
        evaluation 2
        implementation 2
        planning 2
        steps in 2
    profession 1
        characteristic of 13
    research 12
        kinds of 12
        purposes 12
        qualitative 12
        quantitative 12
        scope of 13
Nutrition 5, 201

O

Obsessive-compulsive disorder 184
Obstructive pulmonary disease, chronic 40
Oedipus complex 146
Oncology 132
Oral
    cavity 82
    cholecystogram 85
    glucose tolerance test 78
        management 78
    hypoglycemic agents 78
    stage 170

Organ of corti 139
Organic mental disorders 182
Organic psychosis 182
Ortolani's sign 164, 164f
Ossification 108
Osteoarthritis 114
    causes 114
Osteoblasts 108
Osteoclasts 108
Osteocytes 108
Osteogenesis imperfecta 166
Osteomalacia 115
    causes 115
Osteomyelitis 115
    causes 115
Osteoporosis 115
    types 115
Otitis media 139
    causes 139
Otosclerosis 139
    causes 139
Ovarian cancer 135
Ovaries 197
Oxygen therapy 35

P

Pacemaker 54
    modes of 55
    types of 55
Palmar grasp 150
Pancreas 77
    structure of 77f
Pancreatic cancer 134
Pancreatitis 7, 80
Panic anxiety 184
Paraphilias 193
Parasomnias 192
Parasympathetic nervous system 24
Parathyroid gland 74
    disorders of 74
Parkinsonism 29
Paroxysmal positional vertigo
    benign 140
    causes of benign 140
Patent ductus arteriosus 158
Pediatric nursing 144
Pelvic traction 113
Pelvis 197
    false 197
    true 197
Peptic ulcer 87
    causes 87
Perception, disorders of 179
Percutaneous transluminal coronary angioplasty 58
Pericardial sac 44
Pericarditis 62
    management 62
    signs 62
    symptoms 62
Peripheral nervous system 24
Peritoneal dialysis 103
Periventricular intraventricular hemorrhage 155
Pernicious anemia 123

Personality disorder 186
    causes 186
    classification of 186
Phallic stage 170
Pharynx 34, 82
Pheochromocytoma 76
    causes 76
Phobia 184
    simple 184
    specific 184
Phosphorus 6
Piaget's theory 148
Pituitary gland 70
    disorders of 70
Placenta 199
    previa 8, 204
        complete 204
        partial 204
Placental stage 206
Plasma 120
Platelets 120
Platypelloid pelvis 197
Pleural effusion 40
Pneumonia 4, 40
Pneumothorax 42
Polyarthritis 159
Polycythemia 124
Polymerase chain reaction 143
Polymorphonuclear leukocytes 120
Positive end-expiratory pressure 37
Positive pressure ventilators, types of 37
Post-icteric stage 95
Postpartum disorders 209
Postpartum hemorrhage 209
    causes 209
    primary 209
    types 209
Postpartum infection 210
    causes 210
Postpartum period 209
    changes in 209
Postpartum psychosis 210
Post-term delivery 208
    causes 208
    management 208
Post-transfusion hepatitis 96
Post-traumatic stress disorder 185
Potassium 7, 48
Precipitous labor 208
    causes 208
    management 208
Pregnancy
    induced hypertension 203
        causes 203
    physiological changes in 200
    signs of 200
Pre-icteric stage 95
Prelabor score 205
Premature ventricular contraction 53, 53f
    causes 53
    management 53
    signs 53
    symptoms 53
Pre-renal cause 101
Presbyopia 138

Preschooler
    development of 152
    growth of 152
Presumptive signs 200
Probable signs 200
Prostate cancer 105, 134
Prostatic hyperplasia, benign 105
Prostatitis 105
    signs 105
    symptoms 105
Protein-rich diets 5
Proximal tracheoesophageal fistula 161
Pseudo kidney sign 82
Psoriasis 128
    causes 128
Psychiatric disorders, classification of 179
Psychiatric history 172
Psychiatric nursing 168
Psychiatry
    revolutions in field of 169
    treatments in 176
Psychoactive substances 190
Psychoanalytical theory 169
Psychosexual development, stages of 170
Psychosocial development 146, 170
Psychotherapy 176
    types of 177
Public health model 174
Pulmonary angiography 38
Pulmonary circulation 44
Pulmonary edema 4, 8, 61
    causes 61
    management 61
    signs 61
    symptoms 61
Pulmonary embolism 4, 7, 66, 111
    causes 66
    management 66
    signs 66
    symptoms 66
Pulmonary function test 38
Pulmonary stenosis 158
Pulse oximetry 38
Pyloric stenosis 8, 162
Pyrazinamide 41

R

Radiation therapy 133
    types 133
Raynaud's phenomenon 65
    management 65
    signs 65
    symptoms 65
Recruitment 17
    third-party method 18
Rectal atresia 162
Red blood cells 120
    count, normal 7
Reflexes 150
Refraction 138
Rehabilitation phase 16
Renal
    angiography 101
    calculi 104
        causes 104
        management 105
        surgical management 105
    changes 209
    failure
        acute 101
        chronic 102
    failure causes
        acute 101
        chronic 102
    replacement therapies 102
        continuous 103
    scanning 101
    system 98, 200
Renin angiotensin mechanism 47
Reproductive system 21
Respiratory
    acidosis 4, 39
    alkalosis 4, 5, 39
    distress syndrome 153
    medications 39
    system
        anatomy of 34, 34f
        primary functions 33
        secondary functions 33
Retention enema 86
Retina 137
Retinopathy of prematurity 154
Retrolental fibroplasia 154
Reye's syndrome 155
Rheumatic heart disease 159
Rheumatoid arthritis 114
Rheumatoid factor 111
Rifampicin 41
Ringworm 126
Rinne's test 139
Road traffic accidents 35
Rooting reflex 150
Roving's sign 82
Rule of nine 129, 129f
Russell traction 113

S

Saccular aneurysm 65
Samsonic suicide 188
Schizophrenia 179
    causes 179
    types of 180
School-age
    development of 152
    growth of 152
Sclera 137
Scoliosis 165
Sebaceous glands 127
Seizures 30
    types 31
Sella turcica 70
Sengstaken-Blakemore tube 81
Sensorineural hearing loss 139
Serum
    albumin 7
    bicarbonate 7
    bilirubin
        direct 7
        total 7
    calcium 7
    chloride 7
    cholesterol 7
    creatine 7
    globulin 7
    iron 7
    lipids 49
    lithium, normal 7
    magnesium 7
    phosphorus 7
    potassium 7
    protein 7
    sodium 7
    thyroxine 7
    triiodothyronine 7
    uric acid 7, 111
Sexual disorders 193
Sexual dysfunctions 193
Sheehan's syndrome 210
    causes 210
Shock 8, 131
    cardiogenic 131
    causes 131
    neurogenic 131
    septic 131
    types of 131
Sickle cell anemia 123
Sigmoidoscopy 84
Sinus bradycardia 52
    causes 52
    management 52
    signs 52
    symptoms 52
Sinus tachycardia 51, 52f
Skeletal
    muscle 109
    system 108
    traction 114
Skin 126
    cancer 128, 133
        causes 128
        types 128
    functions of 126
    layers of 127
    structure of 127f
    testing 142
    traction 113
        types of 113
Sleep cycle, normal 191
Sleep disorders 191
    causes of 192
    classification of 192
Sleep-terror disorders 193
Sleep-walking disorder 193
Social phobia 184
Sodium 48
Somatic nervous system 24
Somatoform disorder 185
Somogyi phenomenon 79
Spina bifida 155
    cystica 155
    occulta 155
    types 155
Spinal cord 26
    injury 30
    structure of 26f

Spinal fusion 118
Spinal shock 30
Spontaneous mode 37
Sputum examination 38
Squamous cell
    cancers 95
    carcinoma 128
Squint 137
Stable angina 56
Stevens-Johnson syndrome 143
Stimuli, internal 184
Stokes-Adams syndrome 45
Stomach 82
    cancer 94
    structure of 83f
Strabismus 137
Streptococcal pharyngitis 125
Stress, manifestations of 19
Stroke 28
Subclavian catheter 103
Subcutaneous nodules 159
Subinvolution of uterus 210
    causes 210
    management 210
Substance abuse disorder 189
Suctioning 35
Suctioning nursing care 35
Sudoriferous glands 127
Suicidal ideation 173
Suicide 187
    assessment of 188
    causes 187
    of revenge 188
    types 188
Sulfur 6
Superficial burns 129
Supine hypotensive syndrome 204
Sydenham's chorea 159
Sympathetic nervous system 24
Synovial joints 109
Systemic circulation 44
Systemic lupus erythematosus 142
    causes 142
    types 142

T

Tachycardia, types of ventricular 53
Tay-sachs disease 156
Telehealth 11
Telemedicine 11
Telenursing 11
    purposes of 12
Tensilon test 29, 29f
Testicular cancer 134
Thalassemia 123
Therapeutic communication 174
    techniques 174
Therapeutic community 178
Therapeutic environment 178
Therapeutic impasses 172
Therapeutic relationship 171
    phases of 171
Thoracentesis 8, 38

Thoracic aortic aneurysm 65
    causes 65
    management 65
    signs 65
    symptoms 65
Thromboangiitis obliterans 64
Thrombophlebitis 67
    management 67
    signs 67
    symptoms 67
Thyroid
    function test 72
    gland 71
        disorders of 72
    hormones 72
    medications 72
        throughout pregnancy 72
    scan 72
    stimulating hormone 70
    storm 73
        causes 73
Thyroidectomy 8, 73
Tibial torsion 165
Tic disorder 195
    management 195
Tinea 126
Toddler
    development of 151
    growth of 151
Tokophobia 205
Tonic neck reflex 150
Tonsillectomy 7
Tonsillitis 156
Total hip replacement 117
Total parenteral nutrition 5, 8
Total placenta previa 204
Tourette syndrome 195
Trachea 34
Tracheoesophageal
    atresia 161
    fistula 161
        distal 161
Traction 113
    types of 113
Tragus 139
Truncus arteriosus 159
Tuberculin skin test 38
Tuberculosis 41
    causes 41
Tuning fork test 139

U

Ulcerative colitis 92
    causes 92
Unstable angina 57
Uremic syndrome 102
Ureters 99
Urethra 99
Urinary
    bladder 99
    system, anatomy of 99, 99f
Urine
    analysis 100

    disorder, sweet 77
    sugar in 77
    sweet 77
Uterine fibroids 205
    management 205
Uterus 197, 201

V

Vagina 197, 201
Vanillylmandelic acid 101
Variant angina 57
Varicose vein 8, 67
    management 67
    signs 67
    symptoms 67
Vascular disorders 63
Venous stasis ulcer 67
    management 67
    signs 67
    symptoms 67
Ventilation, continuous mandatory 37
Ventilator settings 37
Ventricular fibrillation 54, 54f
Ventricular septal defect 144, 157
Ventricular tachycardia 53, 53f
Vestibulocochlear nerve 139
Viral disorder 143
Visceral muscle 109
Vitamin 5
    A 6
    B1 6
    B12 6
    B2 6
    B3 6
    B5 6
    B6 6
    B7 6
    B9 6
    C 6
    D 6
    E 6
    K 6
Vitreous humor 138
Vomiting 159
    chronic 131
    of blood 89

W

Weaning 37
Weber's test 139
Wernicke's syndrome 189
White blood cells 120
Wilms' tumor 135
Withdrawal syndrome 189
    simple 189
Womb 197

Y

Yawning 34
Young's formula 8

EU GSPR Authorised Reprsentative
Logos Europe, 9 rue Nicolas Poussin
1700, La Rochelle, France
Phone: +33 (0) 6 67 93 73 78
E-mail: contact@logoseurope.eu

www.ingramcontent.com/pod-product-compliance
Ingram Content Group UK Ltd.
Pitfield, Milton Keynes, MK11 3LW, UK
UKHW050458150426
5217IPUK00025B/1748